George A. Horvath, MD

Neonatal and Pediatric Clinical Pharmacology

Guest Editors

JOHN N. VAN DEN ANKER, MD, PhD
MAX J. COPPES, MD, PhD
GIDEON KOREN, MD

PEDIATRIC CLINICS
OF NORTH AMERICA

www.pediatric.theclinics.com

October 2012 • Volume 59 • Number 5

SAUNDERS an imprint of ELSEVIER, Inc.

W.B. SAUNDERS COMPANY
A Division of Elsevier Inc.

1600 John F. Kennedy Boulevard • Suite 1800 • Philadelphia, Pennsylvania 19103-2899

http://www.theclinics.com

THE PEDIATRIC CLINICS OF NORTH AMERICA Volume 59, Number 5
October 2012 ISSN 0031-3955, ISBN-13: 978-1-4557-4918-8

Editor: Kerry Holland
Developmental Editor: Donald Mumford

The Pediatric Clinics of North America (ISSN 0031-3955) is published bimonthly by Elsevier Inc., 360 Park Avenue South, New York, NY 10010-1710. Months of issue are February, April, June, August, October, and December. Periodicals postage paid at New York, NY and additional mailing offices. Subscription prices are $191.00 per year (US individuals), $444.00 per year (US institutions), $259.00 per year (Canadian individuals), $591.00 per year (Canadian institutions), $308.00 per year (international individuals), $591.00 per year (international institutions), $93.00 per year (US students and residents), and $159.00 per year (international and Canadian residents and students). To receive students/resident rare, orders must be accompanied by name of affiliated institution, date of term, and the signature of program/residency coordinator on institution letterhead. Orders will be billed at individual rate until proof of status is received. Foreign air speed delivery is included in all *Clinics* subscription prices. All prices are subject to change without notice. **POSTMASTER:** Send address changes to *The Pediatric Clinics of North America*, Elsevier Health Sciences Division, Subscription Customer Service, 3251 Riverport Lane, Maryland Heights, MO 63043. **Customer Service: 1-800-654-2452 (US and Canada). From outside of the US and Canada: 1-314-447-8871. Fax: 1-314-447-8029. For print support, E-mail: JournalsCustomerService-usa@elsevier.com. For online support, E-mail: JournalsOnlineSupport-usa@elsevier.com.**

Reprints. For copies of 100 or more, of articles in this publication, please contact the Commercial Reprints Department, Elsevier Inc., 360 Park Avenue South, New York, NY 10010-1710. Tel.: 212-633-3812; Fax: 212-462-1935; E-mail: reprints@elsevier.com.

The Pediatric Clinics of North America is also published in Spanish by McGraw-Hill Inter-americana Editores S.A., Mexico City, Mexico; in Portuguese by Riechmann and Affonso Editores, Rua Comandante Coelho 1085, CEP 21250, Rio de Janeiro, Brazil; and in Greek by Althayia SA, Athens, Greece.

The Pediatric Clinics of North America is covered in *MEDLINE/PubMed (Index Medicus), Excerpta Medica, Current Contents, Current Contents/Clinical Medicine, Science Citation Index, ASCA, ISI/BIOMED,* and *BIOSIS.*

Printed in the United States of America.

GOAL STATEMENT

The goal of the *Pediatric Clinics of North America* is to keep practicing physicians and residents up to date with current clinical practice in pediatrics by providing timely articles reviewing the state-of-the-art in patient care.

ACCREDITATION

The *Pediatric Clinics of North America* is planned and implemented in accordance with the Essential Areas and Policies of the Accreditation Council for Continuing Medical Education (ACCME) through the joint sponsorship of the University Of Virginia School Of Medicine and Elsevier. The University Of Virginia School of Medicine is accredited by the ACCME to provide continuing medical education for physicians.

The University of Virginia School of Medicine designates this enduring material activity for a maximum of 15 *AMA PRA Category 1 Credit*(s)™ for each issue, 90 credits per year. Physicians should only claim credit commensurate with the extent of their participation in the activity.

The American Medical Association has determined that physicians not licensed in the US who participate in this CME enduring material activity are eligible for a maximum of 15 *AMA PRA Category 1 Credit*(s)™ for each issue, 90 credits per year.

Credit can be earned by reading the text material, taking the CME examination online at http://www.theclinics.com/home/cme, and completing the evaluation. After taking the test, you will be required to review any and all incorrect answers. Following completion of the test and evaluation, your credit will be awarded and you may print your certificate.

FACULTY DISCLOSURE/CONFLICT OF INTEREST

The University of Virginia School of Medicine, as an ACCME accredited provider, endorses and strives to comply with the Accreditation Council for Continuing Medical Education (ACCME) Standards of Commercial Support, Commonwealth of Virginia statutes, University of Virginia policies and procedures, and associated federal and private regulations and guidelines on the need for disclosure and monitoring of proprietary and financial interests that may affect the scientific integrity and balance of content delivered in continuing medical education activities under our auspices.

The University of Virginia School of Medicine requires that all CME activities accredited through this institution be developed independently and be scientifically rigorous, balanced and objective in the presentation/discussion of its content, theories and practices.

All authors/editors participating in an accredited CME activity are expected to disclose to the readers relevant financial relationships with commercial entities occurring within the past 12 months (such as grants or research support, employee, consultant, stock holder, member of speakers bureau, etc.). The University of Virginia School of Medicine will employ appropriate mechanisms to resolve potential conflicts of interest to maintain the standards of fair and balanced education to the reader. Questions about specific strategies can be directed to the Office of Continuing Medical Education, University of Virginia School of Medicine, Charlottesville, Virginia.

The faculty and staff of the University of Virginia Office of Continuing Medical Education have no financial affiliations to disclose.

The authors/editors listed below have identified no financial or professional relationships for themselves or their spouse/partner:

Susan M. Abdel-Rahman, PharmD; Luigi Atzori, MD, PhD; Jacob T. Brown, PharmD; Max J. Coppes, MD, PhD (Guest Editor); Kaitlyn Delano, Bsc; Vassilios Fanos, MD; Ryan S. Funk, PharmD, PhD; Kerry Holland, (Acquisitions Editor); Nicoletta Iacovidou, MD; Evelyne Jacqz-Aigrain, MD, PhD; Florentia Kaguelidou, MD, PhD; Gideon Koren, MD, FRCPC, FACMT (Guest Editor); John Lantos, MD; Naomi Laventhal, MD, MA; J. Steven Leeder, PharmD, PhD; B. Ryan Phelps, MD, MPH, AAHIV; Pavla Pokorna, MD; Natella Rakhmanina, MD, FAAP, AAHIVS; Karen Rheuban, MD (Test Editor); Michael Rieder, MD, PhD, FRCPC, FRCP (Glasgow); Robin H. Steinhorn, MD; Aggeliki Syggelou, MD, PhD(c); Beth A. Tarini, MS, MS; Dick Tibboel, MD, PhD; Monique van Dijk, PhD; Annewil van Saet, MD, PhD; Jonathan Wagner, DO; Enno D. Wildschut, MD, PhD; and Theodoros Xanthos, MD.

The authors/editors listed below identified the following professional or financial affiliations for themselves or their spouse/partner:

Maurice J. Ahsman, PharmD, PhD is a consultant for LAP&P Consultants, Leiden (NL).

Walter K. Kraft, MD receives research support from Merck.

John N. van den Anker, MD, PhD (Guest Editor) is a consultant for Reckitt Benckiser, QRxPharma, and GSK, and is on the Advisory Board for Reckitt Benckiser and ENO Pharmaceuticals.

Disclosure of Discussion of Non-FDA Approved Uses for Pharmaceutical Products and/or Medical Devices

The University of Virginia School of Medicine, as an ACCME provider, requires that all faculty presenters identify and disclose any off-label uses for pharmaceutical and medical device products. The University of Virginia School of Medicine recommends that each physician fully review all the available data on new products or procedures prior to clinical use.

TO ENROLL

To enroll in the Pediatric Clinics of North America Continuing Medical Education program, call customer service at 1-800-654-2452 or visit us online at www.theclinics.com/home/cme. The CME program is available to subscribers for an additional fee of $223.00.

Contributors

GUEST EDITORS

JOHN N. VAN DEN ANKER, MD, PhD, FCP, FAAP
Vice Chair of Pediatrics for Experimental Therapeutics and the Evan and Cindy Jones Chair in Pediatric Clinical Pharmacology; Chief, Division of Pediatric Clinical Pharmacology, Children's National Medical Center- Sheikh Zayed Campus for Advanced Children's Medicine; Professor, Departments of Pediatrics, Pharmacology & Physiology, The George Washington University School of Medicine and Health Sciences, Washington, DC; Adjunct Faculty, Intensive Care, Erasmus MC-Sophia Children's Hospital, Rotterdam, The Netherlands

MAX J. COPPES, MD, PhD, MBA
Senior Vice President, Center for Cancer & Blood Disorders, Children's National Medical Center–Sheikh Zayed Campus for Advanced Children's Medicine, Professor of Oncology, Medicine, and Pediatrics, Georgetown University; Clinical Professor of Pediatrics, The George Washington University School of Medicine and Health Sciences, Washington, DC

GIDEON KOREN, MD, FRCPC, FACMT
Director, The Motherisk Program, and the Division of Clinical Pharmacology and Toxicology, The Hospital for Sick Children; Professor of Pediatrics, Pharmacology, Pharmacy and Medical Genetics, The University of Toronto; Professor of Medicine, Pediatrics and Physiology/Pharmacology and the Ivey Chair in Molecular Toxicology, The University of Western Ontario, Toronto, Canada

AUTHORS

SUSAN M. ABDEL-RAHMAN, PharmD
Division of Clinical Pharmacology and Medical Toxicology, Children's Mercy Hospitals and Clinics; Professor, Department of Pediatrics, School of Medicine, University of Missouri-Kansas City, Kansas City, Missouri

MAURICE J. AHSMAN, PharmD, PhD
LAP&P Consultants BV, Leiden, The Netherlands

LUIGI ATZORI, MD, PhD
Professor of Clinical Pathology, Department of Biomedical Sciences, University of Cagliari, Cagliari, Italy

JACOB T. BROWN, PharmD
Postdoctoral Fellow in Pediatric Clinical Pharmacology, Division of Clinical Pharmacology and Medical Toxicology, Children's Mercy Hospitals and Clinics, Kansas City, Missouri

KAITLYN DELANO, BSc
Department of Pharmacology, Faculty of Medicine, University of Toronto; Division of Clinical Pharmacology and Toxicology, The Hospital for Sick Children, Toronto, Ontario, Canada

VASSILIOS FANOS, MD
Professor of Pediatrics; Director, Neonatal Intensive Care Unit, Puericulture Institute and Neonatal Section, AOU Cagliari, University of Cagliari, Cagliari, Italy

RYAN S. FUNK, PharmD, PhD
Postdoctoral Fellow in Pediatric Clinical Pharmacology, Division of Clinical Pharmacology and Medical Toxicology, Children's Mercy Hospitals and Clinics, Kansas City, Missouri

NICOLETTA IACOVIDOU, MD
Assistant Professor of Pediatrics-Neonatology, Medical School, National and Kapodistrian University of Athens, Athens, Greece

EVELYNE JACQZ-AIGRAIN, MD, PhD
Université Paris Diderot, Sorbonne Paris Cité; Department of Pediatric Pharmacology and Pharmacogenetics, Hôpital Robert Debré; INSERM Clinical Investigation Center, Paris, France

FLORENTIA KAGUELIDOU, MD, PhD
Université Paris Diderot, Sorbonne Paris Cité; Department of Pediatric Pharmacology and Pharmacogenetics, Hôpital Robert Debré; INSERM Clinical Investigation Center, Paris, France

GIDEON KOREN, MD, FRCPC, FACMT
Director, The Motherisk Program, The Hospital for Sick Children; Professor of Pediatrics, Pharmacology, Pharmacy and Medical Genetics, The University of Toronto; Professor of Medicine, Pediatrics and Physiology/Pharmacology and the Ivey Chair in Molecular Toxicology; Department of Pharmacology, Faculty of Medicine, University of Toronto; Division of Clinical Pharmacology and Toxicology, The Hospital for Sick Children, The University of Western Ontario, Toronto, Canada

WALTER K. KRAFT, MD, FACP
Associate Professor, Departments of Pharmacology and Experimental Therapeutics, Medicine, and Surgery, Thomas Jefferson University, Philadelphia, Pennsylvania

JOHN LANTOS, MD
Professor of Pediatrics; Director of Pediatric Bioethics, Children's Mercy Bioethics Center, Children's Mercy Hospital, Kansas City, Missouri

NAOMI LAVENTHAL, MD, MA
Assistant Professor, Division of Neonatal-Perinatal Medicine, Department of Pediatrics and Communicable Diseases, University of Michigan School of Medicine, Ann Arbor, Michigan

J. STEVEN LEEDER, PharmD, PhD
Marion Merrell Dow-Missouri Endowed Chair of Pediatric Clinical Pharmacology; Professor of Pediatrics and Pharmacology, Division of Clinical Pharmacology and Medical Toxicology, Department of Pediatrics, Children's Mercy Hospital and Clinics, University of Missouri-Kansas City Schools of Medicine and Pharmacy, Kansas City, Missouri

B. RYAN PHELPS, MD, MPH, AAHIVS
Attending Physician, Division of Infectious Diseases, Children's National Medical Center; Senior Pediatric Care/PMTCT Advisor, USAID Office of HIV/AIDS, Washington, DC

PAVLA POKORNA, MD
Department of Pediatric Surgery, Intensive Care, Erasmus MC-Sophia Children's Hospital, Rotterdam, The Netherlands; Faculty of medicine, Department of Pediatrics, PICU/NICU, Charles University, Prague, Czech Republic

NATELLA RAKHMANINA, MD, PhD, FAAP, AAHIVS
Associate Professor of Pediatrics, Department of Pediatrics, The George Washington University School of Medicine and Health Sciences; Director, Special Immunology Program, Division of Infectious Diseases, Children's National Medical Center, Washington, DC

MICHAEL RIEDER, MD, PhD, FRCPC, FAAP, FRCP (Glasgow)
CIHR-GSK Chain in Paediatric Clinical Pharmacology, Departments of Paediatrics Physiology & Pharmacology and Medicine; Scientist, Robarts Research Institute, Schulich School of Medicine & Dentistry, Western University, London, Ontario, Canada

ROBIN H. STEINHORN, MD
Division Head of Neonatology; Raymond and Hazel Speck Berry Professor of Pediatrics, Department of Pediatrics, The Ann and Robert H. Lurie Children's Hospital of Chicago, Northwestern University, Chicago, Illinois

AGGELIKI SYGGELOU, MD, PhD(c)
Resident in Pediatrics, Medical School, National and Kapodistrian University of Athens, Athens, Greece

BETH A. TARINI, MD, MS
Assistant Professor of Pediatrics and Communicable Diseases, Child Health Evaluation and Research Unit, Department of Pediatrics and Communicable Diseases, University of Michigan School of Medicine, Ann Arbor, Michigan

DICK TIBBOEL, MD, PhD
Medical Director, Intensive Care; Professor of Research, Department of Pediatric Surgery, Erasmus MC-Sophia Children's Hospital, Rotterdam, The Netherlands

JOHN N. VAN DEN ANKER, MD, PhD, FCP, FAAP
Vice Chair of Pediatrics for Experimental Therapeutics and the Evan and Cindy Jones Chair in Pediatric Clinical Pharmacology; Chief, Division of Pediatric Clinical Pharmacology, Children's National Medical Center- Sheikh Zayed Campus for Advanced Children's Medicine; Professor, Departments of Pediatrics, Pharmacology & Physiology, The George Washington University School of Medicine and Health Sciences, Washington, DC; Adjunct Faculty, Intensive Care, Erasmus MC-Sophia Children's Hospital, Rotterdam, The Netherlands

MONIQUE VAN DIJK, PhD
Associate Professor of Quality Care, Department of Pediatric Surgery; Neonatal Intensive Care, Department of Pediatrics, Erasmus MC-Sophia Children's Hospital, Rotterdam, The Netherlands

ANNEWIL VAN SAET, MD, PhD
Department of Pediatric Surgery, Intensive Care, Erasmus MC-Sophia Children's Hospital; Department of Cardio-Thoracic Anesthesiology, Erasmus MC, Rotterdam, The Netherlands

JONATHAN WAGNER, DO
Pediatric Cardiology Fellow, Section of Cardiology, Division of Clinical Pharmacology and Medical Toxicology, Department of Pediatrics, Children's Mercy Hospital and Clinics, University of Missouri-Kansas City School of Medicine, Kansas City, Missouri

ENNO D. WILDSCHUT, MD, PhD
Pediatric-Intensivist, Department of Pediatric Surgery, Intensive Care, Erasmus MC-Sophia Children's Hospital, Rotterdam, The Netherlands

THEODOROS XANTHOS, MD
Moderator MSc, Cardiopulmonary Resuscitation, Medical School, National and Kapodistrian University of Athens, Athens, Greece

Contents

Human development is described by the various anatomic and physiologic changes that occur as the single-celled zygote matures into an adult human being. Concomitant with bodily maturation are changes in the complex interactions between pharmacologic agents and the biologic matrix that is the human body. Profound changes in the manner by which drugs traverse the body during development can have significant implications in drug efficacy and toxicity. Although not a replacement for well-conducted, pediatric, pharmacokinetic studies, an understanding of developmental biology and the mechanisms for drug disposition invariably assists the pediatric clinician with the judicious use of medications in children.

The dose-exposure-response relationship for drugs may differ in pediatric patients compared with adults. Many clinical studies have established drug dose–exposure relationships across the pediatric age spectrum; however, genetic variation was seldom included. This article applies a systematic approach to determine the relative contribution of development and genetic variation on drug disposition and response using HMG-CoA reductase inhibitors as a model. Application of the approach drives the collection of information relevant to understanding the potential contribution of ontogeny and genetic variation to statin dose-exposure-response in children, and identifies important knowledge deficits to be addressed through the design of future studies.

Metabolomics is based on the detailed analysis of metabolites and represents a unique chemical fingerprint of an organism. This approach allows assessing the dynamic behavior of biologic systems with multiple network interactions among individual components. The field of metabolic profiling has rapidly developed over the last decade, with successful applications in various research areas including toxicology, disease diagnosis and classification, pharmacology, and nutrition. This article provides a comprehensive account of existing data in the literature from animal and clinical studies on the use of metabolomics for improved understanding of medical conditions affecting the neonate and the developing human being.

Biomarkers are an important tool for clinicians to detect long-term exposure to a multitude of compounds, including drugs of abuse, alcohol, and environmental toxicants. Using hair and meconium as matrices for biomarker testing provides a longer window of detection than that of blood or urine, providing clinically relevant information on prenatal exposures. The use of biomarkers can aid clinicians in early diagnosis and implementing appropriate interventions. The increasing burden of environmental toxicants has warranted the development of biomarkers for specific compounds, which could decrease exposure in humans.

Adverse drug reactions (ADRs) complicate at least 5% of all courses of therapy for children. Dealing with an ADR requires a stepwise approach in appreciation of the possibility of an ADR, assessment of whether the adverse event in question is drug-related, assessment of causality, assistance in treating the symptoms of the ADR, and dealing with the aftermath of the event. Several new developments likely will improve the ability to assess, evaluate, treat, and prevent ADRs in children. These developments include tools to evaluate causality, laboratory tests to diagnose ADRs, pharmacogenomic approaches to prevent ADRs, and new insights into treating serious ADRs.

The delivery of safe and effective antiretroviral therapy to children and adolescents is crucial to save the lives of millions of children worldwide. The immunologic response to human immunodeficiency infection is closely related to a child's development and creates age-specific parameters for the evaluation of therapeutic response to antiretroviral therapy. Similarly, the development and maturation of organ systems involved in drug absorption, distribution, metabolism, and elimination determines significant changes in the pharmacokinetics of antiretroviral drugs throughout childhood. The authors review the evolution in treatment of pediatric HIV from infancy through adolescence.

The optimal evaluation and use of antibacterial agents that are very frequently prescribed in neonates during various situations such as early- and late-onset invasive infections depend on adapted dose selection, based on population pharmacokinetic/pharmacodynamic modeling and simulation, using approved surrogate biomarkers as pharmacodynamic end points. Data on efficacy can be extrapolated from adult and pediatric data because of comparable mechanistic action of antibiotics in neonates, children, and adults. However, evaluation of efficacy and toxicity in the neonate should always be discussed with regulatory agencies and are highly recommended when feasible.

10% of all pediatric patients receiving ECMO, ECMO therapy is initiated during or after cardiopulmonary resuscitation. Therapeutic hypothermia is frequently used in children after cardiac arrest, despite the lack of randomized controlled trials that show its efficacy. Hypothermia is frequently used in children and neonates during cardiopulmonary bypass (CPB). By combining data from pharmacokinetic studies in children on ECMO and CPB and during hypothermia, this review elucidates the possible effects of hypothermia during ECMO on drug disposition.

Children have been identified as uniquely vulnerable clinical research subjects since the early 1970s. This article reviews the historical underpinnings of this designation, the current regulatory framework for pediatric and neonatal research, and common problems in pediatric research oversight. It also presents 3 areas of pediatric and neonatal research (genomic screening, healthy children donating stem cells, and therapeutic hypothermia for neonates with hypoxic-ischemic encephalopathy) that highlight contemporary challenges in pediatric research ethics, including balancing risk and benefit, informed consent and assent, and clinical equipoise.

PEDIATRIC CLINICS
OF NORTH AMERICA

ISSUE OF RELATED INTEREST

Clinics in Perinatology March 2012 (Volume 39:1)
Evidence-Based Neonatal Pharmacotherapy
Alan R. Spitzer, MD, *Guest Editor*
http://www.perinatology.theclinics.com/issues?issue_key=S0095-5108(11)X0006-4

NOW AVAILABLE FOR YOUR iPhone and iPad

Preface

Neonatal and Pediatric Clinical Pharmacology

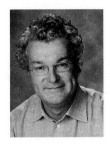 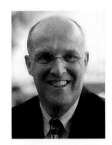 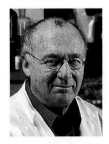

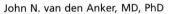

John N. van den Anker, MD, PhD   Max J. Coppes, MD, PhD, MBA   Gideon Koren, MD, FRCPC, FACMT

Guest Editors

"It was the best of times, it was the worst of times, it was the age of wisdom, it was the age of foolishness, it was the epoch of belief, it was the epoch of incredulity, it was the season of Light, it was the season of Darkness, it was the spring of hope, it was the winter of despair, we had everything before us, we had nothing before us, we were all going directly to Heaven, we were all going the other way." Charles Dickens wrote these lines in the midst of the 19th century, yet it is amazing how they still resonate in the beginning of the 21st century, especially for the lives of children all over the world. There have been remarkable advances in the health and well-being of children, contrasted by the devastating influences of war, political unrest, poverty, and relatively new diseases such as HIV/AIDS.

However, even in the so-called developed world, there are still significant unmet medical needs for children. Moreover, the history of drug development is clearly one of neglecting the specific needs of children, by incorrectly assuming that data generated in adults can be applied directly to children. For decades, the needs of infants, children, and adolescents have been ignored in the process of drug development.[1]

In adults, ischemic heart disease, hypertension, Alzheimer's disease, and many types of cancer and other conditions have a high prevalence. If a drug is developed to treat one of these conditions, there are many patients to enroll in clinical trials, and once the drug is approved, the marketplace is large and profitable. For children, there are relatively few patients with any specific diagnosis and thus fewer patients to study, making clinical trials challenging. Furthermore "children" are not one group. Studies might be needed in newborns, infants, toddlers, older children, and adolescents. Each of these subgroups may have different dosing needs, different responses to medications, and different adverse reaction profiles, necessitating different dosage forms for safe and accurate administration. The cost and complexity of studies go up

Pediatr Clin N Am 59 (2012) xv–xviii
http://dx.doi.org/10.1016/j.pcl.2012.07.014
0031-3955/12/$ – see front matter © 2012 Elsevier Inc. All rights reserved.

and, once the studies are completed, the marketplace may be so small that it is economically not viable to produce and distribute the product.

Traditionally, this process rendered children as "therapeutic orphans," and pediatricians have been forced to use medicines with little evidence-based data to support a proper choice of medicines and doses, and without information of what to expect in terms of efficacy and side effects.[2] Tragic outcomes from gray baby syndrome from chloramphenicol and deaths from drug excipients, such as diethylene glycol in elixir of sulfanilamide and benzyl alcohol in intravenous drugs used in newborns, are well-documented examples of the need for scientifically sound and ethically driven pediatric drug development and therapeutics.

In pediatric medicine, the patient may be a preterm infant weighing 400 g or a morbidly obese adolescent weighing as much as 250 kg. Drug doses for these children are often derived by scaling from adult dosages after adjusting for body weight.[3] However, it is well known that the pharmacokinetics of a drug, including drug absorption, distribution, metabolism, and excretion, are substantially different in children as compared to adults, and that the pharmacokinetics change with growth and maturation.[4]

Legislative actions such as the Best Pharmaceuticals for Children Act have raised the priority of pediatric studies through financial incentives and have been remarkably successful over the years.[5] There has been a major response to the Act by the pharmaceutical industry, working in collaboration with academic pediatricians and the FDA. Much needed new data about medicines in children have been developed and old assumptions about doses, efficacy, and side effects of many drugs were shown to be incorrect. Efforts by the *Eunice Kennedy Shriver* National Institute of Child Health and Development to plan and support pediatric investigation as part of the National Institutes of Health roadmap initiative in Clinical and Translational Science Awards and in creating the Pediatric Pharmacology Research Unit Network,[6] and more recently the Specialized Centers in Research in Pediatric Developmental Pharmacology, have been vital in advancing the field of developmental and pediatric pharmacology. Similarly, efforts within the FDA to improve pediatric drug development have been pivotal to move the agenda forward.

One of the critical elements in all human investigation is the assurance of the very highest ethical standards. Indeed, some of the critical elements of human investigation ethical assurance, particularly those related to respect for persons and human autonomy leading to concepts of voluntary informed consent, had been viewed as impediments to having children participate in clinical trials. Issues were raised especially in trials where the prospect of direct benefit to the child has been absent or unlikely. While there always should be an ongoing discussion and consideration of ethical issues as context, science, and society change, there is now a reasonable grounding to allow for pediatric investigation both in the United States and internationally. In fact, as the science of clinical investigation has advanced to allow us to address key issues in therapeutics in children, we have come to realize that the use of medicines in clinical practice not guided by data from good studies in children places children at greater risk than participation in well-designed, ethically conducted clinical trials. The advances in outcomes of children with cancer are a tribute to the value of capturing clinical results of therapies in structured clinical trials.

The future of pediatric therapeutics will depend on our expanding knowledge of disease pathogenesis, the discovery of new drug targets leading to new medicines, the skillful and ethical evaluation of those medicines in children, and the evolution of innovative approaches to support the development of medicines specifically for pediatric diseases. There is clearly a need for more and better trained pediatric clinical investigators, including clinical pharmacologists.

We have entered the era of increased emphasis on "personalized medicine," providing the right drug for the right child based on improved diagnostic specificity and understanding of the net benefit of a specific therapy for a specific patient.[7] A gradual move away from the traditional development of "blockbuster" drugs to more targeted therapeutics is needed, but the costs of drug development will keep on rising and there will be a demand for regulatory change too.

This issue of the *Pediatric Clinics in North America* is devoted to the topic of Neonatal and Pediatric Clinical Pharmacology. The same topic was covered by an issue of *Pediatric Clinics in North America* more than 15 years ago. The increase in knowledge in this area has shown an unprecedented growth in these years, and scientific contributions in this discipline have been published in numerous journals. This underscores the fact that the field of neonatal and pediatric clinical pharmacology has reached adulthood and in the coming years will continue to improve pharmacotherapy further in neonates, infants, children, and adolescents. All articles in this volume have been written by authors who published their pivotal work in this field in recent years.

However, although many important topics are dealt with, it is not possible to cover all aspects of this rapidly expanding field in a single volume. The articles cover a wide area of concerns for those who deal with neonatal and pediatric clinical medicine including updates on pharmacological treatments of HIV, pulmonary hypertension, opioid addiction, infectious diseases in the newborn, and pain-related issues, but also will present state-of-the-art updates on developmental pharmacology, developmental pharmacogenomics, new ways in detecting ADRs, the impact of new treatments such as hypothermia and ECMO on drug disposition, the importance of biomarkers, the emerging field of metabolomics, and ethical issues in neonatal and pediatric clinical trials.

It is clear that the worldwide collaboration among academicians, pharmaceutical industry, and regulatory authorities is critical for the future success of the discipline of neonatal and pediatric clinical pharmacology, but, more importantly, for the health and normal development of neonates, infants, children, and adolescents. All authors have provided not only the latest information in their areas of expertise but also presented the readers with food for thought on the directions their areas are moving toward. We are very grateful to all the authors for the time and effort they have put into writing these in-depth contributions.

John N. van den Anker, MD, PhD
Division of Pediatric Clinical Pharmacology
Children's National Medical Center
Sheikh Zayed Campus for Advanced Children's Medicine
GWU School of Medicine and Health Sciences
111 Michigan Avenue, NW
Washington, DC 20010, USA

Max J. Coppes, MD, PhD, MBA
Center for Cancer & Blood Disorders
Children's National Medical Center
Sheikh Zayed Campus for Advanced Children's Medicine
GWU School of Medicine and Health Sciences
111 Michigan Avenue, NW
Washington, DC 20010, USA

Gideon Koren, MD, FRCPC, FACMT
Division of Clinical Pharmacology and Toxicology
The Hospital for Sick Children, Division of Pediatrics, Pharmacology
Pharmacy and Medical Genetics
The University of Toronto
Division of Medicine, Pediatrics and Physiology/Pharmacology
The Ivey Chair in Molecular Toxicology
The University of Western Ontario
Toronto, Canada

E-mail addresses:
jvandena@childrensnational.org (J.N. van den Anker)
mcoppes@bccancer.bc.ca (M.J. Coppes)
gkoren@sickkids.ca (G. Koren)

REFERENCES

1. Kimland E, Odlind V. Off-label drug use in pediatric patients. Clin Pharmacol Ther 2012;91(5):796–801.
2. Shirkey H. Therapeutic orphans. Pediatrics 1968;72:119–20.
3. Johnson TN. The problems in scaling adult drug doses to children. Arch Dis Child 2008;93:207–11.
4. Kearns GL, Abdel-Rahman SM, Alexander SW, et al. Developmental pharmacology-drug disposition, action and therapy in infants and children. N Engl J Med 2003;349:1157–67.
5. Best Pharmaceuticals for Children Act of 2001, 42 USC 284 et seq as amended.
6. Cohen SN. The Pediatric Pharmacology Research Unit (PPRU) Network and its role in meeting pediatric labeling needs. Pediatrics 1999;104:644–5.
7. Leeder JS, Kearns GL, Spielberg SP, et al. Understanding the relative roles of pharmacogenetics and ontogeny in pediatric drug development and regulatory science. J Clin Pharmacol 2010;5:1377–87.

Erratum

Please note that a correction is needed in an article title in *Pediatric Clinics of North America* 59:4. The correct title of the article by Darius J. Bägli, MDCM, FRCSC is "Is Bladder Dysfunction in Children Science Fiction or Science Fact: Editorial Comment." The publisher apologizes for this error.

http://dx.doi.org/10.1016/j.pcl.2012.09.006
0031-3955/12/$ – see front matter

pediatric.theclinics.com

Pediatric Pharmacokinetics
Human Development and Drug Disposition

Ryan S. Funk, PharmD, PhD[a], Jacob T. Brown, PharmD[a],
Susan M. Abdel-Rahman, PharmD[a,b,*]

KEYWORDS

- Pediatric • Pharmacokinetic • Development • Absorption • Distribution
- Metabolism • Excretion • Transport

KEY POINTS

- Drug disposition is dynamic and can be attributed to developmental physiologic changes.
- An understanding of the anatomic and physiologic changes during development is paramount in predicting age-dependent changes in drug disposition.
- Without a complete understanding of how biology drives drug disposition, pediatric clinical pharmacokinetic studies are a necessity for rational drug use in children.
- Future studies are needed to understand the ontogeny of drug disposition pathways, including the importance of drug transporters, in pediatric clinical pharmacokinetics.

INTRODUCTION

The efficacious use of therapeutic agents is often guided by an understanding of the relationship between dose and exposure (ie, pharmacokinetics [PK]). These relationships vary based on the demographic, genetic, anthropomorphic, and pathologic constitution of the patient being treated. As such, the clinical practitioner is required to understand how these patient-specific factors influence the disposition of drugs in the body. For pediatric practitioners, the process of growth and development overlays these patient-specific factors adding complexity to therapeutic management. In the absence of pediatric PK studies to guide the safe and effective use of medications, pediatric dosing can be guided by knowledge of the anatomic and physiologic factors that govern drug disposition and the developmental patterns that influence these factors.[1]

Disclosure: The authors have no competing financial interests.
[a] Division of Clinical Pharmacology and Medical Toxicology, Children's Mercy Hospitals and Clinics, 2401 Gillham Road, Kansas City, MO 64108, USA; [b] Department of Pediatrics, School of Medicine, University of Missouri-Kansas City, 2464 Charlotte Street, Kansas City, MO 64108, USA
* Corresponding author. Division of Clinical Pharmacology and Medical Toxicology, Children's Mercy Hospitals and Clinics, 2401 Gillham Road, Kansas City, MO 64108.
E-mail address: srahman@cmh.edu

This article links understanding of anatomic and physiologic changes observed during human development to their impact on drug disposition. It discusses developmental changes that can affect the absorption, distribution, metabolism, and excretion (ADME) of therapeutic agents in children. Relevant examples from the literature are discussed and attention is drawn to developmental changes that have yet to be described. Where human data are unavailable, animal data are supplemented to allude to the potential role of ontogeny in drug disposition.

ABSORPTION

Drugs administered by extravascular routes must overcome multiple barriers to reach the systemic circulation. In addition to the physical and chemical processes that affect drug absorption (ie, stability, solubility, permeability), mechanical barriers such as transporter-mediated uptake and efflux are being found to play an important role in regulating the absorption of many drugs. All of these processes are influenced by development, thus influencing the PK profiles of many drugs in children.

Peroral Absorption

Following oral administration, there are several ontogenic factors that influence systemic drug absorption. One of the most prominent is the period of relative achlorhydria observed shortly after birth.[2] Gastric pH influences absorption by 2 mechanisms: permeation and stability. Although the stomach is not a principal site of drug absorption, the decrease in ionization of weakly acidic drugs in the low-pH environment of the stomach can theoretically enhance permeation across the epithelial lining of the stomach. In contrast, a decrease or delay in absorption could be expected for weakly acidic drugs (eg, phenobarbital, phenytoin) under conditions of increased gastric pH in the newborn.[3–5] More importantly, the stomach is an important site of pH-dependent drug degradation, ultimately affecting the amount of intact drug that reaches the small intestine. Perhaps the best-documented example of the impact of development on gastric pH arises with the acid-labile β-lactam antibiotic penicillin, with which plasma concentrations in the neonate reach levels 5 to 6 times those seen in infants and children owing to protection from decomposition (**Fig. 1**A).[6]

In contrast with the permeation-limited absorption of many water-soluble drugs, oral absorption of many lipophilic drugs is limited by their poor solubility in the aqueous digestive fluids. Absorption of drugs in this category often shows significant food effects (eg, enhanced absorption in the fed state).[7] Stimulation of bile acid secretion into the alimentary canal by food results in micellar solubilization of many lipophilic drugs rendering their absorption dependent on biliary function. Despite an increase in circulating bile acid levels in young infants, concentrations of the major bile salts in the intestinal lumen are reduced, likely the result of a decrease in transporter-mediated secretion of bile acids into the biliary canaliculi.[8,9] As a result, clinically significant changes in drug absorption are possible for solubility-limited drugs. This possibility is shown by data on the antiviral pleconaril, a highly lipophilic compound that, in adults, shows a 2-fold increase in exposure with food.[10] Although dose escalation studies in adults revealed a dose-proportional increase in exposure, dose escalation in neonates resulted in no increase in exposure.[11] This failure to increase neonatal drug exposure may reflect restricted bioavailability caused by limited micellar solubilization. If so, then other solubility-limited, lipophilic drugs may have similar saturable absorption profiles in neonates.

In addition to the impact of the gastrointestinal fluid composition on the solubility and permeability of drugs, the rate of gastric emptying (GE) influences the speed at

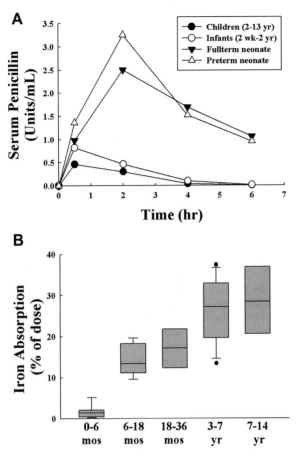

Fig. 1. (*A*) Penicillin plasma concentrations following the oral administration of a single 22,000 units/kg dose in neonates, infants, and children. (*B*) Age-dependent enteral absorption of iron expressed as a percentage of the dose administered.

which drugs are presented to the absorptive surfaces of the small intestine. The rate of GE is prolonged in the first week of life and approaches adult values by 6 to 8 months of age.[4,12] There exists a significant level of developmental variation in GE, in part because a variety of newborn disorders can significantly affect GE rates, among them prematurity, respiratory disease, gastroesophageal reflux disease, and congenital heart disease. Intestinal motility further affects the drug's residence time, thereby serving as another important determinant of the rate and extent of drug absorption.[13] In the young infant, intestinal contractile frequency and amplitude are reduced and highly variable.[14] The overall impact of decreased emptying and motility on drug absorption depends on the dissolution and permeation properties of the formulation. For drugs that are rapidly and completely absorbed within the small intestine, absolute bioavailability in young infants is expected to remain mostly unchanged, although the rate of absorption, and consequently the maximum drug concentration (C_{max}), may be significantly reduced and the time to C_{max} (T_{max}) delayed. Age-dependent changes in the absorption rate constant (k_a) and T_{max} for numerous drugs and nutrients (eg, L(+)-arabinose, phenobarbital, sulfonamides, digoxin, cisapride) support this hypothesis.[4,15]

Attempts to enhance absorption rates in young infants via administration of a prokinetic agent can increase k_a; however, absolute differences in the absorption rate constants between neonates (<30 days of life) and infants (>30 days of life) remain unchanged despite pharmacologic stimulation.[4] These results suggest that additional developmental factors influence the rate of drug absorption in the neonate.

Apart from physicochemical and mechanical forces, phase I and phase II drug metabolizing enzymes (DME) residing in the intestinal tract influence drug absorption. Although only limited data exist on the age-dependent expression of most intestinal DMEs, existing data support a developmental component for at least some of the enzymes. Duodenal biopsies have shown increases in intestinal CYP1A1 and CYP3A with increasing age.[16,17] Thus, drugs metabolized by these pathways are expected to undergo less presystemic intestinal clearance in young children. Among the intestinal phase II enzymes evaluated to date, glutathione S-transferase (GST)–mediated conjugating capacity of the antineoplastic agent busulfan was highest in distal duodenal biopsies from children less than 5 years of age compared with children older than 8 years of age and adolescents.[18] These findings are in accordance with age-dependent changes in the presystemic clearance of this drug, implying that young children may require higher oral doses of drugs that are subject to clearance via glutathione conjugation. With the paucity of data on the ontogeny of intestinal DMEs, further studies are needed to fully examine the influence of development on intestinal drug metabolism.

One of the newest and still emerging fields is the study of the impact of drug transporters on absorption. Transporter proteins expressed along the intestinal tract not only facilitate the uptake of nutrients and drugs across the intestinal epithelium but also limit their absorption by actively pumping them back into the intestinal lumen. As with intestinal DMEs, very few data have been generated on developmental changes in transporter expression, and the studies that have been completed are primarily restricted to the transport of nutrients (ie, SGLT1, GLUT2, PEPT1) in animal models, many of which seem to be maximally expressed shortly after birth.[19] By contrast, the acquisition of iron absorption capacity (mediated by DMT1) increases linearly after birth, reaching adult levels by early childhood (see **Fig. 1B**).[20,21]

Among established drug transporters, it seems that P-glycoprotein (P-gp) is present in the intestine by 1 month of age.[22] Other PK studies provide circumstantial evidence supporting developmental changes in intestinal drug transporter activity. For example, the H_2-receptor antagonist nizatidine (a substrate for intestinal transporters whose activity can be modified by the coadministration of apple juice) shows an age-dependent decrease in apparent oral clearance despite no age dependence on terminal elimination rate constant.[23,24] Even transporters whose expression seems to mature shortly after birth can show age effects.[25] Drugs whose transport is mediated by the intestinal peptide transporter 1 (PEPT1) compete with milk peptides for uptake,[26] and infants on a milk-based diet with condensed feeding frequency likely have milk peptides continuously distributed along the intestinal lumen. Thus, the magnitude of drug-nutrient interactions may be more pronounced in the young infant. An advanced understanding of developmental changes in intestinal transporter activity will facilitate understanding of the potential for drug-drug and drug-nutrient interactions in young children.

Extraoral Absorption

Despite conventional preferences to deliver drugs orally, nonoral routes of administration may be preferred in some settings. As with peroral administration, the absorption of extraorally administered drugs is also subject to developmental variation. The absorption of rectally administered drugs depends in part on drug dissolution profiles within the lower intestinal tract. Rectal formulations with delayed release characteristics (ie, erythromycin, acetaminophen) may experience decreased residence times in young infants owing to an increase in the number of high-amplitude pulsatile contractions of the lower intestine.[27] Preterm neonates have enhanced rectal acetaminophen bioavailability, possibly caused by reductions in presystemic metabolism, intestinal motility, or temperature instability.[28]

Although infrequently used, percutaneous administration can be an efficient means of delivering drugs to children. The increased systemic exposure experienced by children is a product of developmental differences in the neonate and young infant that result in enhanced percutaneous absorption, namely an increased body surface area/mass ratio, higher rates of tissue perfusion, and a higher degree of skin hydration.[29,30] These differences can increase a child's risk of toxicity to topically applied agents even when systemic exposure is not the goal of treatment. Unintended consequences of topical agents have been shown for numerous agents, such as antihistamines, steroids, sulfadiazine, talcum powder, and laundry detergent.[31]

In addition, absorption following intramuscular (IM) injection is considered. Although IM absorption of some drugs in children is reported as erratic, others are efficiently absorbed by this route, which may be explained by increases in capillary density (25%–50%) experienced by the young infant to assist with the metabolic demands of growth and development.[32] Peak plasma concentrations for some drugs (eg, cephalosporins, aminoglycosides) are consequently significantly higher in neonates compared with young children, presumably reflecting a change in the rate of absorption from the site of administration.[33,34]

DISTRIBUTION

Once absorbed into the systemic circulation, the extent to which a drug penetrates extravascular tissues is described by the drug's volume of distribution (V_d). The underlying determinants of drug distribution include the physiologic characteristics of the tissue and the physicochemical and transport properties of the drug. Thus, physiologic changes observed throughout development can have a sizable impact on the distribution properties of a drug.

One of the more prominent changes that influence drug distribution is the fluid composition of the body. Water comprises approximately 80% of a newborn infant's body weight, with fractional decreases over the first 4 months of life to adult levels (approximately 60%) (**Fig. 2A**).[35] Hydrophilic drugs that are mainly restricted to the aqueous fluid compartments (eg, gentamicin, linezolid) consequently have a larger apparent V_d and decreased plasma concentrations in the young infants.[36,37] In conjunction with developmental changes in drug clearance, these children can experience circulating concentrations that fail to adequately meet pharmacodynamic criteria if dose and dosing interval are not adjusted for age.[37–39]

As opposed to total body water, total body fat stores are reduced in infants and approach adult values in the first years of life, with age-dependent fluctuations throughout childhood (see **Fig. 2B**). Based on these changes, it theoretically could be expected that lipophilic drugs would show a lower V_d in infants and young children; however, this is largely not observed, because these drugs tend to freely associate with cellular components in tissues other than adipose. The failure to observe a lower V_d for lipophilic agents in young children may also indicate that additional tissue retention mechanisms compensate for the changes in body composition. A variety of retention mechanisms can facilitate the partitioning and accumulation of drugs in tissue.[40]

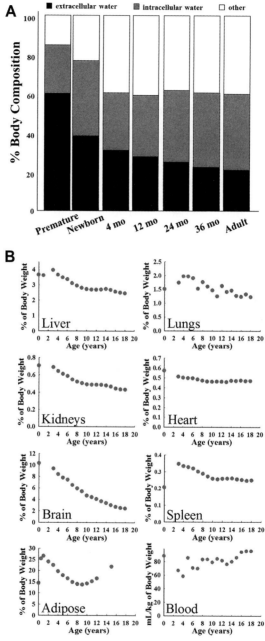

Fig. 2. (*A*) Body water composition as a percentage of body weight in neonates, infants, young children, and adults. (*B*) Age-dependent changes in tissue mass relative to total body weight.

For example, a subset of drugs with extremely large V_d accumulate in tissues through their affinity for acidic subcellular compartments (ie, lysosomes), which are enriched in the liver, lung, heart, brain, and kidneys.[41,42] Thus, age-dependent changes in the mass of these organs relative to total body mass would result in V_d differences with age (see **Fig. 2**B), particularly when blood flow/volume to these tissues is comparable with or greater than that of adults.[43] Although speculative, these changes in fractional organ mass may contribute to changes in the V_d, and future studies addressing the impact of development on tissue retention mechanisms are needed to more thoroughly evaluate their relevance to pediatric pharmacotherapy.

A drug must exist in its free, unbound form to distribute out of the central compartment and into extravascular tissues. Therefore, the apparent V_d of a drug depends not only on its ability to enter and accumulate in tissue but also on the free fraction of the circulating drug. Protein binding depends on the quantity of circulating plasma proteins (eg, α-1-acid glycoprotein [AAG] and albumin), the drug's binding affinity for these proteins, and the presence of endogenous or exogenous substances that compete for binding sites, including free fatty acids, bilirubin, and other drugs.[44–46] Development influences each of these factors, with neonates and young infants experiencing reduced concentration of albumin and AAG, protein isoforms for which drugs have a reduced affinity, and increased circulating concentrations of ligands that can displace drugs from their binding sites.[47] Compared with older children and adults, young infants experience increased free fractions, and thus increased V_d, of many drugs (eg, barbiturates, opioid analgesics).[48,49] The clinical importance of developmental changes in the fractional protein binding of drugs ultimately depends on the therapeutic agent under consideration and its therapeutic index.

Although limited data are available describing the ontogeny of transmembrane proteins responsible for the cellular uptake and efflux of drugs, there is strong biologic evidence to support the assertion of a developmental expression profile. The endogenous substrates for these transport proteins include a variety of substances that are crucial to normal human growth and development (eg, metals, electrolytes, amino acids, nucleotides, lipids, carbohydrates, steroids). Realizing that these substrates are used by different tissues to different extents throughout development, adaptive mechanisms that control transporter expression and activity are likely involved. To date, only limited data from postmortem brain tissue are available, suggesting that P-gp, MRP1 (multidrug resistance protein 1), and BCRP (breast cancer resistance protein) all show distinct anatomic and cellular expression patterns that are developmentally dependent.[50] Such differences may explain changes in the central nervous system (CNS) penetration of drugs that are substrates for these transport proteins; however, other studies suggest that changes in pore density and regional blood flow may account for age-dependent differences in CNS drug penetration.

METABOLISM

In addition to the liver functioning in a variety of life-sustaining synthetic and digestive processes, it also serves as the predominant organ of metabolism for exogenously administered drugs. Hepatic clearance pathways are usually divided into phase I (eg, oxidation, reduction, hydrolysis) and phase II (eg, covalent conjugation) reactions. The DMEs responsible for drug bioconversion are found in multiple tissues other than the liver; however, these extrahepatic sites (with the exception of the intestine) are of minimal significance in overall drug clearance and this article only discusses the liver. As alluded to earlier, an understanding of the ontogeny of DMEs helps to appreciate the potential for drug-drug, drug-nutrient, and drug-gene interactions in children.

Phase I Metabolism

Phase I drug metabolism is typically performed by a group of mixed-function oxidases referred to as the cytochromes P450 (CYPs). These enzymes are highly expressed in the liver; CYP3A4 being the most clinically relevant followed by CYP2D6 > CYP2C >

CYP2E1 > CYP1A2. Although the fetus expresses a high level of CYP3A7, humans undergo an isoform switch shortly after birth and CYP3A7 rapidly decreases coincident with a steady increase in CYP3A4 expression and activity through the first year of life (**Fig. 3**A).[51,52] The clinical implications of this profile can be shown for numerous CYP3A substrates (eg, sildenafil, cisapride) that show marked reductions in half-life during infancy.[15,53,54]

In contrast with CYP3A4, CYP2D6 reaches adult activity levels by 2 weeks of life.[55] For this enzyme, genetic variations seem to have a greater impact on activity than does development. Within the CYP2C family, the 2 predominant isoforms display distinct developmental patterns. CYP2C9 expression and activity in human liver microsomes suggest that, in the early postnatal period (0–5 months), enzyme activity and expression are similar to those of older children (5 months–18 years). In contrast, CYP2C19 expression seems to increase over the first 6 months of life, with a corresponding increase in substrate-specific activity.[56] Interestingly, PK data for the CYP2C9 substrate phenytoin reveals a terminal half-life that decreases from 20 hours at birth to 8 hours at 2 weeks of life.[57,58] Further, intravenous PK data for the CYP2C19 substrate omeprazole have been found to have high clearance rates in the young infant that normalizes in the first 5 years of life.[59,60] The discrepancy between the data observed in vitro and pediatric PK data highlights the complexity of predicting in vivo processes in the growing child based on in vitro data. This assertion is

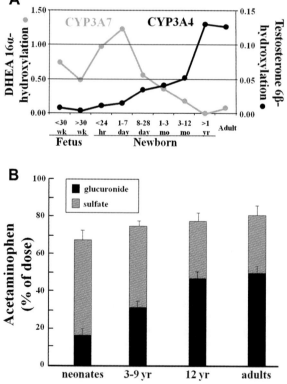

Fig. 3. (A) Developmental changes in the activities of hepatic CYP3A4 and CYP3A7. (B) Sulfate and glucuronide conjugates of acetaminophen as a percent of total dose in newborns, children and adults. DHEA, dehydroepiandrosterone.

reinforced by the finding that CYP2C9 and VKORC1 genotypes explain less of the variability in warfarin dosing for children than they do in adults.[61]

Although not responsible for the metabolism of a large number of marketed drugs, CYP2E1 is important in the metabolism of a variety of anesthetic agents and has been found to be differentially expressed throughout development. Protein and activity levels are negligible in the prenatal period but gradually increase to within 80% of adult levels by the first year of life.[62] CYP1A2 similarly shows negligible levels of activity in the prenatal period and levels in the neonate are 4% to 5% of those found in adults. CYP1A2 activity steadily increases with age to 10% to 15%, 20% to 25%, and 50% to 55% of adult values at 1 to 3 months, 3 to 12 months, and 1 to 9 years of age, respectively.[63]

Phase II Metabolism

The conjugation reactions performed by phase II DMEs serve to increase the water solubility of the drug molecule, thereby facilitating excretion. Multiple gene families, each with multiple isoforms, are involved in these reactions, including uridine 5'-diphosphoglucuronosyltransferases (UGTs), GSTs, N-acetyltransferases (NATs), and sulfotransferases (SULTs).

UGT1A1, involved in the metabolism of acetaminophen, ibuprofen, and warfarin, is absent in the fetal liver but measurable immediately after birth and expressed at adult levels by 3 to 6 months of life.[64] Transcript levels of UGT1A9, involved in the metabolism of ethinyl estradiol, ibuprofen, and acetaminophen, are approximately 44% of those seen in adults at 6 months of life and 64% of the adult values by 2 years of age.[65] Using morphine clearance as a surrogate, the activity of UGT2B7 seems to be low in premature neonates but increases to levels greater than those observed in adults in the first year of life.[66]

SULTs are involved in the biosynthesis and metabolism of multiple endogenous biochemicals including steroid hormones, catecholamines, and thyroid hormone. SULT1A1 seems to be expressed in the fetal liver at levels comparable with those of children and adolescents. In contrast, SULT2A1 shows a significant increase during the first 3 months of life when activity levels comparable with those of adults are achieved.[67] In addition, data on GSTs A1 and A2 (DMEs that facilitate the conjugation of glutathione to the electrophilic centers of endogenous and exogenous substrates) reveal that both enzymes are present in the fetal liver but that adult expression levels are not achieved until 1 to 2 years of life.[68]

Compensatory metabolic pathways are in place for many of the phase I and phase II DMEs that are developmentally dependent. For some drugs, the total function of all relevant compensatory pathways may result in no change in the overall clearance of the drug as a function of age. For other drugs, the compensatory pathways may not be as efficient, resulting in age-dependent reductions in total body clearance. For example, acetaminophen is primarily metabolized via UGT1A6 and SULT1A1, with adults predominantly using the former pathway and newborns the latter (see **Fig. 3B**).[69] Despite compensatory sulfation in young infants, these patients still exhibit an increased half-life compared with children and adolescents.[70] Thus, the clinical relevance of ontogenic variation in DMEs depends, in part, on the presence of compensatory metabolic pathways, the therapeutic index of the drug, and the nature of the metabolites that are formed.

The ontogeny of biologic pathways involved in the metabolism of large-molecular-weight therapeutic agents also needs to be discussed; however, very limited data exist on this topic. Among the limited existing data is the example of antihemophilic factors. Factor VIII, a protein involved in the clotting cascade, shows a shorter half-life in infants and young children 1 to 6 years of age (9.2 hours) compared with in adolescents and adults 10 to 65 years of age (12.2 hours).[71] PK studies on insulin, growth hormone, and erythropoietin all seem to suggest age-dependent changes in clearance as well.[72–77] With the increase in the number of biologic agents being brought to the market and their increased use in children, it will be important to characterize the disposition pathways of these proteins and their ontogeny.

EXCRETION

In addition to maintaining electrolyte and fluid homeostasis, the kidney is the predominant organ responsible for the excretion of drugs and their metabolites. Structural and functional maturation of the kidney occurs throughout childhood and these changes are well described elsewhere.[78–80] Although glomerular filtration rate (GFR) and renal tubular secretion are low in the newborn, they reach and exceed adult levels within the first few years of life (**Fig. 4**A).[81] Such changes contribute to reduced clearance of renally eliminated drugs in the neonate and increased clearance of renally excreted drugs in young children.[82] For example, pharmacokinetic studies of vancomycin indicate that total body clearance averages 1.14 mL/min/kg in neonates (<1 month of

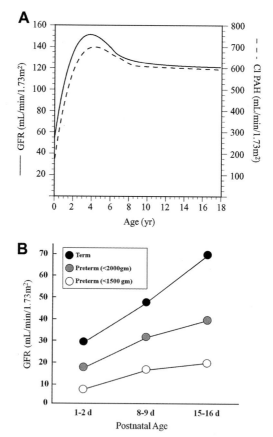

Fig. 4. (A) Age-dependent changes in GFR and p-aminohippurate (PAH) clearance. (B) Postnatal and developmental changes in renal filtration capacity in preterm and term neonates.

age), 1.91 mL/min/kg in infants (1–12 months of age), and 3.17 mL/min/kg in children older than 1 year of age (average age of 5.8 years), compared with 0.92 mL/min/kg in adults with normal renal function.[83,84] These changes in renal clearance often necessitate significant dose modifications for renally cleared drugs.

Compared with the full-term neonate, GFR is significantly reduced in the premature neonate after birth (see **Fig. 4**B).[80] Despite a notable increase in the first 2 weeks of life, GFR in premature neonates remains significantly suppressed compared with full-term neonates, suggesting differences in the maturation of the filtration process in these 2 populations. These observed differences in renal architecture and perfusion with age, both gestational and postnatal, result in clear developmental PK profiles for drugs that are passively and actively cleared by the kidney. For example, fluconazole's protracted half-life in premature infants (88 hours vs 19.5–25 hours in full-term infants) directly affects the dosing recommendations for this antifungal.[85]

In contrast with passive filtration, little is known about renal secretory pathways in children, with the exception of the proteins involved in the tubular secretion of p-aminohippurate (PAH).[80] Among the numerous remaining transporters involved in drug translocation, developmental expression profiles for these proteins have yet to be defined in humans. Studies on transporter expression in rats and mice have shown a clear age dependence that may suggest what will be found for humans.[86–90] In addition, excretion cannot be reviewed without addressing biliary clearance, an often overlooked, but significant, contributor to drug disposition. The first few weeks of life seem to be accompanied by reduced expression of the hepatic transport proteins that facilitate biliary drug clearance.[91] Reduced biliary drug excretion in neonates corresponds with increased fractional urinary excretion of several drugs (eg, ceftriaxone, cefoperazone).[92,93] Depending on the transport proteins involved and the ratio of biliary excretion to total drug clearance, age-dependent changes in biliary secretion may or may not cause clinically significant changes in drug clearance.

SUMMARY

For special populations in which there are only limited data to guide drug dosing, it is crucial for the clinician to understand how underlying physiologic changes within the population can affect drug disposition. In pediatrics, an understanding of the underlying physiologic changes can be garnered through a working knowledge of developmental biology. Through an understanding of the physiologic processes that dictate the disposition properties of a drug, the pediatric clinician can arrive at rational recommendations when selecting and optimizing drug therapy. As long as deficits continue to exist in the understanding of the physiologic processes involved in drug disposition, it will not be possible to fully appreciate the impact of ontogeny on these processes. In many cases, observations made in clinical PK studies will lay the foundation that ultimately expands understanding of the role of developmental changes on drug disposition.

REFERENCES

1. Abdel-Rahman SM, Kauffman RE. The integration of pharmacokinetics and pharmacodynamics: understanding dose-response. Annu Rev Pharmacol Toxicol 2004;44:111–36.
2. Agunod M, Yamaguchi N, Lopez R, et al. Correlative study of hydrochloric acid, pepsin, and intrinsic factor secretion in newborns and infants. Am J Dig Dis 1969; 14(6):400–14.
3. Hogben CA, Schanker LS, Tocco DJ, et al. Absorption of drugs from the stomach. II. The human. J Pharmacol Exp Ther 1957;120(4):540–5.

4. Heimann G. Enteral absorption and bioavailability in children in relation to age. Eur J Clin Pharmacol 1980;18(1):43–50.

5. Milsap RL, Jusko WJ. Pharmacokinetics in the infant. Environ Health Perspect 1994;11(Suppl 102):107–10.

6. Huang NN, High RH. Comparison of serum levels following the administration of oral and parenteral preparations of penicillin to infants and children of various age groups. J Pediatr 1953;42(6):657–8.

7. Parrott N, Lukacova V, Fraczkiewicz G, et al. Predicting pharmacokinetics of drugs using physiologically based modeling–application to food effects. AAPS J 2009;11(1):45–53.

8. Poley JR, Dower JC, Owen CA Jr, et al. Bile acids in infants and children. J Lab Clin Med 1964;63:838–46.

9. Suchy FJ, Balistreri WF, Heubi JE, et al. Physiologic cholestasis: elevation of the primary serum bile acid concentrations in normal infants. Gastroenterology 1981; 80(5 Pt 1):1037–41.

10. Abdel-Rahman SM, Kearns GL. Single oral dose escalation pharmacokinetics of pleconaril (VP 63843) capsules in adults. J Clin Pharmacol 1999;39(6):613–8.

11. Kearns GL, Bradley JS, Jacobs RF, et al. Single dose pharmacokinetics of pleconaril in neonates. Pediatric Pharmacology Research Unit Network. Pediatr Infect Dis J 2000;19(9):833–9.

12. Gupta M, Brans YW. Gastric retention in neonates. Pediatrics 1978;62(1):26–9.

13. Dressman JB, Bass P, Ritschel WA, et al. Gastrointestinal parameters that influence oral medications. J Pharm Sci 1993;82(9):857–72.

14. Berseth CL. Gestational evolution of small intestine motility in preterm and term infants. J Pediatr 1989;115(4):646–51.

15. Kearns GL, Robinson PK, Wilson JT, et al. Cisapride disposition in neonates and infants: in vivo reflection of cytochrome P450 3A4 ontogeny. Clin Pharmacol Ther 2003;74(4):312–25.

16. Stahlberg MR, Hietanen E, Maki M. Mucosal biotransformation rates in the small intestine of children. Gut 1988;29(8):1058–63.

17. Johnson TN, Tanner MS, Taylor CJ, et al. Enterocytic CYP3A4 in a paediatric population: developmental changes and the effect of coeliac disease and cystic fibrosis. Br J Clin Pharmacol 2001;51(5):451–60.

18. Gibbs JP, Liacouras CA, Baldassano RN, et al. Up-regulation of glutathione S-transferase activity in enterocytes of young children. Drug Metab Dispos 1999;27(12):1466–9.

19. Pacha J. Development of intestinal transport function in mammals. Physiol Rev 2000;80(4):1633–67.

20. Gladtke E, Rind H. Iron therapy during childhood. Ger Med Mon 1966;11(11): 438–42.

21. Garrick MD. Human iron transporters. Genes Nutr 2011;6(1):45–54.

22. Fakhoury M, Litalien C, Medard Y, et al. Localization and mRNA expression of CYP3A and P-glycoprotein in human duodenum as a function of age. Drug Metab Dispos 2005;33(11):1603–7.

23. Abdel-Rahman SM, Johnson FK, Gauthier-Dubois G, et al. The bioequivalence of nizatidine (Axid) in two extemporaneously and one commercially prepared oral liquid formulations compared with capsule. J Clin Pharmacol 2003;43(2): 148–53.

24. Abdel-Rahman SM, Johnson FK, Connor JD, et al. Developmental pharmacokinetics and pharmacodynamics of nizatidine. J Pediatr Gastroenterol Nutr 2004; 38(4):442–51.

25. Fanta S, Niemi M, Jonsson S, et al. Pharmacogenetics of cyclosporine in children suggests an age-dependent influence of ABCB1 polymorphisms. Pharmacogenet Genomics 2008;18(2):77–90.
26. Morimoto K, Kishimura K, Nagami T, et al. Effect of milk on the pharmacokinetics of oseltamivir in healthy volunteers. J Pharm Sci 2011;100(9):3854–61.
27. Di Lorenzo C, Flores AF, Hyman PE. Age-related changes in colon motility. J Pediatr 1995;127(4):593–6.
28. van Lingen RA, Deinum JT, Quak JM, et al. Pharmacokinetics and metabolism of rectally administered paracetamol in preterm neonates. Arch Dis Child Fetal Neonatal Ed 1999;80(1):F59–63.
29. Okah FA, Wickett RR, Pickens WL, et al. Surface electrical capacitance as a noninvasive bedside measure of epidermal barrier maturation in the newborn infant. Pediatrics 1995;96(4 Pt 1):688–92.
30. Fluhr JW, Pfisterer S, Gloor M. Direct comparison of skin physiology in children and adults with bioengineering methods. Pediatr Dermatol 2000;17(6):436–9.
31. West DP, Worobec S, Solomon LM. Pharmacology and toxicology of infant skin. J Invest Dermatol 1981;76(3):147–50.
32. Carry MR, Ringel SP, Starcevich JM. Distribution of capillaries in normal and diseased human skeletal muscle. Muscle Nerve 1986;9(5):445–54.
33. Sheng KT, Huang NN, Promadhattavedi V. Serum concentrations of cephalothin in infants and children and placental transmission of the antibiotic. Antimicrob Agents Chemother (Bethesda) 1964;10:200–6.
34. Kafetzis DA, Sinaniotis CA, Papadatos CJ, et al. Pharmacokinetics of amikacin in infants and pre-school children. Acta Paediatr Scand 1979;68(3):419–22.
35. Friis-Hansen B. Water distribution in the foetus and newborn infant. Acta Paediatr Scand 1983;305:7–11.
36. Siber GR, Echeverria P, Smith AL, et al. Pharmacokinetics of gentamicin in children and adults. J Infect Dis 1975;132(6):637–51.
37. Kearns GL, Abdel-Rahman SM, Blumer JL, et al. Single dose pharmacokinetics of linezolid in infants and children. Pediatr Infect Dis J 2000;19(12):1178–84.
38. Noone P, Parsons TM, Pattison JR, et al. Experience in monitoring gentamicin therapy during treatment of serious gram-negative sepsis. Br Med J 1974;1(5906):477–81.
39. Moore RD, Smith CR, Lietman PS. The association of aminoglycoside plasma levels with mortality in patients with gram-negative bacteremia. J Infect Dis 1984;149(3):443–8.
40. Kurz H, Fichtl B. Binding of drugs to tissues. Drug Metab Rev 1983;14(3):467–510.
41. MacIntyre AC, Cutler DJ. The potential role of lysosomes in tissue distribution of weak bases. Biopharm Drug Dispos 1988;9(6):513–26.
42. Yokogawa K, Ishizaki J, Ohkuma S, et al. Influence of lipophilicity and lysosomal accumulation on tissue distribution kinetics of basic drugs: a physiologically based pharmacokinetic model. Methods Find Exp Clin Pharmacol 2002;24(2):81–93.
43. Haddad S, Restieri C, Krishnan K. Characterization of age-related changes in body weight and organ weights from birth to adolescence in humans. J Toxicol Environ Health A 2001;64(6):453–64.
44. Windorfer A, Kuenzer W, Urbanek R. The influence of age on the activity of acetylsalicylic acid-esterase and protein-salicylate binding. Eur J Clin Pharmacol 1974;7(3):227–31.
45. Nau H, Luck W, Kuhnz W. Decreased serum protein binding of diazepam and its major metabolite in the neonate during the first postnatal week relate to increased free fatty acid levels. Br J Clin Pharmacol 1984;17(1):92–8.

46. Rane A, Lunde PK, Jalling B, et al. Plasma protein binding of diphenylhydantoin in normal and hyperbilirubinemic infants. J Pediatr 1971;78(5):877–82.

47. Kanakoudi F, Drossou V, Tzimouli V, et al. Serum concentrations of 10 acute-phase proteins in healthy term and preterm infants from birth to age 6 months. Clin Chem 1995;41(4):605–8.

48. Kingston HG, Kendrick A, Sommer KM, et al. Binding of thiopental in neonatal serum. Anesthesiology 1990;72(3):428–31.

49. Meistelman C, Benhamou D, Barre J, et al. Effects of age on plasma protein binding of sufentanil. Anesthesiology 1990;72(3):470–3.

50. Daood M, Tsai C, Ahdab-Barmada M, et al. ABC transporter (P-gp/ABCB1, MRP1/ABCC1, BCRP/ABCG2) expression in the developing human CNS. Neuropediatrics 2008;39(4):211–8.

51. Lacroix D, Sonnier M, Moncion A, et al. Expression of CYP3A in the human liver–evidence that the shift between CYP3A7 and CYP3A4 occurs immediately after birth. Eur J Biochem 1997;247(2):625–34.

52. Stevens JC, Hines RN, Gu C, et al. Developmental expression of the major human hepatic CYP3A enzymes. J Pharmacol Exp Ther 2003;307(2):573–82.

53. Maya MT, Domingos CR, Guerreiro MT, et al. Comparative bioavailability of two immediate release tablets of cisapride in healthy volunteers. Eur J Drug Metab Pharmacokinet 1998;23(3):377–81.

54. Mukherjee A, Dombi T, Wittke B, et al. Population pharmacokinetics of sildenafil in term neonates: evidence of rapid maturation of metabolic clearance in the early postnatal period. Clin Pharmacol Ther 2009;85(1):56–63.

55. Blake MJ, Gaedigk A, Pearce RE, et al. Ontogeny of dextromethorphan O- and N-demethylation in the first year of life. Clin Pharmacol Ther 2007;81(4):510–6.

56. Koukouritaki SB, Manro JR, Marsh SA, et al. Developmental expression of human hepatic CYP2C9 and CYP2C19. J Pharmacol Exp Ther 2004;308(3):965–74.

57. Bourgeois BF, Dodson WE. Phenytoin elimination in newborns. Neurology 1983;33(2):173–8.

58. Whelan HT, Hendeles L, Haberkern CM, et al. High intravenous phenytoin dosage requirement in a newborn infant. Neurology 1983;33(1):106–8.

59. Jacqz-Aigrain E, Bellaich M, Faure C, et al. Pharmacokinetics of intravenous omeprazole in children. Eur J Clin Pharmacol 1994;47(2):181–5.

60. Faure C, Michaud L, Shaghaghi EK, et al. Intravenous omeprazole in children: pharmacokinetics and effect on 24-hour intragastric pH. J Pediatr Gastroenterol Nutr 2001;33(2):144–8.

61. Nowak-Gottl U, Dietrich K, Schaffranek D, et al. In pediatric patients, age has more impact on dosing of vitamin K antagonists than VKORC1 or CYP2C9 genotypes. Blood 2010;116(26):6101–5.

62. Vieira I, Sonnier M, Cresteil T. Developmental expression of CYP2E1 in the human liver. Hypermethylation control of gene expression during the neonatal period. Eur J Biochem 1996;238(2):476–83.

63. Sonnier M, Cresteil T. Delayed ontogenesis of CYP1A2 in the human liver. Eur J Biochem 1998;251(3):893–8.

64. de Wildt SN, Kearns GL, Leeder JS, et al. Glucuronidation in humans. Pharmacogenetic and developmental aspects. Clin Pharmacokinet 1999;36(6):439–52.

65. Strassburg CP, Strassburg A, Kneip S, et al. Developmental aspects of human hepatic drug glucuronidation in young children and adults. Gut 2002;50(2):259–65.

66. Scott CS, Riggs KW, Ling EW, et al. Morphine pharmacokinetics and pain assessment in premature newborns. J Pediatr 1999;135(4):423–9.
67. Duanmu Z, Weckle A, Koukouritaki SB, et al. Developmental expression of aryl, estrogen, and hydroxysteroid sulfotransferases in pre- and postnatal human liver. J Pharmacol Exp Ther 2006;316(3):1310–7.
68. Strange RC, Davis BA, Faulder CG, et al. The human glutathione S-transferases: developmental aspects of the GST1, GST2, and GST3 loci. Biochem Genet 1985; 23(11–12):1011–28.
69. Miller RP, Roberts RJ, Fischer LJ. Acetaminophen elimination kinetics in neonates, children, and adults. Clin Pharmacol Ther 1976;19(3):284–94.
70. Allegaert K, Van der Marel CD, Debeer A, et al. Pharmacokinetics of single dose intravenous propacetamol in neonates: effect of gestational age. Arch Dis Child Fetal Neonatal Ed 2004;89(1):F25–8.
71. Bjorkman S, Oh M, Spotts G, et al. Population pharmacokinetics of recombinant factor VIII: the relationships of pharmacokinetics to age and body weight. Blood 2012;119(2):612–8.
72. Rosenbaum M, Gertner JM. Metabolic clearance rates of synthetic human growth hormone in children, adult women, and adult men. J Clin Endocrinol Metab 1989; 69(4):820–4.
73. Kearns GL, Kemp SF, Frindik JP. Single and multiple dose pharmacokinetics of methionyl growth hormone in children with idiopathic growth hormone deficiency. J Clin Endocrinol Metab 1991;72(5):1148–56.
74. Brown MS, Jones MA, Ohls RK, et al. Single-dose pharmacokinetics of recombinant human erythropoietin in preterm infants after intravenous and subcutaneous administration. J Pediatr 1993;122(4):655–7.
75. Mortensen HB, Lindholm A, Olsen BS, et al. Rapid appearance and onset of action of insulin aspart in paediatric subjects with type 1 diabetes. Eur J Pediatr 2000;159(7):483–8.
76. Danne T, Lupke K, Walte K, et al. Insulin detemir is characterized by a consistent pharmacokinetic profile across age-groups in children, adolescents, and adults with type 1 diabetes. Diabetes Care 2003;26(11):3087–92.
77. Danne T, Becker RH, Heise T, et al. Pharmacokinetics, prandial glucose control, and safety of insulin glulisine in children and adolescents with type 1 diabetes. Diabetes Care 2005;28(9):2100–5.
78. McCrory WM. Embryonic development and prenatal maturation of the kidney. In: Edelman CM, editor. Pediatric kidney disease. Boston: Little, Brown and Company; 1978. p. 3–25.
79. Spitzer A. Renal physiology and functional development. In: Edelmann CM, editor. Pediatric kidney disease. Boston: Little, Brown and Company; 1978. p. 25–128.
80. John TR, Moore WM, Jeffries JE, editors. Children are different: developmental physiology. 2nd edition. Columbus (OH): Ross Labs; 1978.
81. Hayton WL. Maturation and growth of renal function: dosing renally cleared drugs in children. AAPS PharmSci 2000;2(1):E3.
82. Chen N, Aleksa K, Woodland C, et al. Ontogeny of drug elimination by the human kidney. Pediatr Nephrol 2006;21(2):160–8.
83. Matzke GR, McGory RW, Halstenson CE, et al. Pharmacokinetics of vancomycin in patients with various degrees of renal function. Antimicrobial Agents Chemother 1984;25(4):433–7.
84. Schaad UB, McCracken GH Jr, Nelson JD. Clinical pharmacology and efficacy of vancomycin in pediatric patients. J Pediatr 1980;96(1):119–26.

85. Saxen H, Hoppu K, Pohjavuori M. Pharmacokinetics of fluconazole in very low birth weight infants during the first two weeks of life. Clin Pharmacol Ther 1993; 54(3):269–77.

86. Buist SC, Cherrington NJ, Choudhuri S, et al. Gender-specific and developmental influences on the expression of rat organic anion transporters. J Pharmacol Exp Ther 2002;301(1):145–51.

87. Slitt AL, Cherrington NJ, Hartley DP, et al. Tissue distribution and renal developmental changes in rat organic cation transporter mRNA levels. Drug Metab Dispos 2002;30(2):212–9.

88. Rosati A, Maniori S, Decorti G, et al. Physiological regulation of P-glycoprotein, MRP1, MRP2 and cytochrome P450 3A2 during rat ontogeny. Dev Growth Differ 2003;45(4):377–87.

89. Maher JM, Slitt AL, Cherrington NJ, et al. Tissue distribution and hepatic and renal ontogeny of the multidrug resistance-associated protein (Mrp) family in mice. Drug Metab Dispos 2005;33(7):947–55.

90. Alnouti Y, Petrick JS, Klaassen CD. Tissue distribution and ontogeny of organic cation transporters in mice. Drug Metab Dispos 2006;34(3):477–82.

91. Rollins DE, Klaassen CD. Biliary excretion of drugs in man. Clin Pharmacokinet 1979;4(5):368–79.

92. Rosenfeld WN, Evans HE, Batheja R, et al. Pharmacokinetics of cefoperazone in full-term and premature neonates. Antimicrobial Agents Chemother 1983;23(6): 866–9.

93. Hayton WL, Stoeckel K. Age-associated changes in ceftriaxone pharmacokinetics. Clin Pharmacokinet 1986;11(1):76–86.

Pediatric Pharmacogenomics
A Systematic Assessment of Ontogeny and Genetic Variation to Guide the Design of Statin Studies in Children

Jonathan Wagner, DO[a,b,*], J. Steven Leeder, PharmD, PhD[b]

KEYWORDS

- Pharmacogenomics • Ontogeny • HMG-CoA reductase inhibitors • Statins
- Low-density lipoprotein cholesterol • OATP1B1 • Cytochrome P450 • Pediatrics

KEY POINTS

- The traditional model of clinical drug development is to investigate the effect of statins in populations, and then attempt to apply the data to treat individual patients.
- The problem is further complicated when the population experience is in adults, and the information is to be applied to pediatric patients of different ages.
- There is a need to conduct studies to identify and quantify sources of interindividual variability in statin disposition and response for the management of dyslipidemias in children and adolescents.
- The challenge for the future is to address each of the knowledge deficits identified previously to better characterize the dose-exposure-response relationship in children and adolescents such that the design of future clinical trials will be better informed, increasing the likelihood of clinically useful data and avoiding the mistakes of the past.

There has been extensive reform in pediatric drug labeling accomplished over the past 20 years as a direct result of new federal laws and regulations. In 1994, the Food and Drug Administration (FDA) called for drug manufacturers to determine if existing data were sufficient for pediatric drug labeling.[1] Participation in this endeavor was subpar and, therefore, the FDA Modernization Act was enacted in November 1997. This legislation provided an additional 6-month patent exclusivity to manufacturers that

[a] Section of Cardiology, Children's Mercy Hospital and Clinics, University of Missouri-Kansas City School of Medicine, 2401 Gillham Road, Kansas City, MO 64108, USA; [b] Division of Clinical Pharmacology and Medical Toxicology, Department of Pediatrics, Children's Mercy Hospital and Clinics, University of Missouri-Kansas City School of Medicine, 2401 Gillham Road, Kansas City, MO 64108, USA
* Corresponding author.
E-mail address: jbwagner@cmh.edu

Pediatr Clin N Am 59 (2012) 1017–1037
http://dx.doi.org/10.1016/j.pcl.2012.07.008
0031-3955/12/$ – see front matter © 2012 Elsevier Inc. All rights reserved.
pediatric.theclinics.com

conduct pediatric clinical trials according the FDA parameters.[2] A detailed review of the chronologic events from 1994 to 2002 is provided by Steinbrook.[3] In January 2002, the Best Pharmaceuticals for Children Act provided further opportunities for drug manufacturers to generate data on drugs that were off-patent or patented drugs that had not been studied in children.[4] One year later, the Pediatric Research Equity Act enabled the FDA to require pediatric studies.[5] Overall, the results from this legislation have led to a dramatic increase in pediatric studies on more than 300 drugs and biologic products. The plethora of new information has illuminated the continued challenge of appropriate pediatric drug dosing, efficacy, and safety.

As is widely appreciated in pediatric medicine, the changes that occur as children grow and develop influence the diagnosis and treatment of clinical disease. Merely extrapolating from adult therapeutic data may overlook the influence that developmental changes in expression of genes responsible for drug disposition have on dosing requirements and safety profiles of drugs that have distinct variation from birth until adulthood. Pharmacotherapy in children, like adults, is dependent on clear understanding of the dose-exposure-response relationship of the drug to be administered; however, extrapolation of adult experience to pediatric age groups is complicated by age-associated differences in the pharmacokinetics of several drugs used clinically in children.[6] In the past decade, ontogeny of drug disposition, specifically in the domain of hepatic drug metabolizing enzymes, has been discovered[7]; however, our understanding of genetic variation's impact on drug disposition and efficacy in pediatrics still is lacking.[8,9] As expected though, the difficulty in performing prospective pediatric studies, because of ethical challenges and/or inadequate participation, have limited this greater understanding.

Understanding the relative contribution of ontogeny and genetic variation to observed variability in drug disposition and response in children challenges all parties involved in pediatric drug research. The implementation of pharmacogenetic and pharmacogenomic strategies in children serves as another barrier to improve pediatric drug therapeutics. In the absence of more comprehensive data, a systematic approach has been developed to gather more information about certain drugs, identify knowledge gaps, and design studies to address those deficits. This approach has been used previously to address the dilemma of over-the-counter cough and cold preparations.[10] Our goal in this article was to illustrate the use of this systematic approach to assess current knowledge regarding the effects of ontogeny and genetic variation on the dose-exposure-response of a drug class whose use in pediatrics is anticipated to increase in the near future.

EVOLUTION OF STATIN THERAPY IN CHILDREN

Cardiovascular disease remains the number one cause of mortality in the United States despite significant progress in medical and invasive treatments.[11] Although symptoms typically appear in the fifth and sixth decades of life, atherosclerotic coronary artery disease (CAD) has its origins in childhood. In 1953, autopsies performed on 300 US servicemen in their 20s revealed that more than 75% had evidence of coronary atherosclerosis.[12] Another autopsy study of US soldiers killed in the Vietnam War showed a 45% rate of atherosclerosis.[13] In a subsequent study involving young children and adolescents, fatty streaks, clinically silent precursors to CAD, were observed in the aortas of all children after the age of 3 years and progressed rapidly to coronary involvement by adolescence. Advancement to fibrous plaques mostly occurred in the third to fourth decades.[14] The Pathobiological Determinants of Atherosclerosis in Youth study and the Bogalusa Heart Study noted varying stages of atherosclerosis in young children and youth with elevated low-density lipoprotein cholesterol (LDL) and other risk factors, such as obesity, hypertension, tobacco smoke exposure, and diabetes.[15,16] These landmark studies have highlighted the need for implementing lipid screening and preventive cardiovascular measures during childhood.

The prevalence of total cholesterol (TC) higher than 200 mg/dL has risen to 10% in adolescents.[17] Epidemiologic studies have documented that 75% of children with a TC concentration greater than the 90th percentile have TC concentrations higher than 200 mg/dL in their early twenties.[18] Elevated cholesterol is commonly associated with being overweight or obese. An alarming one-third of 2-year-olds to 19-year-olds in the United States are diagnosed as overweight with a body mass index greater than the 85th percentile for age and sex.[19] A 55-year observational study showed that being overweight in adolescence resulted in a twofold higher relative risk of CAD mortality, independent of adult weight.[20] With the increasing prevalence of overweight children, the prevalence of clinically diagnosed CAD in young to middle-age adults is expected to increase by 5% to 16% by 2035.[21]

In 1992, the National Cholesterol Education Program recommended lipid screening for children with a family history of premature CAD or dyslipidemia and in children with other risk factors, such as obesity, hypertension, and diabetes mellitus.[22] This screening strategy has uncovered more cases of subclinical dyslipidemia that, without screening, would have been unrecognized for decades. More recent data have revealed that using family history alone to select children for lipid screening misses many patients with moderate acquired dyslipidemia and genetic dyslipidemia who may require pharmacologic treatment.[23] Therefore, updated guidelines from the American Academy of Pediatrics now recommend *universal* lipid screening at ages 9 to 11 years, and again at ages 18 to 21 years.[24]

Treatment strategies for dyslipidemia, including lifestyle modifications and pharmacologic therapy, have been well established in adults. In those who fail lifestyle modifications, pharmacologic therapy is commonly implemented. Guidelines for diet and pharmacologic treatment in children have also been established.[24,25] There are several classes of medication available for treatment of dyslipidemia. The 3-hydroxy-3-methyl-glutaryl coenzyme A (HMG-CoA) reductase inhibitors (statins) are now the mainstay of pharmacologic treatment of adult and pediatric dyslipidemia because of their demonstrated efficacy in the primary and secondary prevention of coronary artery disease and relatively mild side-effect profile.[26–30] HMG-CoA reductase inhibitors decrease the hepatic synthesis of cholesterol by blocking the conversion of HMG-CoA to mevalonate, which is the rate-limiting step in cholesterol synthesis (**Fig. 1**). The LDL-C receptor genes respond to this decrease of intracellular sterol by upregulating cell-surface LDL-C receptor expression,[31] which ultimately decreases the serum LDL. Furthermore, the pleiotropic effects of statins include the decrease of inflammatory mediators downstream from HMG-CoA reductase. This pleiotropic effect could ultimately provide efficacy in other disorders of childhood inflammation beyond the scope of dyslipidemia. For example, patients with sickle cell disease can develop oxidative stress and chronic inflammation to their distal vasculature as a result of transient vaso-occlusion and subsequent reperfusion injury.[32] Hoppe and colleagues[33] found that biomarkers of vascular dysfunction, including C-reactive protein and interleukin 6, were decreased in adolescents with sickle cell disease from 50% up to 70% after a 3-week trial of low (20 mg) or moderate (40 mg) doses of simvastatin. Additionally, statins have been used after cardiac transplantation to prevent coronary allograft vasculopathy (CAV). In pediatric cardiac transplantation, the prevalence of CAV is less pronounced compared with adults, but has

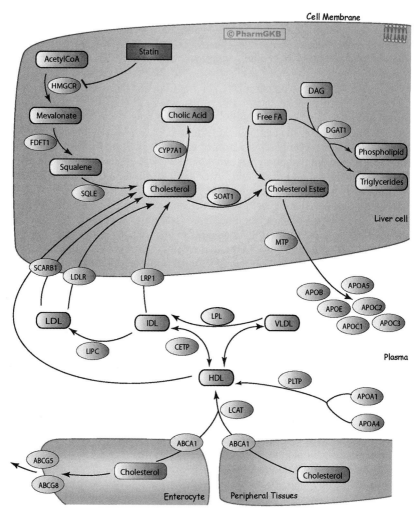

Fig. 1. Cholesterol biosynthesis pathway. Statins as a class inhibit endogenous cholesterol production by competitive inhibition of HMG-CoA reductase (HMGCR), which catalyzes conversion of HMG-CoA to mevalonate, an early rate-limiting step in cholesterol synthesis. The effect of statins is shown in the context of genes involved in the metabolism and transport of plasma lipoproteins that affect atherosclerosis and cardiovascular disease risk. A more detailed description of individual genes and gene products can be found at http://www.pharmgkb.org/pathway/PA2031 (accessed May 14, 2012). (*Courtesy of* Pharmacogenomics Knowledgebase, with permission from PharmGKB and Stanford University.)

been reported to be as high as 17% in one retrospective analysis.[34] LDL levels >100 mg/dL, greater than optimal and near adult treatment range, have been reported in 39% of pediatric patients 1 year after transplantation,[35] which can be secondary to posttransplant steroid and cyclosporine therapy. Addition of pravastatin therapy in pediatric cardiac transplant recipients yielded a lower incidence of CAV.[34] Overall, statins are usually well tolerated and result in a 20% to 50% reduction in cholesterol from baseline.[36] Available information on statin use in pediatrics implies that statins are being used conservatively in children, estimated to be 1:4500 children.[37] However, this crude estimate is likely to underestimate current use, as it is derived from an analysis of Medicaid data from 2000 and a commercial Caremark database from 2004,[38] and preceded the increase in obesity and type 2 diabetes in children that has occurred over the past decade.

There are currently 7 FDA-approved statins: lovastatin, simvastatin, pravastatin, fluvastatin, atorvastatin, rosuvastatin, and pitavastatin. Most statin trials in pediatric subjects have involved lovastatin, simvastatin, and pravastatin.[28] Lovastatin, the first statin developed in the late 1980s, is a lipophilic, semisynthetic inhibitor of HMG-CoA reductase. It is administered as an inactive lactone prodrug and is hydrolyzed in the liver to its active metabolites.[39] Simvastatin, introduced in the early 1990s, is also a lipophilic, semisynthetic inhibitor of HMG-CoA reductase and administered as an inactive lactone prodrug that undergoes carboxylesterase-mediated conversion in the plasma, liver, and intestine to simvastatin acid, which is the active metabolite.[40] Pravastatin, introduced in the early 1990s, is a hydrophilic, semisynthetic inhibitor of HMG-CoA reductase.[41] Because of its hydrophilic nature, it fails to cross the blood-brain barrier, making it a potentially safer alternative for maturing brains in children. Unlike other statins, it is not significantly metabolized by cytochrome P450 enzymes. In fact, the major metabolites are mainly produced in the acidic conditions of the stomach and are inactive.[42]

Most pediatric trials have focused on efficacy of lipid lowering and safety. The most recent double-blind, randomized, placebo-controlled, multicenter trial involving lovastatin (20 mg until week 4 then 40 mg from week 5 until week 24) in 54 postmenarchal females with familial hyperlipidemia between the ages of 10 and 17 years demonstrated a 23% reduction in LDL at 4 weeks and 27% after 24 weeks of treatment. Additionally, there were no clinically significant adverse effects observed between the 2 treatment groups over a 6-month period.[43] The largest double-blind, randomized, placebo-controlled multicenter trial with simvastatin (10 mg titrating up to 40 mg by week 24 continuing until week 48) in children aged 10 to 17 years, by de Jongh and colleagues,[44] demonstrated a 41% reduction in LDL, displaying simvastatin's efficacy in LDL reduction in children as well. There was a small decrease in dehydroepiandrosterone sulfate compared with subjects taking placebo, but no other changes in adrenal, gonadal, or pituitary hormones were observed in the treatment or placebo groups. No serious adverse drug events were reported in either treatment group. Three previous double blind, randomized, placebo-controlled trials have demonstrated an approximate 25% to 35% reduction in LDL with pravastatin use in children, validating its efficacy in this age group.[41,45,46] In addition to lowering LDL and total cholesterol, there is evidence that statin therapy in children with dyslipidemia can reverse increased carotid intima-medial thickness and arterial endothelial dysfunction measured by ultrasound and flow-mediated dilation, respectively,[46,47] which are biomarkers of the atherosclerotic process.[48–54] However, these studies all involved a fixed dose of statin medication, and the effective dose received by each subject (mg per kg) would be expected to vary across the population, and the variability in dose administered alone could contribute to variability in response. For instance, de Jongh and colleagues[44] reported a mean decrease of 41% LDL cholesterol with a standard deviation of 39.2% at 48 weeks of simvastatin therapy, and Wiegman and colleagues[46] reported that pravastatin was associated with a mean decrease in LDL of 24% with a range of 7% to 41%. It is likely that additional factors, specifically ontogeny and genetic variation, will also contribute to variability in statin disposition and response in pediatric patients. These factors are discussed in more detail in this article.

CONTRIBUTIONS OF ONTOGENY AND GENETIC VARIATION IN DRUG DISPOSITION

The relative lack of data regarding pediatric drug disposition is a limiting factor for optimal pediatric drug-dosing strategies to maximize efficacy and minimize the potential for toxicity. Given that the use of statins can be anticipated to increase as a result of mandatory screening programs and difficulty with adherence to dietary and behavioral modifications, the pediatric community should be proactive in establishing therapeutic guidelines before statins are in widespread use. These therapeutic guidelines should be based on solid information concerning the dose-exposure-response relationship in pediatric patients, and studies designed to generate this information should take advantage of existing knowledge related to the contributions of ontogeny and genetic variation. The purpose of the remainder of this review is to present 3 fundamental issues that should be considered when assimilating current knowledge for application to problems related to variability in drug disposition and response in children. This systematic approach is applied to identify knowledge deficits related to the contribution of ontogeny and genetic variation to impact statin disposition and response in children, with implications for the design of future studies to address these knowledge deficits.

Fundamental Issues for Assessing Variability in Drug Disposition in Children

1. Knowledge of gene products that are quantitatively important in the disposition (absorption, distribution, metabolism, and excretion) of the drug(s) of interest

Simvastatin and lovastatin have been 2 of the most commonly studied HMG-CoA reductase inhibitors in the pediatric population. They are both semisynthetic, lipophilic compounds administered as lactone prodrugs[39,55] that are mainly absorbed from the gastrointestinal tract via passive diffusion and are subsequently hydrolyzed to active beta-hydroxy acid forms, simvastatin acid, or lovastatin acid, in the liver.[39] In vivo, approximately 60% to 85% of the simvastatin prodrug is absorbed in the stomach, whereas only 30% of lovastatin prodrug is absorbed.[39,56,57] Owing to their lipophilic nature, simvastatin and lovastatin are more than 95% protein bound in the plasma. Fluvastatin, atorvastatin, and pitavastatin are synthetic, lipophilic (although less than simvastatin and lovastatin) compounds administered in their active form. They are absorbed rapidly via passive diffusion in the gastrointestinal tract secondary to their lipophilic nature and have a bioavailability of 30%, 12%, and 51%, respectively. They are also highly protein bound owing to their lipophilic nature.[39,56,58] Pravastatin remains a popular statin used in childhood and is labeled for use in children older than 8 years. It is a hydrophilic, semisynthetic compound that is administered in its active acidic form. Gastrointestinal absorption is estimated to be 30% to 35% owing to its highly hydrophilic nature and reduced passive diffusion; absolute bioavailability is lower (17%–18%) as a consequence of this incomplete absorption and first-pass metabolism. Because of its hydrophilic nature, it is only 50% protein bound.[39,56] Rosuvastatin is a synthetic, hydrophilic (although less than pravastatin) compound that is administered in its active form. It also undergoes a slower absorption phase owing to its less lipophilic nature, but its protein binding is greater relative to pravastatin.[59,60]

The liver is the major site of action and clearance for all statins used clinically. Hepatic uptake of statins is mediated by influx transporters known as organic anion transporting polypeptides (OATPs; Phase 0), followed by cytochrome P450 (CYP)-mediated oxidative metabolism for most statins (Phase 1), conjugation with glucuronic acid (Phase 2), and excretion of conjugated metabolites in the bile via the multidrug resistance protein (MRP) family of efflux transporters (Phase 3).[56,61] These processes are summarized in **Fig. 2**. Theoretically, any of these steps could be rate-limiting for statin clearance, but animal studies indicate that more comprehensive models that

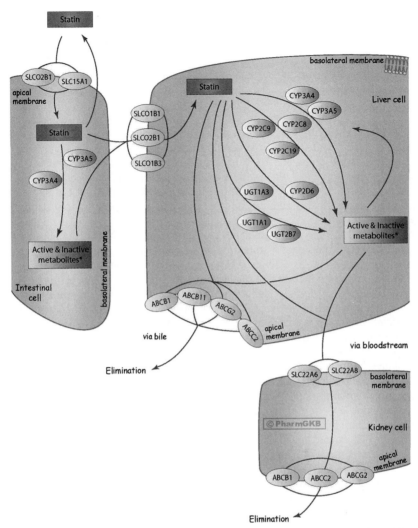

Fig. 2. Genes involved in statin disposition. Cellular uptake of statins is mediated by the *SLCO* and *SLC* gene families of transporters. Once inside cells, phase 1 metabolism of the drugs is mediated by *CYP* members, of which CYP3A4 appears to be most important, in general. Phase 2 conjugation by glucuronosyltransferases (UGTs) is followed by cellular efflux by ABC cassette transporters. Specific details for individual statins is provided in the text, and a more detailed description of individual genes and gene products can be found at http://www.pharmgkb.org/pathway/PA145011108 (accessed May 14, 2012). (*Courtesy of* Pharmacogenomics Knowledgebase, with permission from PharmGKB and Stanford University.)

include hepatic uptake are superior to models based on metabolism alone in predicting in vivo statin clearance from in vitro systems.[62] Each of these 4 steps of statin disposition in liver will be discussed in more detail later in this article. Emphasis will be paid to those processes that are *quantitatively* important in hepatic statin disposition to distinguish those processes that profoundly affect systemic statin exposure in humans from those that are merely *capable* of transporting or metabolizing statins based on data from isolated in vitro systems.

Hepatic uptake

Although statins may gain entry to hepatocytes by passive diffusion, the process is facilitated by a transporter-mediated system. The primary transporter mediating the hepatocellular uptake of statins is OATP1B1, the protein product of the *SLCO1B1* gene, and has been the subject of several comprehensive reviews.[56,61,63] For pitavastatin, OATP1B3 (*SLCO1B3* gene product) has been reported to play a minor role, but uptake primarily occurs by OATP1B1-mediated transport.[61,64] Additionally, fluvastatin and rosuvastatin have been shown to be substrates of OATP1B3 and OATP2B1-mediated transport.[63,65,66] Although simvastatin and lovastatin can inhibit OATP1B1-mediated transport,[67] OATP1B1 appears less important for cellular uptake of these agents relative to other statins because of their highly lipophilic nature and greater role for passive diffusion.[68]

Inhibitors of OATP1B1 are of great utility to gain insight into the functional importance of OATP1B1-mediated statin uptake. For example, concurrent administration of a potent inhibitor of OATP1B1 would be expected to increase the systemic exposure (as determined by an increase in total area under the curve [AUC]) for those statins that rely on OATP1B1 for hepatic drug uptake. Theoretically, the greater the increase in AUC in the presence of inhibitor, the greater the role of OATP1B1 in mediating hepatic drug uptake, as reduced entry into the liver is accompanied by an increase in the statin concentration circulating in plasma; if a particular statin is not dependent on OATP1B1 for cellular uptake, the AUC will not be affected by the presence of an inhibitor. The quantitative importance of OATP1B1 for statin uptake in vivo has been established using rifampin, a known inhibitor of OATP1B1 and OATP1B3 in vitro. For example, concurrent administration of a single 600-mg dose of rifampin resulted in a sixfold increase in the AUC of atorvastatin acid compared with atorvastatin alone.[69] Cyclosporine, a potent inhibitor of OATP1B1 and CYP3A4, increased atorvastatin AUC 7-fold to 15-fold, fluvastatin AUC 3-fold to 4-fold, lovastatin AUC 20-fold, pravastatin AUC 5-fold to 10-fold, pitavastatin AUC 5-fold, rosuvastatin AUC 7-fold, and simvastatin AUC 3-fold to 8-fold (reviewed in Niemi and colleagues[63]). The potential contribution of CYP3A4 inhibition to the increased AUC of statins associated with cyclosporine is considered to be minor at best, given that rosuvastatin, pravastatin, and pitavastatin are excreted unchanged and are not significantly metabolized by CYP3A4.[70] Pravastatin, a very hydrophilic compound that does not have significant passive diffusion capabilities, had a 10-fold increase in AUC when given in pediatric patients on immunosuppressive therapy containing cyclosporine compared with patients receiving pravastatin for familial hypercholesterolemia,[71] documenting the importance of OATP1B1-mediated transport of pravastatin into the hepatocyte. The effect of cyclosporine on rosuvastatin AUC (sevenfold increase), another hydrophilic compound, is consistent with an important role for OATP1B1 in hepatic uptake.[72] Cumulatively, the data from studies with inhibitor studies provide convincing evidence that the OATP1B1 transporter is a critically important determinant of drug disposition for most of the statins. This quantitative importance of *SLCO1B1* is also confirmed by pharmacogenetic studies, as described later in this article.

Phase 1 metabolism

Current evidence indicates that cytochrome P450 3A4 (CYP3A4) is the primary pathway for statin metabolism. Exceptions include pravastatin, pitavastatin, and rosuvastatin, which do not undergo significant CYP-mediated metabolism,[58,61,64] and fluvastatin, which is a substrate for CYP2C9, based on both in vitro and in vivo data.[73–75] Although in vitro reaction phenotyping studies suggest that CYPs 2C8, 2C9, 2C19, 2D6, 3A4, and 3A5 are *capable* of metabolizing various statins, CYP3A4 appears to be primarily responsible for the metabolism of simvastatin, lovastatin, and atorvastatin,[76–78] with CYP2C8 contributing to the metabolism of some statins. The quantitative importance of CYP3A4-dependent metabolism is illustrated by a 90% decrease in simvastatin acid metabolism in the presence of CYP3A4/5 inhibitor troleandomycin in vitro,[78] and by in vivo pharmacokinetic studies in which concurrent administration of CYP3A4 inhibitors, such as itraconazole results in 15- to 19-fold increases simvastatin and lovastatin AUC.[56,79–81] A more modest 47% increase in atorvastatin AUC is observed with coadministered itraconazole.[82] Administration of CYP3A4 inhibitors has no significant effect on clearance of pravastatin, fluvastatin, rosuvastatin, or pitavastatin, consistent with the limited role of CYP3A4 in the metabolism of these compounds.[70]

Phase 2 metabolism

Conjugation with glucuronic acid catalyzed by uridine 5'-diphospho-glucuronosyl-transferase (UDP) glucuronosyl transferases (UGTs) is the primary route by which statins and statin metabolites are further metabolized in hepatocytes.[83,84] The open acid forms of the statins are glucuronidated by UGT to form an acyl glucuronide that subsequently cyclizes to form a lactone ring. This process of lactonization is a common metabolic pathway for all statins in the open acid form, and results in a loss of pharmacologic activity. Statin lactones can be converted back to the open acid forms by carboxyl esterase and subject to further metabolism or excretion into the urine or bile; lactones can also be directly metabolized by cytochrome P450.[61] Fujino and colleagues[85] demonstrated that the statin lactones are more rapidly metabolized by cytochrome P450 than the statin open acids. Concurrent administration of gemfibrozil, a fibrate that inhibits cytochrome P450 and UGT-mediated metabolism of simvastatin and atorvastatin, has been reported to increase the AUC of simvastatin acid, but not the lactone form, consistent with an inhibitory effect on the lactonization of simvastatin acid in vivo.[86] Overall, the contribution of UGT-dependent metabolism is considered to be substantially less than the role of CYPs.[85] Other statins, such as pravastatin, rosuvastatin, and pitavastatin, undergo excretion in their intact form and do not undergo extensive cytochrome P450 or UGT-mediated metabolism.

Phase 3 cellular efflux

Efflux of the conjugated statin metabolites occurs via several efflux transporters located on the canalicular membrane of the hepatocyte (see **Fig. 2**). The biliary excretion of statins is mediated by multiple transporters, including multidrug resistance associated protein 2 (MRP2; *ABCC2*), multidrug resistance 1 (MDR1; *ABCB1*), breast cancer resistance protein (BCRP; *ABCG2*), and bile salt exporting pump (BSEP; *ABCB11*). There is insufficient information to determine the quantitative importance of efflux transporters as determinants of the systemic exposure to statins.

When all phases of hepatocellular uptake and metabolism are considered, OATP1B1 appears to be a crucial determinant of statin drug disposition. Furthermore, CYP3A4 activity, and to a lesser extent CYP2C8, contribute to the disposition of statins that are substrates for CYP-mediated metabolism (eg, simvastatin, lovastatin, and atorvastatin). However, when a clinical cassette microdosing study design was used to investigate the relative contribution of OATP1B1 and CYP3A4 toward atorvastatin disposition, AUC was increased 12-fold following inhibition of OATP1B1 by rifampin, but was unaffected by inhibition of CYP3A4 by itraconazole.[87] Thus, hepatic uptake by OATP1B1 appears to be the rate-limiting step in atorvastatin hepatic clearance.

2. Identification of allelic variation in the genes of interest that are associated with functional consequences in vivo

The solute carrier organic anion transporter (SLCO) gene family codes for OATP transporters,[88] and the effect of genetic variation on statin disposition has been the subject of considerable interest.[63] SLCO1B1 is expressed exclusively in the liver and its major role is drug and xenobiotic transport into the hepatocyte. The observation of extreme "high outliers" (n = 4 of 84 healthy male volunteers) in a pharmacokinetic study of pravastatin[89] was subsequently attributed to 2 single-nucleotide variants (SNVs) in SLCO1B1, −11187G>A in the promoter region and c.521T>C in exon 5, which were associated with a 50% reduction of nonrenal clearance.[90] This effect was independently confirmed by haplotype analysis, in which heterozygous carriers of SLCO1B1*15B (containing the 388A>G and 521T>C variants) had a mean pravastatin AUC 0 to 12 hours that was 93% higher compared with noncarriers, and heterozygous carriers of the *17 haplotype (containing the −11187G>A, 388A>G, and 521T>C variants) had 130% higher AUC compared with noncarriers.[91] Multiple SLCO1B1 haplotypes have now been described and haplotype frequencies vary across geographic regions. The combined frequency of low activity SLCO1B1*5 and *15 haplotypes is 15% to 20% in Europeans, 10% to 15% in Asians, and approximately 2% in sub-Saharan Africans, whereas the *1B haplotype, which is generally considered to be associated with higher activity, ranges in frequency from 26% in Europeans to up to 77% in sub-Saharan Africans.[63] The functional consequence of the SLCO1B1 haplotype on statin AUC generally follows the dependence of individual statins on OATP1B1 for cellular uptake. Heterozygosity for SLCO1B1*5 and *15 haplotypes is associated with an approximately 3-fold increase in AUC for simvastatin acid, and 2.5-fold and 2-fold increases for atorvastatin and pravastatin, respectively; fluvastatin AUC appears to be least affected by SLCO1B1 genotype.[63] The effect of rifampin on atorvastatin AUC is also dependent on SLCO1B1 genotype with a ninefold increase in AUC associated with the fully functional SLCO1B1 521TT genotype compared with a fourfold increase in AUC in subjects who are homozygous for the 521CC genotype associated with reduced transporter expression.[92] Thus, pharmacogenetic studies support a critical role for OATP1B1/SLCO1B1 in statin disposition.

Allelic variation in SLCO1B1 has important implications for drug safety, as the increased systemic exposure associated with reduced activity haplotypes has the potential to increase the risk of myopathy in statin-treated patients. This relationship has been demonstrated by the STRENGTH (Statin Response Examined by Genetic Haplotype Markers) trial, in which heterozygosity for a noncoding SNV in linkage disequilibrium with c.521T>C SNV was associated with a 4.5-fold increase in risk of myopathy, and increase to 16.9 in subjects homozygous for the SNV.[93]

The relationship between genetic variation in phase 1 metabolism and statin disposition is limited relative to SLCO1B1 pharmacogenetics and cellular uptake. Although CYP3A4 activity is highly variable in humans, genetic determinants of the observed variability remain unclear.[94] Recently, Wang and colleagues[95] identified an SNV in intron 6 of CYP3A4 (rs35599367 C>T) that has now been designated the CYP3A4*22 allele. This variant was associated with 1.7-fold and 2.5-fold decreases in CYP3A4 expression and activity in heterozygous and homozygous carriers, respectively. In patients receiving stable doses of either atorvastatin, simvastatin, and lovastatin, individuals with a CYP3A4*22 allele required a 0.2-fold to 0.6-fold lower dose of statin therapy for lipid control, consistent with decreased CYP3A4 activity and reduced statin clearance. This effect has been replicated by Elens and colleagues,[96] who studied 80 patients treated with simvastatin and observed that patients either homozygous or heterozygous for CYP3A4*22 had a 0.25-mmol/L and 0.29-mmol/L reduction in total and LDL cholesterol, respectively, compared with those with homozygous wild type. Thus, allelic variation in CYP3A4 also appears to influence the pharmacodynamic impact of statins that are dependent on this CYP for their metabolism. The CYP2C9*3 allele has a much more dramatic effect on CYP2C9 activity, and patients homozygous for the *3 allele had threefold lower clearance of the active fluvastatin enantiomer, but reduction in serum cholesterol was not related to CYP2C9 genotype.[97]

Although phase 2 metabolism has a more limited impact on statin disposition compared with cellular uptake or phase 1 metabolism, recent work suggests that UGT allelic variants may have a modest effect on statin activity. Lactonization of atorvastatin has been attributed to UGT1A3, and the UGT1A3*2 allele has been associated with increased lactonization activity.[98] The lactone has reduced clinical effect, and a study conducted in 23 healthy volunteers demonstrated that homozygosity of the UGT1A3*2 allele was accompanied by a 1.7-fold and 2.7-fold increase in AUC of atorvastatin lactone and 2-hydroxyatorvastatin lactone, respectively, compared with those homozygous for UGT1A3*1 allele. Furthermore, increase lactone formation correlated with a decreased effect on total and LDL cholesterol lowering from baseline.[99]

The functional consequence of genetic variation in phase 3 efflux transporters is limited relative to the role of cellular uptake. Studies of allelic variation in ABCC2 reveal a dependence on the SLCO1B1 genotype.[100] Allelic variation in ABCB1 does not appear to have any significant role in the interindividual variability in the pharmacokinetics of fluvastatin, pravastatin, lovastatin, and rosuvastatin.[101] The ABCG2 c.421C>A variant has been associated with reduced transport activity in vitro,[102] and the AUC of atorvastatin, fluvastatin, simvastatin lactone, and rosuvastatin is reported to be 72%, 72%, 111%, and 144% greater in subjects with a c.421AA genotype compared with the wild-type c.421CC genotype group,[103,104] but no significant impact on simvastatin acid or pravastatin pharmacokinetics.[103]

3. Knowledge of the developmental profile (ontogeny) of key pathways involved in drug disposition

As presented previously, SLCO1B1 and CYP3A4 have emerged as the primary determinants of statin disposition based on studies conducted in adults. Relative to drug metabolism, considerably less is known about the ontogeny of transporters (influx and efflux) during human development. Nevertheless, knowledge of ontogeny is essential for proper application and interpretation of pharmacogenetic data, as genotype-phenotype relationships are only apparent once the gene is expressed, and are most stable when the gene is fully expressed. A comprehensive analysis of transporter mRNA expression in mice of different ages and developmental stages using next-generation mRNA sequencing analysis revealed that the expression of transporters in liver is both age-specific and isoform-specific.[105] Of the 15 SLCO genes in mice, only 5 were expressed in liver, with 2 (Slco1a4 and Slco1b2) being included in an adolescent-enriched group of transcripts, and 3 (Slco1a1, Slco2a1, and Slco2b1) have adult-enriched patterns of expression. Slco1b2 is considered to be the mouse homolog of human SLCO1B1 and SLCO1B3, and showed a biphasic developmental profile with expression increasing rapidly after birth, peaking during adolescence (10–20 days postnatal age) and declining during the transition from adolescence to adulthood before eventually returning to adolescent levels of expression. The ontogeny of SLCO1B1 in humans is not known, but if its ontogeny is as complex as mouse *Oatp1b2*, the functional consequence of *SLCO1B1* genetic variation in children may be difficult to assess across the developmental spectrum. Indeed, only one small pharmacokinetic/pharmacogenetic trial in children has been published to date. In 21 children with familial hyperlipidemia who received pravastatin, the *SLCO1B1* −11187GA genotype appeared to have the opposite effect from that observed in adults. Children with the variant SNV had an 81% *lower* peak pravastatin concentration (Cmax) and 74% lower AUC compared with children with the wild-type (−11187GG) genotype in marked contrast to published adult experience in which the variant genotype was associated with higher AUC values. Additionally, patients with the c.521T>C genotype had a 49% lower peak plasma pravastatin concentration and 26% lower AUC, but these differences did not achieve statistical significance.[106] This study suffers from a small number of children with the variant genotype, and genotype-phenotype relationships could also be confounded by concurrent administration of cyclosporine in the patients who had cardiac transplantation included in the study. However, the changes in Cmax and AUC are opposite to what would be expected if cyclosporine was inhibiting residual transporter function in patients with the variant genotypes. Clearly, these preliminary findings need to be replicated in a larger group of patients, and the potential effect of age (ontogeny) taken into consideration.

The ontogeny of CYPs and UGTs in humans appears to occur in distinct patterns.[7] *CYP3A4* is a member of a gene locus that contains 3 other members, *CYP3A5, CYP3A7,* and *CYP3A43*. The ontogeny of *CYP3A7* is characteristic of the Group 1 pattern of expression proposed by Hines[7]: high expression in fetal liver followed by decreasing expression after birth, and minimal expression in adults. CYP3A5 protein and activity can be detected in fetal and postnatal liver, and genetic variation is a more important determinant of variability in expression than ontogeny. The developmental trajectory of CYP3A4 follows the Group 3 pattern of expression in which functional CYP3A4 activity is minimal in fetal liver, but increases after birth. In vitro studies conducted with a large panel of postmortem pediatric liver tissues indicates that CYP3A7 activity in the first week of postnatal life is comparable to that observed in fetal liver, and declines by an order of magnitude over the first year of life. In contrast, CYP3A4 activity is low at birth, demonstrates modest increases in activity over the first month, but remains less than that observed in adult level between 1 and 10 years of age.[107] These in vitro data imply that CYP3A7 may be the dominant CYP3A isoform in the first year of life, with CYP3A4 assuming increasing importance thereafter. In vivo data are consistent with acquisition of functional CYP3A4 activity after birth and through the first year of life. Pharmacokinetic studies with midazolam, which is considered to be a prototypic CYP3A4 substrate, and cisapride in neonates, consistently indicate that clearance increases with postnatal age.[108] Similarly, an investigation of sildenafil pharmacokinetics in newborns revealed that a threefold increase in drug clearance over the first week of life was accompanied by an increase in the formation of the CYP3A4-dependent *N*-desmethyl metabolite.[109] A longitudinal phenotyping study conducted in infants 2 weeks to 12 months of age also supported maturation of CYP3A4 through an increase in N-demethylated metabolites of the cough suppressant dextromethorphan.[110] Estimates of weight-adjusted drug clearance (mL/min/kg) for CYP3A4 substrates generally are higher in younger children, necessitating higher weight-adjusted (mg/kg) doses than adults to achieve similar target concentrations[108]; however, these differences tend to be less pronounced when clearance (and dose) are adjusted for body surface area. For example, allometric scaling of sildenafil clearance indicates that adult levels are achieved by the end of the first week of life.[109] Complicating a clearer understanding of the ontogeny of drug metabolism is that liver mass as a percentage of total body mass changes throughout childhood, being higher (3.5%, range 2.1%–4.7%) in children 2 years of age compared with 2.2% (range 1.8%–2.8%) in individuals older than 18 years.[111] The issue of ontogeny is further confounded by the possibility that the pattern of metabolites formed by children may differ from that observed in adults, as has been reported recently for sirolimus, a substrate of CYP3A4 and CYP3A5.[112] To our knowledge, the ontogeny of statin metabolism has not been investigated to date.

CYP2C9 ontogeny is relevant to fluvastatin metabolism and also demonstrates a Group 3 developmental profile. Similar to CYP3A4, estimates of weight-adjusted drug clearance and dose requirement are higher in young children than adults, but these differences largely disappear when developmental differences in organ size are taken into consideration.[108]

SUMMARY

Based on the American Academy of Pediatrics guidelines, approximately 0.8% of adolescents 12 to 17 years old with dyslipidemia may qualify for pharmacologic treatment. This translates into approximately 200,000 12-year-olds to 17-year-olds eligible for statin therapy.[113] Given the ongoing childhood obesity epidemic, and the increased incidence of dyslipidemia associated with obesity, it is anticipated that the number of children and adolescents identified with dyslipidemia will continue to increase and some of these may ultimately require statin therapy. With the potential for increased use of statins in children and adolescents, it is imperative that we have improved understanding of the developmental characteristics affecting the pharmacokinetics and pharmacodynamics of statins in these pediatric populations. Simply extrapolating pediatric dosing guidelines from adult dose-exposure-response relationships fails to recognize the complexity of growth and developmental changes in pediatric patients, and the clinical implications for drug efficacy or adverse drug effects.[6] Interestingly, a recent study demonstrated that genetic risk scores derived from 95 SNVs associated with blood lipids in adults explained twice as much of the total variance in high-density lipoprotein cholesterol, LDL-cholesterol, and total cholesterol in 3-year-old to 6-year old children compared with adults.[114] On the one hand, it is encouraging that genetic markers of risk derived from adult data are also applicable to children, but the data also imply that additional factors influence lipid levels in children and adults, and environmental factors cannot be ignored.

From the perspective of statin treatment, as summarized previously, available data from adult studies implicate hepatocellular uptake via OATP1B1 and CYP3A4-dependent metabolism as critical determinants of statin disposition. This analysis also identified important knowledge deficits relevant for pediatric investigations. First, the ontogeny of *SLCO1B1* in humans is unknown, and therefore it is not possible to predict the influence that developmental differences in OATP1B1 expression may have on statin systemic exposure at different ages/developmental stages. Second, without this information, it is difficult to predict the effect of allelic variation in *SLCO1B1* on statin system exposure in pediatric populations, as illustrated by the limited pediatric data to date,[106] nor when genotype-phenotype relationships observed in adults will become apparent in children. It is interesting to note in this regard that genotype-phenotype relationships for *ABCB1* were not apparent in children younger than 8 years old, but were observed in children 8 years of age and older.[115] Thus, genotype-aided pharmacokinetic studies are warranted in children and adolescents to resolve this matter and determine if age-related differences in the dose-exposure relationship are present. Finally, modeling studies suggest that

Table 1
Drug distribution of Food and Drug Administration–approved statins

Statin (Year of Approval)	Phase 0	Phase 1	Phase 2	Phase 3
Lovastatin (1987)	Passive diffusion OATP1B1 (minor)	3A4	UGT	BCRP
Simvastatin (1991)	Passive diffusion OATP1B1 (minor)	3A4	UGT	BCRP(lactone)
Pravastatin (1991)	OATP1B1	3A4 (minor)	UGT (minor)	MRP2 MDR1 (minor) BCRP (minor) BSEP (minor)
Fluvastatin (1993)	OATP1B1	2C9	?	BCRP
Atorvastatin (1996)	OATP1B1	3A4	UGT	BCRP
Rosuvastatin (2003)	OATP1B1 OATP1B3 (minor) OATP2B1 (minor)	3A4 (minor)	UGT (minor)	BCRP
Pitavastatin (2009)	OATP1B1 OATP1B3 (minor)	3A4 (minor)	UGT (minor)	MDR2 BCRP MRP2

Abbreviations: BCRP, breast cancer resistance protein; BSEP, bile salt exporting pump; MDR, multi-drug resistance; MRP, multidrug resistance protein; OATP, organic anion transporting polypeptide; UGT, glucuronosyltransferase.

OATP1B1 activity is the primary determinant of plasma statin concentration, whereas intracellular statin concentrations are determined by CYP and efflux transporter activity.[62] Thus, one cannot ignore the potential for developmental or pharmacogenetic differences in CYP3A4 activity to influence the inhibitory effects of statins on cholesterol biosynthesis.

The traditional model of clinical drug development is to investigate the effect of statins in populations, and then attempt to apply the data to treat individual patients (**Table 1**). The problem is further complicated when the population experience is in adults, and the information is to be applied to pediatric patients of different ages. Therefore, there is a need to conduct studies to identify and quantify sources of interindividual variability in statin disposition and response for the management of dyslipidemias in children and adolescents. The challenge for the future is to address each of the knowledge deficits identified previously to better characterize the dose-exposure-response relationship in children and adolescents, such that the design of future clinical trials will be better informed, increasing the likelihood of clinically useful data and avoiding the mistakes of the past.[116]

REFERENCES

1. Food and Drug Administration. Specific requirements on content and format of labeling for human prescription drugs: revision of "pediatric use" subsection in the labeling: final rule (21 C.F.R. part 201). Fed Regist 1994;59:64240–50.
2. Food and Drug Modernization Act of 1997, Pub. L 105–115, Nov. 21, 1997.
3. Steinbrook R. Testing medications in children. N Engl J Med 2002;347:1462–70.
4. Best Pharmaceuticals for Children Act, Pub. L 107–109, Jan. 4, 2002.
5. Pediatric Research Equity Act of 2003, S.650, Jan. 7, 2003.

6. Rodriguez W, Selen A, Avant D, et al. Improving pediatric dosing through pediatric initiatives: what have we learned. Pediatrics 2008;121:530–9.

7. Hines RN. The ontogeny of drug metabolism enzymes and implications for adverse drug events. Pharmacol Ther 2008;118:250–67.

8. Leeder JS, Kearns GL. The challenges of delivering pharmacogenomics into clinical pediatrics. Pharmacogenomics J 2002;2:141–3.

9. Leeder JS. Developmental and pediatric pharmacogenomics. Pharmacogenomics 2003;4:331–41.

10. Leeder JS, Kearns GL, Spielberg SP, et al. Understanding the relative roles of pharmacogenetics and ontogeny in pediatric drug development and regulatory science. J Clin Pharmacol 2010;50:1377–87.

11. Lloyd-Jones D, Adams RJ, Brown TM, et al. Heart disease and stroke statistics—2010 update: a report from the American Heart Association. Circulation 2010;121:e46–215.

12. Enos WF, Holmes RH, Beyer J. Coronary disease among United States soldiers killed in action in Korea; preliminary report. J Am Med Assoc 1953;152:1090–3.

13. McNamara JJ, Molot MA, Stremple JF, et al. Coronary artery disease in combat casualties in Vietnam. JAMA 1971;216:1185–7.

14. Holman RL, Mc GH Jr, Strong JP, et al. The natural history of atherosclerosis: the early aortic lesions as seen in New Orleans in the middle of the 20th century. Am J Pathol 1958;34:209–35.

15. McGill HC Jr, McMahan CA. Determinants of atherosclerosis in the young. Pathobiological Determinants of Atherosclerosis in Youth (PDAY) Research Group. Am J Cardiol 1998;82:30T–6T.

16. Newman WP 3rd, Freedman DS, Voors AW, et al. Relation of serum lipoprotein levels and systolic blood pressure to early atherosclerosis. The Bogalusa Heart Study. N Engl J Med 1986;314:138–44.

17. Hickman TB, Briefel RR, Carroll MD, et al. Distributions and trends of serum lipid levels among United States children and adolescents ages 4-19 years: data from the Third National Health and Nutrition Examination Survey. Prev Med 1998;27:879–90.

18. Lauer RM, Clarke WR. Use of cholesterol measurements in childhood for the prediction of adult hypercholesterolemia. The Muscatine Study. JAMA 1990;264:3034–8.

19. Ogden CL, Carroll MD, Flegal KM. High body mass index for age among US children and adolescents, 2003-2006. JAMA 2008;299:2401–5.

20. Must A, Jacques PF, Dallal GE, et al. Long-term morbidity and mortality of overweight adolescents. A follow-up of the Harvard Growth Study of 1922 to 1935. N Engl J Med 1992;327:1350–5.

21. Bibbins-Domingo K, Coxson P, Pletcher MJ, et al. Adolescent overweight and future adult coronary heart disease. N Engl J Med 2007;357:2371–9.

22. American Academy of Pediatrics. National Cholesterol Education Program (NCEP): highlights of the report of the Expert Panel on Blood Cholesterol Levels in Children and Adolescents. Pediatrics 1992;89:495–501.

23. Ritchie SK, Murphy EC, Ice C, et al. Universal versus targeted blood cholesterol screening among youth: the CARDIAC project. Pediatrics 2010;126:260–5.

24. Expert panel on integrated guidelines for cardiovascular health and risk reduction in children and adolescents: summary report. Pediatrics 2011;128(Suppl 5):S213–56.

25. Kavey RE, Allada V, Daniels SR, et al. Cardiovascular risk reduction in high-risk pediatric patients: a scientific statement from the American Heart Association

Expert Panel on Population and Prevention Science; the Councils on Cardiovascular Disease in the Young, Epidemiology and Prevention, Nutrition, Physical Activity and Metabolism, High Blood Pressure Research, Cardiovascular Nursing, and the Kidney in Heart Disease; and the Interdisciplinary Working Group on Quality of Care and Outcomes Research: endorsed by the American Academy of Pediatrics. Circulation 2006;114:2710–38.

26. Baigent C, Keech A, Kearney PM, et al. Efficacy and safety of cholesterol-lowering treatment: prospective meta-analysis of data from 90,056 participants in 14 randomised trials of statins. Lancet 2005;366:1267–78.

27. O'Gorman CS, Higgins MF, O'Neill MB. Systematic review and metaanalysis of statins for heterozygous familial hypercholesterolemia in children: evaluation of cholesterol changes and side effects. Pediatr Cardiol 2009;30:482–9.

28. Eiland LS, Luttrell PK. Use of statins for dyslipidemia in the pediatric population. J Pediatr Pharmacol Ther 2010;15:160–72.

29. Mills EJ, Wu P, Chong G, et al. Efficacy and safety of statin treatment for cardiovascular disease: a network meta-analysis of 170,255 patients from 76 randomized trials. QJM 2011;104:109–24.

30. Tonelli M, Lloyd A, Clement F, et al. Efficacy of statins for primary prevention in people at low cardiovascular risk: a meta-analysis. CMAJ 2011;183:E1189–202.

31. Belay B, Belamarich PF, Tom-Revzon C. The use of statins in pediatrics: knowledge base, limitations, and future directions. Pediatrics 2007;119:370–80.

32. Hebbel RP. Special issue of Microcirculation: examination of the vascular pathobiology of sickle cell anemia. Foreword. Microcirculation 2004;11:99–100.

33. Hoppe C, Kuypers F, Larkin S, et al. A pilot study of the short-term use of simvastatin in sickle cell disease: effects on markers of vascular dysfunction. Br J Haematol 2011;153:655–63.

34. Mahle WT, Vincent RN, Berg AM, et al. Pravastatin therapy is associated with reduction in coronary allograft vasculopathy in pediatric heart transplantation. J Heart Lung Transplant 2005;24:63066.

35. Singh TP, Naftel DC, Webber S, et al. Hyperlipidemia in children after heart transplantation. J Heart Lung Transplant 2006;25:1199–205.

36. Waters DD. What the statin trials have taught us. Am J Cardiol 2006;98:129–34.

37. Greer FR, Daniels SR. In reply: statin use in children in the United States. Pediatrics 2008;122:1408.

38. Lasky T. Statin use in children in the United States [letter to the editor]. Pediatrics 2008;122:1406–7.

39. Williams D, Feely J. Pharmacokinetic-pharmacodynamic drug interactions with HMG-CoA reductase inhibitors. Clin Pharmacokinet 2002;41:343–70.

40. Mauro VF. Clinical pharmacokinetics and practical applications of simvastatin. Clin Pharmacokinet 1993;24:195–202.

41. Hedman M, Neuvonen PJ, Neuvonen M, et al. Pharmacokinetics and pharmacodynamics of pravastatin in children with familial hypercholesterolemia. Clin Pharmacol Ther 2003;74:178–85.

42. Hatanaka T. Clinical pharmacokinetics of pravastatin: mechanisms of pharmacokinetic events. Clin Pharmacokinet 2000;39:397–412.

43. Clauss SB, Holmes KW, Hopkins P, et al. Efficacy and safety of lovastatin therapy in adolescent girls with heterozygous familial hypercholesterolemia. Pediatrics 2005;116:682–8.

44. de Jongh S, Ose L, Szamosi T, et al. Efficacy and safety of statin therapy in children with familial hypercholesterolemia: a randomized, double-blind, placebo-controlled trial with simvastatin. Circulation 2002;106:2231–7.

45. Knipscheer HC, Boelen CC, Kastelein JJ, et al. Short-term efficacy and safety of pravastatin in 72 children with familial hypercholesterolemia. Pediatr Res 1996; 39:867–71.

46. Wiegman A, Hutten BA, de Groot E, et al. Efficacy and safety of statin therapy in children with familial hypercholesterolemia: a randomized controlled trial. JAMA 2004;292:331–7.

47. de Jongh S, Lilien MR, op't Roodt J, et al. Early statin therapy restores endothelial function in children with familial hypercholesterolemia. J Am Coll Cardiol 2002;40:2117–21.

48. Celermajer DS, Sorensen KE, Gooch VM, et al. Non-invasive detection of endothelial dysfunction in children and adults at risk of atherosclerosis. Lancet 1992; 340:1111–5.

49. Pauciullo P, Iannuzzi A, Sartorio R, et al. Increased intima-media thickness of the common carotid artery in hypercholesterolemic children. Arterioscler Thromb 1994;14:1075–9.

50. Tonstad S, Joakimsen O, Stensland-Bugge E, et al. Risk factors related to carotid intima-media thickness and plaque in children with familial hypercholesterolemia and control subjects. Arterioscler Thromb Vasc Biol 1996;16: 984–91.

51. Mietus-Snyder M, Malloy MJ. Endothelial dysfunction occurs in children with two genetic hyperlipidemias: improvement with antioxidant vitamin therapy. J Pediatr 1998;133:35–40.

52. Jarvisalo MJ, Jartti L, Nanto-Salonen K, et al. Increased aortic intima-media thickness: a marker of preclinical atherosclerosis in high-risk children. Circulation 2001;104:2943–7.

53. de Jongh S, Lilien MR, Bakker HD, et al. Family history of cardiovascular events and endothelial dysfunction in children with familial hypercholesterolemia. Atherosclerosis 2002;163:193–7.

54. Wiegman A, de Groot E, Hutten BA, et al. Arterial intima-media thickness in children heterozygous for familial hypercholesterolaemia. Lancet 2004;363:369–70.

55. Duggan DE, Vickers S. Physiological disposition of HMG-CoA-reductase inhibitors. Drug Metab Rev 1990;22:333–62.

56. Neuvonen PJ, Backman JT, Niemi M. Pharmacokinetic comparison of the potential over-the-counter statins simvastatin, lovastatin, fluvastatin and pravastatin. Clin Pharmacokinet 2008;47:463–74.

57. Vickers S, Duncan CA, Chen IW, et al. Metabolic disposition studies on simvastatin, a cholesterol-lowering prodrug. Drug Metab Dispos 1990;18:138–45.

58. Wensel TM, Waldrop BA, Wensel B. Pitavastatin: a new HMG-CoA reductase inhibitor. Ann Pharmacother 2010;44:507–14.

59. Luvai A, Mbagaya W, Hall AS, et al. Rosuvastatin: a review of the pharmacology and clinical effectiveness in cardiovascular disease. Clin Med Insights Cardiol 2012;6:17–33.

60. Soran H, Durrington P. Rosuvastatin: efficacy, safety and clinical effectiveness. Expert Opin Pharmacother 2008;9:2145–60.

61. Shitara Y, Sugiyama Y. Pharmacokinetic and pharmacodynamic alterations of 3-hydroxy-3-methylglutaryl coenzyme A (HMG-CoA) reductase inhibitors: drug-drug interactions and interindividual differences in transporter and metabolic enzyme functions. Pharmacol Ther 2006;112:71–105.

62. Watanabe T, Kusuhara H, Maeda K, et al. Physiologically based pharmacokinetic modeling to predict transporter-mediated clearance and distribution of pravastatin in humans. J Pharmacol Exp Ther 2009;328:652–62.

63. Niemi M, Pasanen MK, Neuvonen PJ. Organic anion transporting polypeptide 1B1: a genetically polymorphic transporter of major importance for hepatic drug uptake. Pharmacol Rev 2011;63:157–81.

64. Fujino H, Saito T, Ogawa S, et al. Transporter-mediated influx and efflux mechanisms of pitavastatin, a new inhibitor of HMG-CoA reductase. J Pharm Pharmacol 2005;57:1305–11.

65. Ho RH, Tirona RG, Leake BF, et al. Drug and bile acid transporters in rosuvastatin hepatic uptake: function, expression, and pharmacogenetics. Gastroenterology 2006;130:1793–806.

66. Kitamura S, Maeda K, Wang Y, et al. Involvement of multiple transporters in the hepatobiliary transport of rosuvastatin. Drug Metab Dispos 2008;36:2014–23.

67. Hsiang B, Zhu Y, Wang Z, et al. A novel human hepatic organic anion transporting polypeptide (OATP2). Identification of a liver-specific human organic anion transporting polypeptide and identification of rat and human hydroxymethylglutaryl-CoA reductase inhibitor transporters. J Biol Chem 1999;274:37161–8.

68. Sirtori CR. Tissue selectivity of hydroxymethylglutaryl coenzyme A (HMG CoA) reductase inhibitors. Pharmacol Ther 1993;60:431–59.

69. Lau YY, Huang Y, Frassetto L, et al. Effect of OATP1B transporter inhibition on the pharmacokinetics of atorvastatin in healthy volunteers. Clin Pharmacol Ther 2007;81:194–204.

70. Neuvonen PJ, Niemi M, Backman JT. Drug interactions with lipid-lowering drugs: mechanisms and clinical relevance. Clin Pharmacol Ther 2006;80: 565–81.

71. Hedman M, Neuvonen PJ, Neuvonen M, et al. Pharmacokinetics and pharmacodynamics of pravastatin in pediatric and adolescent cardiac transplant recipients on a regimen of triple immunosuppression. Clin Pharmacol Ther 2004;75: 101–9.

72. Simonson SG, Raza A, Martin PD, et al. Rosuvastatin pharmacokinetics in heart transplant recipients administered an antirejection regimen including cyclosporine. Clin Pharmacol Ther 2004;76:167–77.

73. Scripture CD, Pieper JA. Clinical pharmacokinetics of fluvastatin. Clin Pharmacokinet 2001;40:263–81.

74. Transon C, Leemann T, Dayer P. In vitro comparative inhibition profiles of major human drug metabolising cytochrome P450 isozymes (CYP2C9, CYP2D6 and CYP3A4) by HMG-CoA reductase inhibitors. Eur J Clin Pharmacol 1996;50: 209–15.

75. Transon C, Leemann T, Vogt N, et al. In vivo inhibition profile of cytochrome P450TB (CYP2C9) by (+/-)-fluvastatin. Clin Pharmacol Ther 1995;58:412–7.

76. Lennernas H. Clinical pharmacokinetics of atorvastatin. Clin Pharmacokinet 2003;42:1141–60.

77. Prueksaritanont T, Gorham LM, Ma B, et al. In vitro metabolism of simvastatin in humans: identification of metabolizing enzymes and effect of the drug on hepatic P450s. Drug Metab Dispos 1997;25:1191–9.

78. Prueksaritanont T, Ma B, Yu N. The human hepatic metabolism of simvastatin hydroxy acid is mediated primarily by CYP3A, and not CYP2D6. Br J Clin Pharmacol 2003;56:120–4.

79. Kivisto KT, Kantola T, Neuvonen PJ. Different effects of itraconazole on the pharmacokinetics of fluvastatin and lovastatin. Br J Clin Pharmacol 1998;46:49–53.

80. Neuvonen PJ, Jalava KM. Itraconazole drastically increases plasma concentrations of lovastatin and lovastatin acid. Clin Pharmacol Ther 1996;60:54–61.

81. Neuvonen PJ, Kantola T, Kivisto KT. Simvastatin but not pravastatin is very susceptible to interaction with the CYP3A4 inhibitor itraconazole. Clin Pharmacol Ther 1998;63:332–41.
82. Jacobson TA. Comparative pharmacokinetic interaction profiles of pravastatin, simvastatin, and atorvastatin when coadministered with cytochrome P450 inhibitors. Am J Cardiol 2004;94:1140–6.
83. Fujino H, Yamada I, Shimada S, et al. Metabolic fate of pitavastatin, a new inhibitor of HMG-CoA reductase: human UDP-glucuronosyltransferase enzymes involved in lactonization. Xenobiotica 2003;33:27–41.
84. Prueksaritanont T, Subramanian R, Fang X, et al. Glucuronidation of statins in animals and humans: a novel mechanism of statin lactonization. Drug Metab Dispos 2002;30:505–12.
85. Fujino H, Saito T, Tsunenari Y, et al. Metabolic properties of the acid and lactone forms of HMG-CoA reductase inhibitors. Xenobiotica 2004;34:961–71.
86. Prueksaritanont T, Zhao JJ, Ma B, et al. Mechanistic studies on metabolic interactions between gemfibrozil and statins. J Pharmacol Exp Ther 2002;301:1042–51.
87. Maeda K, Ikeda Y, Fujita T, et al. Identification of the rate-determining process in the hepatic clearance of atorvastatin in a clinical cassette microdosing study. Clin Pharmacol Ther 2010;90:575–81.
88. Hagenbuch B, Meier PJ. Organic anion transporting polypeptides of the OATP/SLC21 family: phylogenetic classification as OATP/SLCO superfamily, new nomenclature and molecular/functional properties. Pflugers Arch 2004;447:653–65.
89. Ogawa K, Hasegawa S, Udaka Y, et al. Individual difference in the pharmacokinetics of a drug, pravastatin, in healthy subjects. J Clin Pharmacol 2003;43:1268–73.
90. Nishizato Y, Ieiri I, Suzuki H, et al. Polymorphisms of OATP-C (SLC21A6) and OAT3 (SLC22A8) genes: consequences for pravastatin pharmacokinetics. Clin Pharmacol Ther 2003;73:554–65.
91. Niemi M, Schaeffeler E, Lang T, et al. High plasma pravastatin concentrations are associated with single nucleotide polymorphisms and haplotypes of organic anion transporting polypeptide-C (OATP-C, SLCO1B1). Pharmacogenetics 2004;14:429–40.
92. He YJ, Zhang W, Chen Y, et al. Rifampicin alters atorvastatin plasma concentration on the basis of SLCO1B1 521T>C polymorphism. Clin Chim Acta 2009;405:49–52.
93. SEARCH, Collaborative, Group, Link E, Parish S, Armitage J, et al. SLCO1B1 variants and statin-induced myopathy—a genomewide study. N Engl J Med 2008;359:789–99.
94. Lamba JK, Lin YS, Schuetz EG, et al. Genetic contribution to variable human CYP3A-mediated metabolism. Adv Drug Deliv Rev 2002;54:1271–94.
95. Wang D, Guo Y, Wrighton SA, et al. Intronic polymorphism in CYP3A4 affects hepatic expression and response to statin drugs. Pharmacogenomics J 2010;11:274–86.
96. Elens L, Becker ML, Haufroid V, et al. Novel CYP3A4 intron 6 single nucleotide polymorphism is associated with simvastatin-mediated cholesterol reduction in the Rotterdam Study. Pharmacogenet Genomics 2011;21:861–6.
97. Kirchheiner J, Kudlicz D, Meisel C, et al. Influence of CYP2C9 polymorphisms on the pharmacokinetics and cholesterol-lowering activity of (–)-3S,5R-fluvastatin and (+)-3R,5S-fluvastatin in healthy volunteers. Clin Pharmacol Ther 2003;74:186–94.

98. Riedmaier S, Klein K, Hofmann U, et al. UDP-glucuronosyltransferase (UGT) polymorphisms affect atorvastatin lactonization in vitro and in vivo. Clin Pharmacol Ther 2010;87:65–73.

99. Cho SK, Oh ES, Park K, et al. The UGT1A3*2 polymorphism affects atorvastatin lactonization and lipid-lowering effect in healthy volunteers. Pharmacogenet Genomics 2012;22(8):598–605.

100. Niemi M, Arnold KA, Backman JT, et al. Association of genetic polymorphism in ABCC2 with hepatic multidrug resistance-associated protein 2 expression and pravastatin pharmacokinetics. Pharmacogenet Genomics 2006;16: 801–8.

101. Keskitalo JE, Kurkinen KJ, Neuvonen M, et al. No significant effect of ABCB1 haplotypes on the pharmacokinetics of fluvastatin, pravastatin, lovastatin, and rosuvastatin. Br J Clin Pharmacol 2009;68:207–13.

102. Imai Y, Nakane M, Kage K, et al. C421A polymorphism in the human breast cancer resistance protein gene is associated with low expression of Q141K protein and low-level drug resistance. Mol Cancer Ther 2002;1:611–6.

103. Keskitalo JE, Pasanen MK, Neuvonen PJ, et al. Different effects of the ABCG2 c.421C>A SNP on the pharmacokinetics of fluvastatin, pravastatin and simvastatin. Pharmacogenomics 2009;10:1617–24.

104. Keskitalo JE, Zolk O, Fromm MF, et al. ABCG2 polymorphism markedly affects the pharmacokinetics of atorvastatin and rosuvastatin. Clin Pharmacol Ther 2009;86:197–203.

105. Cui JY, Gunewardena SS, Yoo B, et al. RNA-Seq reveals different mRNA abundance of transporters and their alternative transcript isoforms during liver development. Toxicol Sci 2012;127(2):592–608. http://dx.doi.org/10.1093/toxsci/kfs107.

106. Hedman M, Antikainen M, Holmberg C, et al. Pharmacokinetics and response to pravastatin in paediatric patients with familial hypercholesterolaemia and in paediatric cardiac transplant recipients in relation to polymorphisms of the SLCO1B1 and ABCB1 genes. Br J Clin Pharmacol 2006;61:706–15.

107. Stevens JC, Hines RN, Gu C, et al. Developmental expression of the major human hepatic CYP3A enzymes. J Pharmacol Exp Ther 2003;307: 573–82.

108. de Wildt SN. Profound changes in drug metabolism enzymes and possible effects on drug therapy in neonates and children. Exp Opin Drug Metab Toxicol 2011;7:935–48.

109. Mukherjee A, Dombi T, Wittke B, et al. Population pharmacokinetics of sildenafil in term neonates: evidence of rapid maturation of metabolic clearance in the early postnatal period. Clin Pharmacol Ther 2009;85:56–63.

110. Blake MJ, Gaedigk A, Pearce RE, et al. Ontogeny of dextromethorphan O- and N-demethylation in the first year of life. Clin Pharmacol Ther 2007;81:510–6.

111. Johnson TN, Tucker GT, Tanner MS, et al. Changes in liver volume from birth to adulthood: a meta-analysis. Liver Traspl 2005;12:1481–93.

112. Filler G, Bendrick-Peart J, Strom T, et al. Characterization of sirolimus metabolites in pediatric solid oral organ transplant recipients. Pediatr Transplant 2009;13:44–53.

113. Ford ES, Li C, Zhao G, et al. Concentrations of low-density lipoprotein cholesterol and total cholesterol among children and adolescents in the United States. Circulation 2009;119:1108–15.

114. Tikkanen E, Tuovinen T, Widén E, et al. Association of known loci with lipid levels among children and prediction of dyslipidemia in adults/clinical perspective. Circ Cardiovasc Genet 2011;4:673–80.

115. Fanta S, Niemi M, Jönsson S, et al. Pharmacogenetics of cyclosporine in children suggests an age-dependent influence of ABCB1 polymorphisms. Pharmacogenet Genomics 2008;18:77–90.
116. Benjamin DK, Smith PB, Jadhav P, et al. Pediatric antihypertensive trial failures. Hypertension 2008;51:834–40.

Metabolomics in the Developing Human Being

Aggeliki Syggelou, MD, PhD(c)[a,1], Nicoletta Iacovidou, MD[a,1],
Luigi Atzori, MD, PhD[b], Theodoros Xanthos, MD[a],
Vassilios Fanos, MD[c,*]

KEYWORDS

- Metabolomics • Neonate • Prenatal health • Childhood

KEY POINTS

- The first results on metabolomics are available in perinatology and pediatrics and can help in defining an atlas of metabolic alterations in different conditions and pathologies.
- Metabolomics could rapidly become mainstream in diagnosing and subsequently managing pathologic conditions.
- The availability of information through the analysis of noninvasively collected fluid, such as urine, makes it extremely appealing.
- For neonatology in particular the extended and specific amount of data generated by metabolomics could allow personalized nutritional and therapeutic interventions.
- This approach blazes a revolutionary trail from reductionist medicine to holistic medicine, from descriptive medicine to predictive medicine, and from an epidemiologic perspective to a personalized approach.

INTRODUCTION

The "omics" technologies (genomics, transcriptomics, proteomics, and metabolomics) have impacted the life sciences considerably over the last decade. Starting with genomics at the DNA level, transcriptomics at the RNA level, proteomics at the protein level, and metabolomics at the metabolite level, these scientific technologies are based on the postgenomic activity, assess biologic function at the level of cellular organization, and offer unique insights into small molecule regulation and signaling.[1] It is well known that all cells of the human body are in constant and variable communication with the fluid compartments of the body. This communication helps the cell

The authors declare no conflict of interest.
[a] Medical School, National and Kapodistrian University of Athens, Mikras Asias 75, Athens 11527, Greece; [b] Department of Biomedical Sciences, University of Cagliari, 4 Via Porcell, Cagliari 09124, Italy; [c] Neonatal Intensive Care Unit, Puericulture Institute and Neonatal Section, AOU Cagliari and University of Cagliari, Via Ospedale 119, Cagliari 09134, Italy
[1] These two authors shared authorship.
* Corresponding author.
E-mail address: vafanos@tin.it

metabolites, peptides, and proteins to be part of a dynamic process in which they are either released from cells or taken up by cells from bodily fluids by a variety of mechanisms: normal excretion, transmembrane diffusion, or transport (**Fig. 1**). At least to a certain extent, the biochemical and protein-based changes occurring within cells and organs are reflected in bodily fluids.[2]

Metabolomics is not a novel approach to health and disease; one can find the basic idea of "omics" already appreciated by ancient Greeks who believed that changes in tissue and biologic fluids were early signs of pathology, and thus were capable of serving as indicators of disease processes. In 1506 Ullrich Pinder, in his book *Epiphanie Medicorum*, describes the possible medical value of different colors, smells, and taste of urine.[3] The "omics" technologies allow clinicians to study what causes these different smells and colors as they discover that the differences represent quite complex changes in the biologic system. Aristotle wrote that "the whole is not represented by the sum of its components." In our setting this means that the behavior of complex systems (systems biology) cannot be predicted from the properties of its individual components.

DEFINITION

The study of metabolites in biologic systems, referred to as "metabolomics," primarily involves the study of metabolism. The word "metabolism" derives from the Ancient Greek *metabole*, meaning "change."[4] This new "omic" discipline is based on the detailed analysis of metabolites, which are all the endogenous intracellular and

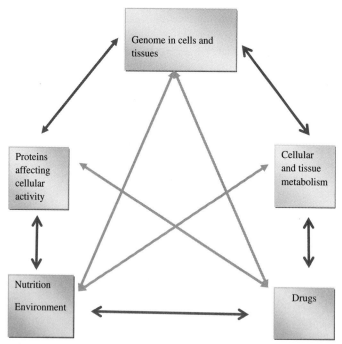

Fig. 1. Dynamic interactions of the several pathways. (*Adapted from* Christians U, Albuisson J, Klawitter J. The role of metabolomics in the study of kidney diseases and in the development of diagnostic tools. In: Edelstein CL, editor. Biomarkers of kidney disease. 1st edition. London: Elsevier Inc; 2011; with permission.)

extracellular compounds produced by the organism.[2] In other terms, the advent of metabolomics, in which all of the metabolites in a given tissue or biofluid are examined, reveals the personal metabolic identity and the metabolites found in biologic fluids are "a snapshot of the chemical fingerprints that specific cellular processes leave behind."[5,6]

Metabolomics can also be defined as the study of the complete set of metabolites of low or intermediate molecular weight (including amino acids, organic acids, sugars, fatty acids, lipids, steroids, small peptides, vitamins, and so forth), reflecting physiology, developmental, or pathologic state of cell, tissue, organ, or organism. "Metabolome" refers to the complete set of all metabolites of an organism or system,[7] whereas the "genome" refers to the complete set of a system's genes. As such, metabolomics provides the opportunity to directly or indirectly assess molecular mechanisms through molecular markers or biomarkers. A biomarker is defined as "a characteristic that is objectively measured and evaluated as an indicator of normal biologic processes, pathogenic processes or pharmacologic responses to therapeutic intervention."[8] It may be part of a single molecular entity but it can also be a group of several molecular entities, as in a molecular pattern or fingerprint. To shed light on this novel science called metabolomics, investigators claim that the metabolome is a quantitative descriptor of all endogenous low-molecular-weight components in a biologic sample, such as urine or plasma. Each cell type and biologic fluid has a characteristic set of metabolites that reflects the organism under particular environmental conditions and that fluctuates according to physiologic demands. The same investigators explain the difference between metabolomics and metabonomics and report that metabolomics is "the comprehensive quantitative analysis of all the metabolites of an organism or a specific biologic sample," whereas metabonomics are "the quantitative measurement over time of the metabolic responses of an individual or population to a disease, drug, treatment or other challenge."[8–10] Metabolomics has to be distinguished from the common pharmacologic use of the term "metabolite" for the degradation of a drug or conjugation products of pharmaceutical agents or xenobiotica.[11]

From 2009 to 2011, more than 5000 manuscripts have been published on this topic, with a dramatic increase in comparison with the previous years (2000–2003, 125 papers; 2004–2006, about 1000 papers; 2006–2008, about 2700 papers).

ADVANTAGES OF THIS "OMICS" TECHNOLOGY

The genotype of a patient can be substantially considered a static parameter and defines the risk or probability of reacting to a disease, drug, or environmental challenge in a certain way. However, the phenotype more closely reflects clinical reality at a given moment.[2] The "omics" studies aim at shedding light on the phenotype of a cell, tissue, or organism through the full spectrum of metabolites present and allow to combine constitutive aspects (eg, genes) and environmental factors (eg, diet, xenobiotics, and drugs). A critical challenge for biology and medicine is to achieve a more open-minded approach of the complex cellular systems as a whole. Thus metabolomics reflect a dynamic behavior of biologic systems with multiple networks of interactions among individual components.[12] Moreover, endogenous metabolites of a biofluid can describe the cellular phenotype, which in response to endogenous or exogenous stimuli, such as hormones, drugs, food, and chemicals, may induce biologic reactions, connecting genomics, transcriptomics, and proteomics and thus changing completely the way of studying and interpreting some cellular processes of diseases. Not long ago, the scientific world was mainly interested in understanding disease complexity by analyzing the significance of a single part or observing the microscopic world with the firm belief that genes are the only powerful discovery tools (eg, DNA analysis at gene level).[1] By contrast, metabolomics describes the metabolic status of the human being and represents an open system influenced by either genotype–phenotype or genotype–environment interactions.

Metabolomic studies are typically performed in biofluids (urine, plasma, cerebrospinal fluid [CSF], maternal milk, or saliva) or tissues (kidney, liver, gut, or brain).[13] Urine contains important information on the overall metabolic state of an individual[14] and has a unique biochemical composition that is affected by multiple parameters, such as genotype, physiologic and pathologic conditions, environment, nutrition, drugs, and so forth. Urine is easy to collect, using simple, noninvasive or painless techniques. In neonates it can be collected using a cotton ball or by the "catch up" technique.[12,15–18] Detailed analysis of the urinary metabolite patterns may help predict clinical presentations, allow for early detection of certain conditions and help monitor a patient's disease progression, treatment response and/or organ recovery.[2]

Understanding the biochemical and pathophysiologic mechanisms underlying the response of a biologic system to endogenous or exogenous stimuli may be the first step required to predict the type of response (in terms of efficacy and safety) of an organism to a specific pharmacologic or nonpharmacologic intervention, thus leading closer to providing "personalized medicine." The development of individualized treatment regimens, optimized for the metabolic status of the patient, is a major goal of medicine in general[18] and of neonatology in particular in the twenty-first century.[19,20] The right therapy for the right patient, minimizing the side effects and maximizing the benefits, is the dream of every physician.[21–23]

Metabolomics has the advantage of a limited number of variables (molecules being measured) compared with the approximately 25,000 genes tested in genomics, the approximately 85,000 transcripts assessed in transcriptomics, and the more than 10,000,000 proteins measured in proteomics. Metabolomics monitors only 1400 to 3000 metabolites and yet provides detailed information about the metabolic activity, reflecting the downstream changes in the genome, transcriptome, and proteome of an individual. The relatively small number of variables may be one of the major advantages of metabolomics compared with other "omics" sciences.[24] Most of these metabolites participate in specific biochemical pathways, such as glycolysis, Krebs cycle, and lipid or amino acid metabolism; signal pathways, such as transmitters and hormones; and specific pathobiochemical processes, such as oxidative stress. Moreover, changes in specific metabolite patterns may reflect changes in real-time pathways and processes, thus making it easy to detect derangements that might have occurred and pointing out certain metabolic reactions.[2]

The diverse composition of metabolites provides a wide range of physicochemical characteristics including molecular weight, hydrophobicity/hydrophilicity, acidity/basicity, and boiling point. The range of molecular weight, from 1 amu (proton) to greater than 1500 amu (eg, gangliosides, lipids, and small peptides), is significantly lower than that observed for proteins, transcripts, and genes. Hydrophobicity/hydrophilicity ranges from polar metabolites, such as low-molecular-weight amino acids to high-molecular-weight nonpolar lipids. Volatility ranges from low boiling point metabolites present in breath including isoprene and carbon dioxide, to high-molecular-weight lipids. The complex interaction between these diverse components is extremely challenging and covers a wide range of biochemical reactions of the human body.[25]

Finally, metabolomics studies are readily available, because most large academic centers have expertise in analytical chemistry, statistics, and bioinformatics. As in all "omics" sciences, metabolomics is a multidisciplinary science involving clinicians, cell biologists, analytical chemists, clinical pharmacologists, biochemists, and statisticians.[24]

HOW A STUDY ON METABOLOMICS IS DESIGNED
Collection of Samples

Mammalian biologic samples are complex and contain metabolites and low- and high-concentration matrix components. Immediately after collection of tissues, cells, urine, or other fluids, the temperature is reduced to subzero levels and samples stored at $-80°C$.[4] Urine from healthy mammals has very low protein content and preparation steps are simple and normally involve dilution and analysis.[25] Blood requires an extra step of preparation to allow separation of serum or plasma at $4°C$ before freezing and storage. The most complex and experimentally difficult systems to extract for metabolomics analysis are tissues; usually more than 30 mg of tissue is required. Homogenization and mechanical or chemical lysis of cell walls is required to allow the release of metabolites.[26]

Metabolic Pattern Analysis

Two important steps are required in planning an "omics" protocol: experimental technique and multivariate data analysis. The study design (adequate sample size and the statistical analysis strategy) should be carefully planned to detect small differences in metabolic profiles in a population with wide biologic variation. As soon as the biofluids have been collected and prepared with specific attention to uniform methods, nuclear magnetic resonance (NMR) spectroscopy, gas chromatography–mass spectrometry, and liquid chromatography–mass spectrometry are the main experimental tools used to measure global sets of metabolites in biologic samples.[12] Targeted (a priori) and untargeted (a posteriori) methods can be used with metabolomics. The first is hypothesis testing; the second, more innovative, is hypothesis generating.[27]

Two distinct methods for metabolomic analysis exist at present: the first one is global metabolomics, which refers to true biomarker discovery and evaluates known or unknown biomarkers indicative of intracellular metabolism; the second method, metabolic fingerprinting, reflects the ways intracellular metabolism affects the external environment by consumption and secretion of metabolites.[28] In both methods, all results are validated using samples collected from different patient cohorts, using independent validation data sets.[24]

After data collection, raw data are converted into biologic knowledge. This requires rigorous biostatistics. Univariate analyses, such as t test, analysis of variance, Mann-Whitney U test, Wilcoxon signed-rank test, and logistic regression, are applied to identify metabolites as potential biomarkers that are capable of differentiating between groups (eg, patients with vs those without a certain disease). These univariate tests are typically used individually to globally screen all of the measured metabolites for an association with a disease, which is where the multiple comparison problems may potentially arise. In the absence of correction for the number of comparisons, testing of multiple hypotheses causes an increase in the probability of obtaining statistically false-positive results. Several statistical methods exist for correction of multiple testing, including the Bonferroni correction, Benjamin-Hochberg false discovery rate, and the Westfall-Young method.[29–31] When strong evidence on a subset of metabolites is found, further testing is performed to validate their plausibility in target-specific studies, often with more detailed phenotypes (eg, subtypes or stages of a disease). Multivariate analyses are important in metabolomics studies because they can reduce the variability of the data and combine complex interactions, because multiple biomarkers rather than one by itself are more likely to be specific for interpretation of a derangement.

Among hundreds of metabolites, variables influencing the projection are selected. Metabolomics is focused to find the key metabolites that are able to characterize pathology; response to a therapeutic intervention; or nutritional modification (scale-free networks). In a simple way it can be considered like a bar code. Modern analytical technologies allow for the identification of patterns that confer significantly more information than the measurement of a single parameter, much as a bar code contains more information than a single number.[31] When a metabolomics protocol is designed a clear research goal should be set, and a quantitative hypothesis to be tested statistically should be identified.[24] Due to the enormous amount of generated data, complex bioinformatic tools, experts in statistics, biochemistry, physics and biotechnology are required.

CLINICAL APPLICATIONS
Metabolomics: New Biomarkers of Prenatal Health

Metabolomic studies in obstetrics and gynecology are not a novel concept. Since the 1960s, studies have reported the important role of specific metabolites in the dynamic interactions among fetus, placenta, and mother.[32] Several studies highlight the strong correlation of biomarkers found in amniotic fluid, in the placenta, or other biofluids of pregnant mothers with fetal malformations (FM), preterm delivery (PTD), premature rupture of membranes (PROM), prediagnostic gestational diabetes mellitus (GDM), and preeclampsia (PE). In a recent paper by Diaz and coworkers,[33] plasma and urine samples were collected at amniocentesis and metabolites' association with prenatal disorders was analyzed. All pregnant women were more than 35 years old or had other medical conditions necessitating amniocentesis. One hundred and ninety-eight plasma and urine samples (only 61 subjects consented for donation of urine and plasma) were collected in total and NMR spectroscopy was applied for the experimental signaling of metabolites. In the FM group, increase in glucogenic amino acids valine and isoleucine and threonine in urine and plasma was reported. Other metabolites, *cis*-aconite, an intermediate of the tricarboxylic acid cycle (TCA), and hypoxanthine indicating ATP degradation were found in high levels in both biofluids; both metabolites are indicative of fetal stress. Finally, choline, which plays an important role in homocysteine metabolism, is highly excreted in FM maternal urine, whereas two other biomarkers *N*-methyl-2-pyridone-5-carboxamide and *N*-methylnicotinamide, products of abnormal nucleotide metabolism, are similarly found in large amounts in the urine samples of the FM group. The latter urine metabolites are also indicative of other prenatal disorders, such as PE, hypoxia, chromosomal disorders, and PTD (choline) or prediagnostic GDM (*N*-methyl-2-pyridone-5-carboxamide, *N*-methylnicotinamide). Maternal plasma in the FM group showed lower plasma betaine and trimethylamine-*N*-oxide concentrations.[33] Other investigators reported that amniotic fluid is a reliable biofluid for detection of multiple prenatal disorders. Amniotic fluid samples were obtained from pregnant women aged 13 to 42 years undergoing amniocentesis during the second trimester of pregnancy (14–25 weeks of gestation). Samples were classified in six groups: (1) the healthy pregnancy; (2) pre-PTD (women who gave birth before 37 weeks of gestation); (3) prediagnostic GDM; (4) FM; (5) PROM; and (6) chromosomal disorders. For the disorders studied, amniotic fluid biomarkers seemed to have the best predictive value for FM. Metabolites analysis showed that malformed fetuses have large needs in glucose, whereas glucolysis is enhanced resulting in glucose and lactate increases. The decrease in the glucogenic amino acids alanine, isoleucine, glutamate, phenylalanine, tyrosine, and valine may be an indication of their enhanced preferential use in gluconeogenesis compared with other amino acids, such as glycine, glutamine, serine, and threonine. A high glutamine level reflects kidney disorders, whereas increased glycine and serine suggest a disturbance in choline and amino acid metabolism. Decrease in leucine and R-oxoisovalerate and the marked increase in ascorbate are indicative of abnormal amino acid biosynthesis in the FM group. For the prediagnostic GDM group, amniotic fluid analysis reported an increase in glucose and a decrease in acetate, creatinine, formate, glutamate, glycine, proline, serine, taurine, formate, and creatinine, suggesting changes in amino acids biosynthesis. In the pre-PTD group, the marked increase in allantoin, a marker of oxidative stress, and a decrease in *myo*-inositol, promoter of fetal lung maturation, was reported.[34]

Preeclampsia

Metabolic profiling has revealed that lipid and ketone body concentrations are lower in women with PE.[35] Kenny and colleagues[36] performed a two-phase study on the metabolomic signature of PE. In the first phase, plasma samples were collected at 15 ± 1 weeks of gestation from women who subsequently developed PE during their pregnancy. In the second phase, the results were validated with the findings of plasma samples of a different group with similar characteristics. An overlap of 14 metabolites was found; thus, a significant metabolic fingerprint was reported to be relevant to the early prediction of subsequent PE. Odibo and colleagues[37] also highlighted the importance of PE-specific metabolomic signature. A prospective cohort of pregnant women who subsequently developed PE and a control group with normal pregnancy outcome were followed-up from the first-trimester of pregnancy to delivery. Maternal blood was obtained at 11 to 14 weeks of gestation and 40 acylcarnitine species (C2–C18 saturated, unsaturated, and hydroxylated) and 32 amino acids were analyzed by liquid chromatography–tandem mass spectrometry. Four metabolites (hydroxyhexanoylcarnitine, alanine, phenylalanine, and glutamate) were significantly higher in women who subsequently developed PE, findings that highlight the first trimester "omics" role in the early diagnosis and prediction of PE.

A recent paper by Heazell and coworkers[38] reviewed the "omics" response of the normal and preeclamptic placental tissue to different oxygen levels. They demonstrated that placental tissue from uncomplicated pregnancies cultured in 1% oxygen (hypoxia) had metabolic similarities to explants from PE pregnancies cultured at 6% oxygen (normoxia). Nevertheless, the investigators suggested that more light should be shed on certain metabolites, such as lipids, glutamate, and glutamine, and metabolites related to tryptophan, leukotriene, and prostaglandin, because they too may play an important role in the metabolic profile of PE.

Horgan and coworkers[39] in a similar study compared placental features seen in small for gestational age (SGA) cases and controls. Placental tissue from both groups was cultured in 1% (hypoxic), 6% (normoxic), and 20% (hyperoxic) oxygen. Metabolic footprints were analyzed and 574 metabolites showed significant difference between SGA and normal pregnancies at one or more oxygen concentrations. SGA explant media cultured under hypoxic conditions was observed, on a univariate level, to exhibit the same metabolic signature as controls cultured under normoxic conditions in 49% of the metabolites of interest, suggesting that SGA tissue is adjusted to hypoxic conditions in vivo. Glycerophospholipid and tryptophan metabolism were highlighted as areas of particular interest.

Two recent cross-sectional metabolomics studies reported the importance of an amniotic fluid metabolic signature for preterm labor (PL) with or without intra-amniotic infection or inflammation (IAI). More specifically, two large groups of women with spontaneous PL and intact membranes were followed retrospectively. Amniotic fluids were collected and classified in three smaller groups based on the pregnancy outcome: (1) PL but delivery at term, (2) PL with PTD but no IAI, and (3) PL with IAI.

Amniotic fluid biomarkers successfully predicted the pregnancy outcome in both groups with PL and with or without IAI. Interestingly, a decrease in amniotic fluid carbohydrates was associated with PTD with or without IAI, whereas an increase in amino acid metabolites is a unique feature of PTL with IAI. The opposite was true in patients with PL who delivered at term where carbohydrates, such as mannose, galactose, and fructose, were found in small amounts in the amniotic fluid, whereas amino acids, such as alanine, glutamine, and glutamic acid, were detected in low levels. This altered amniotic fluid composition was mainly explained by the presence of bacteria, which use carbohydrates as nutrients, and the catabolic state of the septic fetus. Two metabolites, methyladenine and diamino pimelic acid, components of bacterial processes and bacterial wall, respectively, were highlighted as the most significant biomarkers in this setting, in group classification.[40,41]

Metabolomics in Nonhuman Models

Metabolomics analysis performed in nonhuman models also can shed light on the metabolic profile of the fetus and neonate with certain clinical conditions. A recent paper highlighted the plasma metabolome of fetal sheep brain after inflammatory-induced exposure. The fetal sheep were injected with *Escherichia coli* lipopolysaccharide (LPS) or saline injection by the umbilical vein and subsequently fetal blood was collected at specified time intervals. Postmortem, the white and gray matter were assessed. Within the first 3 days, LPS exposure caused hypoxia and a significant increase of the Krebs cycle intermediates, and alanine and lactate, and a subsequent decrease in hexoses; oxysteroles (24-hydroxycholesterol-24OHC, 25-hydroxycholesterol-25OHC), 12S-HETE, and spermidine increased after LPS administration, peaking at 6 hours. Moreover, 6 to 9 days later there was a delayed opposite effect of LPS on energy metabolites, hyperoxia, and elevation of sphingomyelins, kynurenine, 3-hydroxykynurenine, putrescine, and asymmetric dimethylarginine (ADMA), the latter ones known to be responsible markers and mediators of inflammation. The role of oxysteroles in proapoptotic pathways of the white matter and the role of ADMA in the regulation of microvascular tone and the endothelial function were highlighted as the metabolic profile of the relevant brain injury.[42]

Metabolic studies in newborn piglets, which underwent hypoxia and then reoxygenation with different oxygen concentrations, revealed the strong association of different resuscitation patterns with metabolic changes. Three different groups of hypoxic newborn piglets received, respectively, 100% oxygen for 60 minutes, 21% oxygen for 60 minutes, 100% oxygen for 15 minutes, and then 21% oxygen for 45 minutes. Plasma parameters (eg, lactate, low pH, and base deficit) were not correlated with the duration of hypoxia; prolonged hypoxia revealed a low level of free and total carnitine, required for normal mitochondrial function, cellular antioxidant activity, and an increase in long-chain acylcarnitines, which have toxic potential. Reoxygenation with different oxygen concentrations showed that hyperoxia was associated with a slower decline of Krebs cycle intermediates and an increase in lanosterole (product of ineffective cholesterol synthesis) and oxysteroles, both indicative of acute neuronal damage.[43]

Atzori and coworkers[44] have recently described metabolomics in urine samples from newborn piglets undergoing hypoxia followed by resuscitation with different oxygen concentrations (ranging from 18% to 100%). Despite reoxygenation, 7 out of 10 piglets became asystolic and died. The most significant urine metabolites, which were different between these discriminating groups, were urea, creatinine, malonate, methylguanidine, and hydroxyisobutyric acid. Malonate, urea, and creatinine are known metabolites in neurologic and renal disorders, aerobic metabolism, and cell death. Metabolomics may predict mortality postasphyxia.

...tribution Center
...roads Drive
MD 21113

...GISTRATION NUMBER 12457811-3

FIRST CLASS MAIL
US POSTAGE PAID
HANOVER, PA 17331
PERMIT #4

FIRST CLASS

\#
ACCOUNT 1941632-2 EPED OCT12
GEORGE A HORVATH, MD
211 N EDDY ST
SOUTH BEND IN 46617-2808

Beckstrom and coworkers[45] reported the role of metabolites in perinatal asphyxia in another nonhuman model. After hysterectomy, umbilical cord was clamped in a *Macaca nemestrina* model and blood was collected before and 15 or 18 minutes after cord occlusion followed by postnatal sampling at 5 minutes of age. Metabolomics analysis with comprehensive two-dimensional gas chromatography with time-of-flight mass spectrometry method revealed 50 metabolites with the greatest change preasphyxia to postasphyxia. Fifteen of the 50 metabolites were significantly elevated in response to asphyxia, 10 of which remained significantly different compared with control animals. Similarly, lactate and creatinine were strongly identified as biomarkers used clinically to assess the degree of hypoxic-ischemic injury caused by perinatal asphyxia and new metabolites including succinic acid and malate (intermediates in the Krebs cycle) and arachidonic acid (a brain fatty acid and inflammatory marker) were increased, implying a disruption in metabolic pathways.

NMR-based metabolomics analysis was performed in an experimental model of septic rats versus control group. Sepsis was induced by cecal ligation and puncture and lung tissue, bronchoalveolar lavage (BAL) fluid, and serum samples were obtained. The increase in alanine concentration in lung tissue and serum samples of septic rats resulted from enhanced pyruvate metabolism and transamination to alanine by the Cori cycle as previously shown in sepsis.[46] Creatine, which was found elevated in lung tissue, BAL, and serum, is a nitrogenous organic acid involved in inflammatory responses.[47] An increase in phosphoethanolamine in the serum of septic rats could indicate cell damage and phospholipid degradation.[48] The increase in serum acetoacetate might be related to enhanced fatty acid oxidation in septic rats.[49] The decreased serum level of formate in septic rats indicates an increased biosynthesis of purine nucleotides in sepsis.[50] *Myo*-inositol, which was found in high levels in lung tissue, but in low concentrations in the BAL, plays critical roles in endotoxin-induced vascular smooth muscle hypocontractility.[51,52]

A similar nonhuman model study reported the metabolic changes during birth transition. Postterm primates gave birth by hysterotomy and prebirth blood samples followed by eight time-points postbirth samples were obtained and analyzed. One hundred metabolites were identified during this transition. Of these 100 metabolites, 23 demonstrated significant change during the first 72 hours postbirth. Of note, four intermediates of the TCA cycle (α-ketoglutaric acid, fumaric acid, malic acid, and succinyl-CoA) were found elevated, which is in accordance with the transition of the neonate from a hypoxic environment in utero to an oxygen-rich one postbirth. *Myo*-inositol and glutaminic acid, which are both correlated with hypoxic ischemic encephalopathy, were similarly elevated in serum samples. *Myo*-inositol is a precursor for inositol phospholipids and glutamic acid is involved in metabolic pathways, such as urea cycle, or serves as a central nervous system signaling molecule for neuronal apoptosis.[53]

Liu and coworkers[54] have recently highlighted the metabolomics application in an experimental protocol of brain injury and hypothermia. Neonatal rat brain slices were divided into three groups, and in the first group 45-minute oxygen-glucose deprivation with a 3 hourly mild hypothermia (32°C) was applied. In the second group, oxygen-glucose deprivation was followed by hypothermia after a 15-minute delay. Total normothermia (37°C) was applied in the control group. Hypothermia was followed by a 3-hour normothermic recovery. "Omics" analysis reported that the final ATP levels, severely decreased at normothermia, equally recovered by immediate and delayed hypothermia and cell death was greater with normothermia and delayed hypothermia, compared with immediate hypothermia; thus, the two hypothermia-treated groups totally restored their initial high-energy phosphates, whereas large differences in early cell death were observed. This implies that the ATP levels do not always reflect the cellular function, and more data are needed to direct optimal cooling temperatures, duration, and rewarming regimens.

In an experimental study in newborn rats, a gentamicin-induced nephrotoxicity was associated with a distinct pattern of urinary metabolites. In particular, 14 parameters were significantly modified by gentamicin administration, including glucose, galactose, N-acetylglucosamine, myo-inositol, butanoic acid, and 3-hydroxybutyrate, all which were increased about threefold, and citrulline, pseudouridine, which elevated at lower levels.[55]

In another study preterm pigs, used as infant models, were given control treatment or broad-spectrum antibiotics just after birth by cesarean section. A close link between the antibiotic treatment, the presence of necrotizing enterocolitis, and the identified urinary metabolites was described, suggesting that urine metabolome could serve as an early biomarker for and subsequent progression of necrotizing enterocolitis in preterm neonates.[56]

Neonatology

"Omics" studies in neonatology suggest that metabolic profiling can indeed play an important role in detecting multiple diseases of the neonatal period. Investigators report the variable application of metabolomics, using biofluids with noninvasive techniques, mainly urine sampling. Dessì and colleagues[57] have recently reported results on metabolomics analysis in urine samples collected from intrauterine growth restricted and appropriate for gestational age babies on the first and fourth day of life. Alterations of three metabolic pathways were highlighted: (1) arginine and proline; (2) the urea cycle; and (3) glycine, serine, and threonine. Urine creatinine and myo-inositol were in high levels, the latter one representing a low fetal insulin production. Taken together all these observations indicate that the major effects of intrauterine growth restriction are on the brain and kidney and are associated with metabolites further involved in the metabolic syndrome. The same investigators described a distinct metabolic profile depending on the type of delivery. Twenty newborns delivered by caesarian section or spontaneous labor underwent metabolomics analysis; their metabolic fingerprint was quite different. Allantoin, betaine, and glycine were significantly higher in newborns born spontaneously than those born by caesarean section. A similar study in piglets showed that piglets born after a caesarian section had a metabolomics profile indicative of hepatic steatosis.[58,59]

Data from our group suggest that metabolomics may predict the postmaturation of preterm and term neonates. The differences in urine metabolites at birth (mainly tyrosine metabolism, tyrosine, tryptophan, phenylalanine biosynthesis, urea cycle, arginine, and proline metabolism) reveal that gestational age has a strong effect on the metabolic profile of the neonate (**Fig. 2**).[60] Similarly, in a small study including newborns with respiratory distress syndrome, BAL fluid was obtained before and after surfactant administration, during mechanical ventilation, and at each extubation time point. Metabolomics analysis showed that 10 (undecane, decanoic acid, dodecanoic acid, hexadecanoic acid, octadecanoic acid, hexadecanoic acid methyl ester, 9-octadecanoic acid, tetracosanoic acid, myristic acid, and phosphate) out of 25 metabolites were overexpressed in neonates who required ventilation after surfactant treatment. Thus, metabolomics profiling of the BAL fluid may be a promising diagnostic tool for future management of neonates with respiratory distress syndrome.[61]

Urine "omics" profiling in preterm newborns may predict the persistent patency of ductus arteriosus in the first 3 to 4 days of life,[62] whereas human milk of a mother who had a PTD might serve as a biofluid for early detection of metabolic intermediates and drugs.[63] Clear differences between the metabolic profile of human breast milk and

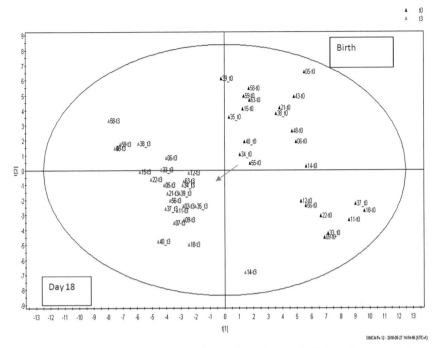

Fig. 2. Postnatal maturation in preterm infants. The red arrow indicates the postnatal maturation of metabolome from day 1 to day 18.

the different brands of formula milk used for preterm infants were observed. In particular, the role of the metabolites choline, lactose, *myo*-inositol, maltose, 9,12-octadecadienoic acid, and 9-octadecadienoic acid was found to be preponderant in differentiating the various types of milk. The results of this study, although still in preliminary form, represent a first step toward optimizing formula milk.[64]

Preliminary data on metabolomics show characteristic profiles for monochorionic and bichorionic twins[65] and for neonates with bronchiolitis of similar severity.[66] All these findings may suggest a potential role for metabolomic monitoring of neonates suffering from a wide range of disorders.

Banupriya and colleagues[67] studied the metabolomics signature of perinatal asphyxia and attempted to correlate the urine biomarkers with asphyxia-mediated death. Twenty asphyxiated and 20 healthy newborn males were enrolled and the urine ratios of malondialdehyde (MDA):creatinine, uric acid:creatinine, and protein:creatinine were evaluated in combination with Apgar scores and hypoxic-ischemic encephalopathy. The multivariate analysis revealed that urinary parameters were significantly associated with the stage of hypoxic-ischemic encephalopathy and Apgar scores. Thus, during asphyxia the urinary excretion rate of uric acid, MDA, and proteins was higher and this has the potential of serving as a biochemical marker for evaluating the severity of asphyxia and possibly predicting outcome.[1]

Finally, metabolomics may shed light on congenital metabolic diseases.[68] Some investigators applied untargeted mass spectrometry–based metabolomics to the methylmalonic acidemia and propionic acidemia. Two acylcarnitine metabolites and numerous unidentified species differentiate methylmalonic acidemia and propionic acidemia. Many metabolites that do not appear in any public database, and that remain unidentified, varied significantly among normal, methylmalonic acidemia, and propionic acidemia. This proof-of-concept study demonstrates that metabolomics may be useful for metabolic disease diagnosis and clinical evaluation.[69]

Childhood

Recently, investigators reported that urine metabolites, such as creatine, glycine, betaine/trimethylamine-N-oxide, citrate, succinate, and acetone, are age-dependent and decrease with age in healthy children. All but creatinine decreased with age. These findings reveal some of the confounding factors that have to be taken into account in applying metabolomics in children.[70,71]

Slupsky[72] considers metabolomic analysis the best method for early diagnosis of pneumonia in childhood and for the detection of its cause. In children with severe pneumonia versus community controls, Laiakis and colleagues[73] confirmed that metabolomics in matched urine and plasma samples have a potential big role in improving diagnostics in childhood pneumonia. Six metabolites (uric acid, hypoxanthine, glutamic acid, L-tryptophan, L-histidine, and adenosine-59-diphosphate [ADP]) were overlapped in children with pneumonia. Plasma uric acid, hypoxanthine, and glutamic acid were higher, whereas plasma L-tryptophan, known for its immunoregulatory effects, and ADP, which activates the platelets for effective hemostasis and blood aggregation, were found to be lower in patients compared with control subjects. Urine uric acid and L-histidine were also found in low levels and this was interpreted as a renal retention of these metabolites to serve as antioxidant and anti-inflammatory mediators. This "omics" study highlighted the host response to lung infection through antioxidant mechanisms, inflammatory pathways, and energy metabolism.

Thus, urinary metabolomics has considerable potential to improve diagnostics for childhood pneumonia: today it is possible to diagnose childhood pneumonia quickly, identify its cause, and monitor the return to normality in the course of an effective antibiotic therapy. This is possible because specific microbes produce unique urinary metabolite patterns in their hosts. Interesting prospects are expected also in the study of bronchiolitis.[66]

Oresic and coworkers[74] investigated changes in the serum metabolome in children who later progressed to type 1 diabetes. Fifty-six children who progressed to type 1 diabetes, and 73 control subjects who remained nondiabetic and permanently autoantibody negative, were enrolled. All children who developed diabetes had low serum levels of succinic acid and phosphatidylcholine at birth, reduced levels of triglycerides and antioxidant ether phospholipids throughout the follow up, and increased levels of proinflammatory lyso phosphatidylcholines several months before autoantibody positivity. The lipid changes were not attributable to HLA-associated genetic risk. Moreover, low levels of ketoleucine and high levels of glutamic acid were followed by the appearance of insulin and glutamic acid decarboxylase autoantibodies. All these findings may shed light on the disease pathogenesis and may serve as a novel tool for type 1 diabetes prevention strategies. In a previous study, urine from children and adolescents with type 1 diabetes was collected and "omics" analysis revealed high levels of citrate, alanine, lactate, and hippurate in children with diabetes compared with the unaffected individuals.[75] According to a similar study, the increased urine citrate, alanine, and hippurate might be the result of the increased glomerular filtration or the transport mechanisms at the tubular level.[76]

One can also analyze the metabolic fingerprint of the exhaled air of children with severe or intermittent asthma (breathomics). Exhaled breath condensate from children with asthma and control subjects was analyzed by NMR spectroscopy. Acetylated and oxidized compounds were detected in the exhaled breath condensate of children with asthma, revealing the potential role of these metabolites in lung pathology.[77] Two

Table 1
Fields of application of metabolomics in newborns and infants and examples of discriminant or involved metabolites (personal experience)

Clinical Condition	Main Results
Gestational age	Discrimination between term, late preterm, and preterm newborns. Important metabolites: alanine, citrate, creatinine, creatine, and dimetylglicine.
Postnatal age	Recognition of metabolic postnatal maturation (see **Fig. 2**).
Type of delivery	Discrimination between spontaneous delivery and caesarean section. Important metabolites: allantoin, betaine, and glycine.
Perinatal asphyxia	Prediction of death, early or late response to resuscitation (see **Fig. 3**). Important metabolites: urea, creatinine, malonate, metilghuanidine, uric acid, hypoxanthine, and malonyladeide.
Intrauterine growth restriction ✓	Discrimination of intrauterine growth restriction compared with control subjects. Six metabolites: creatine, creatinine, myoinositol, sarcosine, betaine, and succinate.
Persistent patent ductus arteriosus and treatment with nonsteroidal anti-inflammatory drugs ✓	Prediction with urine at birth of newborns with persistent patent ductus arteriosus. Important metabolites: metabolism of glucose and tyrosine.
Renal diseases ✓	Discrimination between control subjects and subjects with renal diseases. Nine metabolites: hyppurate, tryptophane, phenylanine, malate, tyrosine, hydrossibutirrate, N-acetyl-glutammate, tryptophan, and proline.
Respiratory distress syndrome	Evaluation of metabolites before and after surfactant.[a] Important metabolites: undecane, decanoic acid, dodecanoic acid, hexadecanoic acid, octadecanoic acid, hexadecanoic acid methyl ester, 9-octadecanoic acid, tetracosanoic acid, myristic acid, and phosphate.
Bronchiolitis	Very preliminary data.
Young adults (24 y) born extremely low birth weight	With a blind urine sample it is possible to attribute the birthweight (<1000 or >3000 g) 24 y after birth. Alterations of metabolism of arginine, proline, purine, pirimidine, istidine, β-alanine, and urea cycle.
Twins	Differentiation between monochorionic and dichorionic twins. Important metabolites: galactitol, N-acetylcysteine, N-acetylglutamate, N-acetyltyrosine, metilguanidine, N-dimethylformamide, and 5-hydroxyindol-3-acetate.
Chronic lung disease	Preliminary, unpublished data.
Human milk and formula	Evaluation of maturation, determination of drugs, and nicotine in human milk. Evaluation of biologic impact of formula. Important metabolites: choline, phospocholine, creatine, and creatine.

[a] Determination in BAL fluid.

other studies reported metabolite differences in the urine of children with severe asthma when compared with the urine of healthy control subjects, specifically a decreased excretion of urocanic acid, methylimidazoleacetic acid, and a metabolite resembling the structure of an Ile-Pro fragment.[78,79] These findings were correlated with immunity response to inflammation and histamine metabolism in asthma, and may someday lead to better therapeutic strategies in patients with respiratory diseases (ie, helping to pinpoint molecular targets for new drugs for asthma).

Several studies have reported on certain biomarkers in plasma or urine indicative of acute kidney injury.[80–84] Atzori and coworkers[85] managed to discriminate children with nephrouropathies (renal dysplasia, vesicoureteral reflux, urinary tract infection, and acute kidney injury) from healthy children through urine metabolic profiling. In particular, renal cortex pathology has been associated with alterations of purine, pyridine, and urea cycle.

Analysis of volatile organic compounds in exhaled breath may be used for the assessment of airway inflammation in children with cystic fibrosis. Specifically, C5-C16 hydrocarbons and N-methyl-2-methylpropylamine, products of lung inflammation and oxidative stress, were detected as the characteristic discriminating features for cystic fibrosis.[86] Therefore, volatile organic compounds in exhaled breath may soon become a new, noninvasive technique to study airway inflammation and oxidative stress in patients with cystic fibrosis.

Finally, specific biomarkers have been identified in the CSF of children with influenza- associated encephalopathy. Overall, two metabolites with particular molecular weight, which were not recorded in the database of the registered chemical and natural substances, were identified and may in the future help the early diagnosis of influenza-associated encephalopathy.[87]

Adulthood

Urine metabolomic analysis in young adults born with a low birth weight suggests the presence of neutrophil gelatinase-associated lipocalin, predictive of chronic kidney

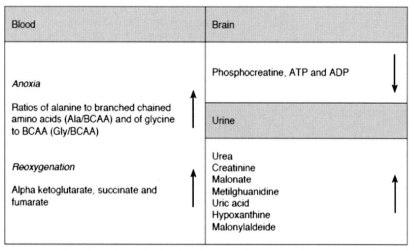

Fig. 3. The panel of altered metabolites in urine, blood, and brain in experimental models of asphyxia. (*Data from* Atzori L, Noto A, Barberini L, et al. Metabolomics in perinatal renal asphyxia. In: Fanos V, Chevalier RL, Faa G, et al, editors. Developmental nephrology: from embryology to metabolomics. 1st edition. Quartu S. Elena (Italy): Hygeia Press; 2011. p. 181–93.)

disease. This protein is able to carry small lipophilic molecules between cells in the body and its concentration in urine and plasma rises with acute kidney injury. Differences in the two groups were related to the alterations in the arginine and proline metabolism, in the purine and pyrimidine metabolism, in the hystidine and alanine metabolism, and with the TCA cycle.[88] The low-birth-weight metabolic profiles reported, in particular the presence of neutrophil gelatinase–associated lipocalin in the urine, may serve as a marker for the presence of a subclinical pathologic process in the kidney.

Differences between term and preterm young adults were also confirmed by other preliminary data indicative of persisting alterations in metabolic pathways initiated in early life. The most marked differences, such as elevated methylamines and acetylglycoproteins and lower hippurate, were reported in preterm young adults **(Table 1)**.[89]

SUMMARY

The first results on metabolomics are available in perinatology and pediatrics and can help in defining an atlas of metabolic alterations in different conditions and pathologies **(Fig. 3**, see **Table 1)**. Metabolomics could rapidly become mainstream in diagnosing and subsequently managing pathologic conditions. The availability of information through the analysis of noninvasively collected fluid, such as urine, makes it extremely appealing. For neonatology in particular the extended and specific amount of data generated by metabolomics could allow personalized nutritional and therapeutic interventions. This approach blazes a revolutionary trail from reductionist medicine to holistic medicine, from descriptive medicine to predictive medicine, and from an epidemiologic perspective to a personalized approach.[23]

REFERENCES

1. Atzori L, Noto A, Barberini L, et al. Metabolomics in perinatal renal asphyxia. In: Fanos V, Chevalier RL, Faa G, et al, editors. Developmental nephrology: from embryology to metabolomics. 1st edition. Quartu S. Elena (Italy): Hygeia Press; 2011. p. 181–93.
2. Edelstein CL, editor. Biomarkers of kidney disease. 1st edition. London (England): Elsevier Inc; 2011.
3. Nicholson JK, Lindon JC. Systems biology: metabonomics. Nature 2008;455: 1054–6.
4. Villas-Boas SG, Nielsen J, Smedsgaard J, et al, editors. Metabolome analysis: an introduction. Hoboken (NJ): Wiley Blackwell; 2007.
5. Lindon JC, Nicholson JK. Spectroscopic and statistical techniques for information recovery in metabonomics and metabolomics. Annu Rev Anal Chem (Palo Alto Calif) 2008;1:45–69.
6. Want EJ, Wilson ID, Gika H, et al. Global metabolic profiling procedures for urine using UPLC-MS. Nat Protoc 2010;5:1005–18.
7. Oliver SG, Winson MK, Kell DB, et al. Systematic functional analysis of the yeast genome. Trends Biotechnol 1998;16:373–8.
8. Biomarkers Definition Working Group. Biomarkers and surrogate endpoints: preferred definitions and conceptual framework. Clin Pharmacol Ther 2001;69: 89–95.
9. Nicholson JK. Global systems biology, personalized medicine and molecular epidemiology. Mol Syst Biol 2006;2:52.
10. Holmes E, Wilson ID, Nicholson JK. Metabolic phenotyping in health and disease. Cell 2008;134:714–7.

11. Sieber M, editor. Evaluation of 1H NMR- and GC/MS-based metabonomics for the assessment of liver and kidney toxicity. Evaluation of 1H NMR- and GC/MS-based metabonomics for the assessment of liver and kidney toxicity. Dissertation zur Erlangung des naturwissenschaftlichen Doktorgrades der Julius-Maximilians-Universität Würzburg. 2009.

12. Fanos V, Antonucci R, Barberini L, et al. Clinical application of metabolomics in neonatology. J Matern Fetal Neonatal Med 2012;25(Suppl 1):104–9.

13. Coen M, Holmes E, Lindon JC, et al. NMR-based metabolic profiling and metabonomic approaches to problems in molecular toxicology. Chem Res Toxicol 2008; 21:9–27.

14. Atzori L, Antonucci R, Barberini L, et al. Metabolomics: a new tool for the neonatologist. J Matern Fetal Neonatal Med 2009;22(Suppl 3):50–3.

15. Fell JM, Thakkar H, Newman DJ, et al. Measurement of albumin and low molecular weight proteins in the urine of newborn infants using a cotton wool ball collection method. Acta Paediatr 1997;86:518–22.

16. Cuzzolin L, Mangiarotti P, Fanos V. Urinary PGE(2) concentrations measured by a new EIA method in infants with urinary tract infections or renal malformations. Prostaglandins Leukot Essent Fatty Acids 2001;64:317–22.

17. Agostiniani R, Mariotti P, Cataldi L, et al. Role of renal PGE2 in the adaptation from foetal to extrauterine life in term and preterm infants. Prostaglandins Leukot Essent Fatty Acids 2002;67:373–7.

18. Wilson ID. Drugs, bugs, and personalized medicine: pharmacometabonomics enters the ring. Proc Natl Acad Sci U S A 2009;106:14187–8.

19. Antonucci R, Atzori L, Barberini L, et al. Metabolomics: the "new clinical chemistry" for personalized neonatal medicine. Minerva Pediatr 2010;62(3 Suppl 1): 145–8.

20. Fanos V, Yurdakök M. Personalized neonatal medicine. J Matern Fetal Neonatal Med 2010;23(Suppl 3):4–6.

21. Baraldi E, Carraro S, Giordano G, et al. Metabolomics: moving towards personalized medicine. Ital J Pediatr 2009;35:30.

22. Kroemer HK, Meyer zu Schwabedissen HE. A piece in the puzzle of personalized medicine. Clin Pharmacol Ther 2010;87:19–20.

23. Fanos V. Cells, the tree, medicines and the tailor. Editorial. Curr Pharm Des 2012; 18(21):2995.

24. Weiss RH, Kim K. Metabolomics in the study of kidney diseases. Nat Rev Nephrol 2011;8:22–33.

25. Dunn WB, Broadhurst DI, Atherton HJ, et al. Systems level studies of mammalian metabolomes: the roles of mass spectrometry and nuclear magnetic resonance spectroscopy. Chem Soc Rev 2011;40:387–426.

26. Wu H, Southam AD, Hines A, et al. High-throughput tissue extraction protocol for NMR- and MS-based metabolomics. Anal Biochem 2008;372:204–12.

27. Patti GJ, Yanes O, Siuzdak G. Innovation: metabolomics: the apogee of the omics trilogy. Nat Rev Mol Cell Biol 2012;13:263–9.

28. Kell DB, Brown M, Davey HM, et al. Metabolic footprinting and systems biology: the medium is the message. Nat Rev Microbiol 2005;3:557–65.

29. Westfall PH, Young SS, editors. Resampling-based multiple testing: examples and methods for P-value adjustment. New York: John Wiley & Sons; 1993.

30. Benjamini Y, Drai D, Elmer G, et al. Controlling the false discovery rate in behavior genetics research. Behav Brain Res 2001;125:279–84.

31. Perpiñá Tordera M. Complexity in asthma: inflammation and scale free networks. Arch Bronconeumol 2009;45:459–65.

32. Mori M. Study of protein biosynthesis in fetus and placenta. I. Incorporation of C-14-amino acids into the human placenta. Am J Obstet Gynecol 1965;93: 1164–71.

33. Diaz SO, Pinto J, Graça G, et al. Metabolic biomarkers of prenatal disorders: an exploratory NMR metabonomics study of second trimester maternal urine and blood plasma. J Proteome Res 2011;10:3732–42.

34. Graca G, Duarte IF, Barros AS, et al. Impact of prenatal disorders on the metabolic profile of second trimester amniotic fluid: a nuclear magnetic resonance metabonomic study. J Proteome Res 2010;9:6016–24.

35. Horgan RP, Clancy OH, Myers JE, et al. An overview of proteomic and metabolomic technologies and their application to pregnancy research. BJOG 2009; 116:173–81.

36. Kenny LC, Broadhurst DI, Dunn W, et al, Screening for pregnancy endpoints consortium. Robust early pregnancy prediction of later preeclampsia using metabolomic biomarkers. Hypertension 2010;56:741–9.

37. Odibo AO, Goetzinger KR, Odibo L, et al. First-trimester prediction of preeclampsia using metabolomic biomarkers: a discovery phase study. Prenat Diagn 2011;31:990–4.

38. Heazell AE, Brown M, Worton SA, et al. Review: the effects of oxygen on normal and pre-eclamptic placental tissue–insights from metabolomics. Placenta 2011; 32(Suppl 2):S119–24.

39. Horgan RP, Broadhurst DI, Dunn WB, et al. Changes in the metabolic footprint of placental explant-conditioned medium cultured in different oxygen tensions from placentas of small for gestational age and normal pregnancies. Placenta 2010; 31:893–901.

40. Romero R, Mazaki-Tovi S, Vaisbuch E, et al. Metabolomics in premature labor: a novel approach to identify patients at risk for preterm delivery. J Matern Fetal Neonatal Med 2010;23:1344–59.

41. Beecher CW. Metabolomic studies at the start and end of the life cycle. Clin Biochem 2011;44:518–9.

42. Keller M, Enot DP, Hodson MP, et al. Inflammatory-induced hibernation in the fetus: priming of fetal sheep metabolism correlates with developmental brain injury. PLoS One 2011;6:e29503.

43. Solberg R, Enot D, Deigner HP, et al. Metabolomic analyses of plasma reveals new insights into asphyxia and resuscitation in pigs. PLoS One 2010; 5:e9606.

44. Atzori L, Xanthos T, Barberini L, et al. A metabolomic approach in an experimental model of hypoxia-reoxygenation in newborn piglets: urine predicts outcome. J Matern Fetal Neonatal Med 2010;23(Suppl 3):134–7.

45. Beckstrom AC, Humston EM, Snyder LR, et al. Application of comprehensive two-dimensional gas chromatography with time-of-flight mass spectrometry method to identify potential biomarkers of perinatal asphyxia in a non-human primate model. J Chromatogr A 2011;1218:1899–906.

46. Gore DC, Jahoor F, Hibbert J, et al. Except for alanine, muscle protein catabolism is not influenced by alterations in glucose metabolism during sepsis. Arch Surg 1995;130:1171–6.

47. Bolton CF. Sepsis and the systemic inflammatory response syndrome: neuromuscular manifestations. Crit Care Med 1996;24:1408–16.

48. Vulimiri SV, Misra M, Hamm JT, et al. Effects of mainstream cigarette smoke on the global metabolome of human lung epithelial cells. Chem Res Toxicol 2009;22: 492–503.

49. Singer M, De Santis V, Vitale D, et al. Multiorgan failure is an adaptive, endocrine-mediated, metabolic response to overwhelming systemic inflammation. Lancet 2004;364:545–8.

50. McClay JL, Adkins DE, Isern NG, et al. (1)H nuclear magnetic resonance metabolomics analysis identifies novel urinary biomarkers for lung function. J Proteome Res 2010;9:3083–90.

51. Sotoda Y, Negoro M, Wakabayashi I. Involvement of decreased myo-inositol transport in lipopolysaccharide-induced depression of phosphoinositide hydrolysis in vascular smooth muscle. FEBS Lett 2002;519:227–30.

52. Izquierdo-García JL, Nin N, Ruíz-Cabello J, et al. A metabolomic approach for diagnosis of experimental sepsis. Intensive Care Med 2011;37(2):2023–32.

53. Beckstrom AC, Tanya P, Humston EM, et al. The perinatal transition of the circulating metabolome in a nonhuman primate. Pediatr Res 2012;71:338–44.

54. Liu J, Litt L, Segal MR, et al. Outcome-related metabolomic patterns from 1H/31P NMR after mild hypothermia treatments of oxygen-glucose deprivation in a neonatal brain slice model of asphyxia. J Cereb Blood Flow Metab 2011;31:547–59.

55. Hanna M, Segar S, Teesch L, et al. Metabolomics markers of nephrotoxicity in newborn rats. Poster presented at PAS/ASPR 2011. Denver (CO), April 30-May 3, 2011.

56. Jiang P, Berri T, Ladegaard Jensen M, et al. Urine metabolome of preterm neonates with treatment of antibiotics. Presented at the Metabomeeting 2011. Helsinki, September 25–28, 2011. Poster 54.

57. Dessì A, Atzori L, Noto A, et al. Metabolomics in newborns with intrauterine growth retardation (IUGR): urine reveals markers of metabolic syndrome. J Matern Fetal Neonatal Med 2011;24(Suppl 2):35–9.

58. Hyde MJ, Griffin JL, Herrera E, et al. Delivery by caesarean section, rather than vaginal delivery, promotes hepatic steatosis in piglets. Clin Sci (Lond) 2009;118:47–59.

59. Ciccarelli S, Atzori L, Noto A, et al. Spontaneous vs cesarean delivery: a metabolomic point of view [abstract]. J Matern Fetal Neonatal Med 2011;24:I–II.

60. Atzori L, Antonucci R, Barberini L, et al. 1H NMR-based metabolomic analysis of urine from preterm and term neonates. Front Biosci (Elite Ed) 2011;3:1005–12.

61. Fabiano A, Gazzolo D, Zimmermann LJ, et al. Metabolomic analysis of bronchoalveolar lavage fluid in preterm infants complicated by respiratory distress syndrome: preliminary results. J Matern Fetal Neonatal Med 2011;24(Suppl 2):55–8.

62. Atzori L, Barberini L, Lussu M, et al. Metabolomics and patent ductus arteriosus diagnosis: is 1H-NMR (nuclear magnetic resonance) spectroscopy of urine at birth predictive as ultrasound? [abstract]. J Matern Fetal Neonatal Med 2011;24(Suppl):I.

63. Marincola FC, Reali A, Barberini L, et al. NMR metabolic target analysis of the aqueous human breast extract [abstract]. J Matern Fetal Neonatal Med 2011;24:V.

64. Marincola FC, Noto A, Reali A, et al. Metabolomic study (aqueous and lipidic extract) of breast milk and formula milk for preterm babies. Proceedings XX European Workshop on Neonatology, Tallin June 1012 [abstract 11]. J Neonatal Perinatal Med 2012;5(2):194–5.

65. Noto A, Paladini L, Paladini A, et al. Metabolomics in twins at birth. Proceedings XX European Workshop on Neonatology, Tallin June 1012 [abstract 12]. J Neonatal Perinatal Med, in press.

66. Atzei A, Atzori L, Moretti C, et al. Metabolomics in paediatric respiratory diseases and bronchiolitis. J Matern Fetal Neonatal Med 2011;24(Suppl 2):59–62.

67. Banupriya C, Ratnakar P, Doureradjou N, et al. Can urinary excretion rate of malondialdehyde, uric acid and protein predict the severity and impending death in perinatal asphyxia? Clin Biochem 2008;41:968–73.

68. Ricquier D. Inherited metabolic diseases: benefits of metabolomics. Med Sci (Paris) 2005;21:512–6 [in French].

69. Wikoff WR, Gangoiti JA, Barshop BA, et al. Metabolomics identifies perturbations in human disorders of propionate metabolism. Clin Chem 2007;53:2169–76.

70. Gu H, Pan Z, Xi B, et al. 1H NMR metabolomics study of age profiling in children. NMR Biomed 2009;22:826–33.

71. Fanos V, Barberini L, Antonucci R, et al. Metabolomics in neonatology and pediatrics. Clin Biochem 2011;44:452–4.

72. Slupsky CM. NMR-based analysis of metabolites in urine provides rapid diagnosis and etiology of pneumonia. Biomark Med 2010;4:195–7.

73. Laiakis EC, Morris GA, Fornace AJ, et al. Metabolomic analysis in severe childhood pneumonia in the Gambia, West Africa: findings from a pilot study. PLoS One 2010;5(9):e12655.

74. Oresic M, Simell S, Sysi-Aho M, et al. Dysregulation of lipid and amino acid metabolism precedes islet autoimmunity in children who later progress to type 1 diabetes. J Exp Med 2008;205:2975–84.

75. Zuppi C, Messana I, Tapanainen P, et al. Proton nuclear magnetic resonance spectral profiles of urine from children and adolescents with type 1 diabetes. Clin Chem 2002;48:660–2.

76. Costacou T, Ferrel RE, Ellis D, et al. Haptoglobin genotype and renal function decline in type 1 diabetes. Diabetes 2009;58:2904–9.

77. Carraro S, Rezzi S, Reniero F, et al. Metabolomics applied to exhaled breath condensate in childhood asthma. Am J Respir Crit Care Med 2007;175:986–90.

78. Saude EJ, Skappak CD, Regush S, et al. Metabolomic profiling of asthma: diagnostic utility of urine nuclear magnetic resonance spectroscopy. J Allergy Clin Immunol 2011;127:757–64.

79. Mattarucchi E, Baraldi E, Guillou C. Metabolomics applied to urine samples in childhood asthma; differentiation between asthma phenotypes and identification of relevant metabolites. Biomed Chromatogr 2012;26:89–94.

80. Mishra J, Dent C, Tarabishi R, et al. Neutrophil gelatinase-associated lipocalin (NGAL) as a biomarker for acute renal injury after cardiac surgery. Lancet 2005;365:1231–8.

81. Dent CL, Ma Q, Dastrala S, et al. Plasma neutrophil gelatinase-associated lipocalin predicts acute kidney injury, morbidity and mortality after pediatric cardiac surgery: a prospective uncontrolled cohort study. Crit Care 2007;11:R127.

82. Bennett M, Dent CL, Ma Q, et al. Urine NGAL predicts severity of acute kidney injury after cardiac surgery: a prospective study. Clin J Am Soc Nephrol 2008; 3:665–73.

83. Al-Ismaili Z, Palijan A, Zappitelli M. Biomarkers of acute kidney injury in children: discovery, evaluation, and clinical application. Pediatr Nephrol 2011;26: 29–40.

84. Washburn KK, Zappitelli M, Arikan AA, et al. Urinary interleukin-18 is an acute kidney injury biomarker in critically ill children. Nephrol Dial Transplant 2008;23: 566–72.

85. Atzori L, Antonucci R, Barberini L, et al. 1H NMR-based metabolic profiling of urine from children with nephrouropathies. Front Biosci (Elite Ed) 2010;2:725–32.

86. Robroeks CM, van Berkel JJ, Dallinga JW, et al. Metabolomics of volatile organic compounds in cystic fibrosis patients and controls. Pediatr Res 2010;68:75–80.

87. Kawashima H, Oguchi M, Ioi H, et al. Primary biomarkers in cerebral spinal fluid obtained from patients with influenza-associated encephalopathy analyzed by metabolomics. Int J Neurosci 2006;116:927–36.

88. Atzori L, Mussap M, Noto A, et al. Clinical metabolomics and urinary NGAL for the early prediction of chronic kidney disease in healthy adults born ELBW. J Matern Fetal Neonatal Med 2011;24:40–3.

89. Modi N, Hyde MJ, Parkinson J, et al. European workshop on neonatology September 2010 [abstract]. J Neonatal Perinatal Med 2010;3(3):254.

Emerging Biomarkers of Intrauterine Neonatal and Pediatric Exposures to Xenobiotics

Kaitlyn Delano, BSc[a,b], Gideon Koren, MD, FRCPC, FACMT[a,b,*]

KEYWORDS

- Biomarker • Drugs • Alcohol • Pediatric • Screening

KEY POINTS

- Biomarkers of exposure can provide clinically relevant information to assist in diagnosis or in evaluation of the severity of chemical exposure, leading to optimal management.
- Using hair and meconium as matrices for biomarkers allows for a longer window of detection of exposures to xenobiotics including drugs, alcohol, and environmental chemicals.
- The use of biomarkers of alcohol that provide more reliable information concerning prenatal ethanol exposure than maternal self-reports aids in the diagnosis of fetal alcohol spectrum disorder.
- Numerous biomarkers are available to detect intrauterine exposure to drugs of abuse, which is associated with many adverse outcomes for fetus, child, and mother.
- Development of environmental toxicant biomarkers provides clinicians with tools to detect long-term, low-level exposures in humans, which may have detrimental effects to their offspring.

INTRODUCTION

There are multiple definitions available for a biomarker, specific to how the biomarker is used. The official National Institutes of Health definition of a biomarker is "a characteristic that is objectively measured and evaluated as an indicator of normal biologic processes, pathogenic processes, or pharmacologic responses to a therapeutic intervention.[1]" In the context of detecting external toxins after exposure during intrauterine life, biomarkers are critical, because many chemicals may not exist any more in the blood or urine of the neonate. Consequently, without the availability of appropriate

[a] Department of Pharmacology, University of Toronto, 1 King's College Circle, Toronto, Ontario M5S 1A8, Canada; [b] Division of Clinical Pharmacology and Toxicology, The Hospital for Sick Children, 555 University Avenue, Toronto, Ontario M5G 1X8, Canada
* Corresponding author.
E-mail address: gkoren@sickkids.ca

Pediatr Clin N Am 59 (2012) 1059–1070
http://dx.doi.org/10.1016/j.pcl.2012.07.005
0031-3955/12/$ – see front matter © 2012 Elsevier Inc. All rights reserved.

biomarkers, even potential toxic intrauterine exposures may be missed. Therefore, biomarkers must be able to generate relevant preclinical or clinical interpretations.[2] The sensitivity and specificity of a biomarker are important, because biomarkers too sensitive or nonspecific may not detect exposures or effects that are clinically relevant.[3]

In this review, we focus on biomarkers of internal dose, a subtype of biomarkers of exposure, which indicate the occurrence and extent of exposure to a compound or its metabolite(s).[3] Measuring the amount of the compound or metabolite in a matrix allows for a measurement of the exposure, rather than only estimating it.[3] By using biomarkers of both the compound and metabolite(s), more information concerning the exposure can be gathered and more accurate interpretations can be made by the clinician. When available, using multiple biomarkers in conjunction may provide more clinically relevant information about the exposure.

Illicit substance use in pregnancy is associated with significant maternal and neonatal morbidity and economic burdens to the health care system.[4] Despite a potential increase in substance abuse during pregnancy, it remains underdiagnosed or completely undiagnosed, putting both the fetus and the mother at risk for long-term sequelae.[5] Maternal self-report has been commonly used in the past to assess potential fetal exposure, but has been found to be unreliable and not correlate with exposure.[6] Using biomarkers to detect use of drugs, alcohol, or environmental toxins can help determine the optimal management of the child.

HAIR AND MECONIUM AS MATRICES FOR IN UTERO BIOMARKERS

Most often, blood and urine are used to test for drug and alcohol use or exposure. Although these 2 matrices are well established, they provide information on only very recent use or exposure, because of the short elimination half-lives of most drugs of abuse.[7,8] Longer-term, chronic exposure is not detected using blood or urine, requiring alternative matrices to capture this type of exposure. Hair and meconium, in neonates, have emerged as novel matrices that provide a wider window of detection. These 2 matrices can be tested to assess prenatal exposure to chemicals, including those resulting from maternal usage.

Hair

Hair follicle development occurs because of ectodermal and mesodermal interactions during epidermal development, beginning at approximately the eighth week of development.[9] The base of the follicle, the dermal papilla, is derived from the mesodermal mesenchyme of the dermis, whereas the remainder of the hair follicle is derived from the ectoderm.[9] The pigmentation of hair and skin is caused by melanocytes, which develop from the neural crest cells.[9] Melanin pigments, eumelanin and pheomelanin, are synthesized and stored in the melanosomes. Eumelanin produces brown and black hair, whereas pheomelanin is responsible for red and blond hair. The proportion of these 2 melanin pigments is what dictates the final color of human hair.[10] The appearance of hair follicles occurs at around the 10th week of fetal development, and continued differentiation results in the formation of various components of the follicle.[9]

Three types of glands are associated with the hair follicle: sebaceous, apocrine, and sweat glands. The sebaceous gland, responsible for the production of sebum, develops on the side of the follicle and is associated with capillary networks, similar to the hair follicle. Sebum is composed of free and combined fatty acids and unsaponifiable material (eg, cholesterol and waxes).[9,11] Apocrine glands secrete an oily, colorless substance directly into the follicle, and are localized in the axilla, eyelids, and external auditory meatus.[11] Sweat glands, located on most of the body surface, produce sweat, comprising mainly water and salts.[11]

Hair growth occurs in a 3-phase cycle, consisting of anagen, catagen, and telogen phases.[11] The anagen phase represents hair production and begins at the 15th week of fetal development, and the scalp of the fetus is completely covered with anagen phase follicles between the 18th and 20th week of gestation.[9] This phase is characterized by a rapid proliferation of matrix cells, which fill the follicle bulb, extending through epithelial cells.[9] The matrix cells are then keratinized, forming the strand of hair.[11] Growth of the hair continues until expression of epidermal growth factors, resulting in apoptosis of follicular keratinocytes and melanocytes, or the catagen phase. During the catagen phase, the bottom of the hair fiber is fully keratinized. At this point, the hair follicle is dormant and in the telogen phase. In respect to a neonate, the first full cycle of hair growth is complete between the 24th and 28th week of development, with the next cycle starting soon after the first one is completed.[9] Consequently, biomarkers present in hair at birth reflect exposure to toxins during the third trimester, and are able to be tested until approximately 3 months after birth. Therefore, if there is hair present after birth, the window of detection is relatively long.

In children (and adults), the hair growth cycle continues, with each phase having a distinct length of time. The growth of each hair follicle is independent, with approximately 85% of all head hair follicles in the anagen phase (growing phase) at any given time.[11] The remainder of hair follicles are not in the growing phase, and this must be taken into account when interpreting any nonneonatal hair results, because drug incorporation does not occur during the resting phase.

Routes of incorporation of compounds into hair include direct incorporation of a chemical via the capillary networks of the hair follicle, as a result of secretions from the sebaceous and sweat glands, and as a result of environmental or external exposure.[12] Measuring and interpreting biomarkers in hair must properly take these different routes of incorporation into account.

The many factors that determine the concentration of a drug in hair should also be considered. These factors include hair color (melanin content), physicochemical properties of the drug, and cosmetic treatment of hair.[13] For example, it has been found that drugs preferentially incorporate into darker hair, most likely because of the relative amounts of eumelanin.[10] Also, physicochemical properties including lipophilicity, basicity, and membrane permeability affect the ability of drugs to incorporate into hair. Generally, basic, lipophilic drugs tend to accumulate more readily into hair samples than more acidic or polar drugs.[12] Cosmetic treatment of hair has been found to decrease hair concentrations of drugs, mainly because of increased hair damage and the removal of hair color pigment.[13] Hair damage causes drug molecules to be lost more easily from the matrix, whereas removal of pigment reduces the amount of melanin to which the drugs are bound.[13] As a result, clinical interpretations of drug concentrations in hair must take these factors into account.

Hair samples are typically collected from the posterior vertex, because hair from this area of the scalp shows the most constant rate of growth.[11] Analysis of hair provides long-term information on an individual's drug use or exposure. Taking advantage of the uniform growth rate of human hair, approximately 1 cm/mo, it is possible to segment hair samples to more accurately assess the time and pattern of use or exposure.[7] The window of detection for nonneonatal hair samples is therefore dependent on hair length.

Meconium

The first few bowel movements of a neonate are composed of meconium.[14] This highly complex matrix begins to form approximately during the 12th week of gestation and consists of water, gastrointestinal tract epithelial cells, bile acids and salts, enzymes, sugars, lipids, intestinal secretions, and swallowed amniotic fluid.[15] Fetal swallowing of amniotic fluid is the mechanism believed to concentrate compounds within meconium as fetal urine is deposited into the amniotic fluid and is subject to swallowing again.[15] Determining factors of drug incorporation into meconium and the extent of their concentration are mainly determined on the ability of the drug to cross the placenta. Most drugs are able to transfer across the placenta, and the rate of transfer is then determined by molecule size, ionization state, lipophilicity, and protein binding.[15] Because most drugs are small enough to transfer via passive diffusion, the major limiting factor, in terms of drug transport to the fetus, is placental blood flow.[16] Once meconium is formed in the fetal intestine, it is considered a physically static matrix, becoming a record of fetal exposure to the drugs in question during the second and third trimesters of pregnancy.[17] A positive meconium test indicates intrauterine exposure during the second and third trimesters, but is unable to show time or pattern of use.[18]

Dose-response relationships are difficult to determine using meconium samples, mainly because of urine contamination. If fetal exposure occurs close to term and the compound is incorporated into the urine, contamination of meconium can occur once urine is evacuated into a soiled diaper.[15] This situation increases the sensitivity of meconium testing because of the increased compound levels in the sample. However, it could affect the ratio of drugs and metabolites in the sample, and the development of dose-response relationships.

Collection of meconium specimens is easy and noninvasive. Because it is discarded material and there is usually sufficient quantity for analysis, this matrix is practical and useful.[14] Ninety-nine percent of infants pass their first meconium within 48 hours, giving this matrix a wider window of detection than blood or urine.[15] Once 48 hours have passed, it is necessary to evaluate the texture and odor of the sample to determine whether it still meconium or has changed to postnatal feces. The time allowed for sample collection, 2 days, may be seen as limited, but if the neonate is at high risk for drug or alcohol in utero exposure and in hospital care, obtaining a viable sample is not problematic. Collected samples should be minimally 0.5 g, to provide sufficient sample for all analyses. Storage of samples for analysis should be at -20°C or -80°C.[15]

BIOMARKERS FOR ALCOHOL USE

Alcohol exposure during pregnancy can have many serious consequences for the offspring, including birth defects and deficits in cognitive performance and mental development.[19,20] The fetal alcohol spectrum disorder (FASD) is an umbrella term, which describes the consequences associated with prenatal alcohol exposure.[6] Affecting approximately 1% of all live births in North America, FASD is a major social and economic burden, which can be minimized by early diagnosis and disease management.[21] The clinical presentation of the disease is inconsistent, some lacking evidence of central nervous system neurodevelopment abnormalities.[15] Typically, for the definite diagnosis of FASD, confirmation of prenatal ethanol exposure is needed because some of the characteristics of the disease, in particular physical, may be absent.[8]

Detection of ethanol or its aldehyde has a limited window because they are both rapidly cleared from the blood. A lack of relationship between maternal ethanol consumption and maternal ethanol levels also limits their use to provide an objective analysis.[22] Ethanol itself is not readily incorporated into matrices because of its volatile nature, limiting the window of detection to the hours leading up to delivery, when many alcohol-dependent mothers may not drink.[23] Two biomarkers, fatty acid ethyl esters (FAEEs) and ethyl glucuronide (EtG), have been established and are currently used to detect exposure or use of alcohol.

FAEEs

FAEEs are nonoxidative metabolites of ethanol, formed through the esterification of ethanol with endogenous fatty acids or fatty acyl-coenzyme A (CoA).[23] These reactions are catalyzed by FAEE synthase or microsomal acyl-CoA:ethanol O-acetyltransferase.[19] In particular, FAEE synthase is present in almost all human tissues, with activity being detected in the heart, liver, lungs, adipose tissue, gall bladder, and pancreas.[23] Depending on the carbon chain length and the location of the double bond, different species of FAEEs can be formed.[8] Most FAEEs are transported by albumin within the blood, and once free, are readily broken down by cellular structures in the blood, liver, and pancreas.[23] Unlike ethanol, FAEEs persist in the body for more than a day after significant alcohol consumption, and are able to accumulate in various matrices.[22] Also in contrast to ethanol, FAEEs are readily metabolized by the placenta and thus do not cross.[8] This characteristic indicates that FAEE levels present in meconium represent fetal ethanol metabolism and thus fetal exposure to ethanol.[17,18]

Several individual FAEEs are analyzed in samples to detect alcohol exposure or use. Interindividual variation in the amount of specific FAEEs formed can result from genetic variations in the enzymes responsible for FAEE formation, the amounts of specific fatty acids in different diets, the degree of alcohol exposure or consumption, and FAEE synthase enzyme kinetics.[8,15,22] Ethyl palmitate, oleate, stearate, and linoleate are the predominate FAEEs found in meconium of ethanol-exposed neonates.[23] The cumulative level of select FAEEs is measured because this provides a redundancy system, resulting in higher efficiency, sensitivity, and specificity.[15,24]

In several studies looking at baseline FAEE levels, infants born to women who did not drink alcohol during pregnancy had low FAEE levels.[25] Because the body produces some ethanol during normal metabolism, FAEEs are detected in individuals who do not consume alcohol, thus requiring a clear cutoff value specific to the matrix for differentiation between heavy-drinking and non drinking individuals.[26]

With respect to meconium, the positive cutoff of cumulative FAEE levels was established at 2 nmol/g meconium.[24] This cutoff has 100% sensitivity and 98.4% specificity for detection of heavy fetal alcohol exposure.[27] However, this cutoff value does not allow differentiating between neonates born to non drinkers and social drinkers.[24] An important limitation of FAEE meconium testing is that samples excreted later in the postpartum period have higher levels of FAEEs than samples collected earlier for the same infant because of de novo production of alcohol from carbohydrates in the meconium.[28] This situation could lead to false-positive FAEE results, and it is recommended to collect meconium samples within 24 hours to ensure that FAEE results properly reflect in utero ethanol exposure.

The FAEE cutoff value for adult hair was established to be 50 ng/g hair, but at this level would identify not only heavy drinkers but some social drinkers too.[29] Hair FAEE results between 20 and 50 ng/g hair indicate moderate levels (ie, social) of drinking.[8] This FAEE cutoff provides optimal sensitivity and specificity, both 90%.[19] Hair care products can result in increased FAEE levels by causing localized FAEE production on the scalp.[29] Differentiating between external and incorporated FAEEs may not be necessary in neonatal hair samples, because the use of hair care products in neonates is not relevant. To confirm FAEE results in adult hair, a secondary confirmatory test is needed, as discussed later.

EtG

EtG is a minor metabolite of ethanol, formed when ethanol is glucuronidated with activated glucuronic acid instead of water.[10] Although EtG testing lacks sensitivity in detecting moderate or social drinkers, it is highly specific for heavy alcohol use.[30] EtG measurements are used to confirm hair FAEE results. As mentioned earlier, increased hair FAEE levels can reflect alcohol abuse, social drinking, or use of ethanol-containing hair care products.[29] EtG can help rule out ambiguous FAEE results caused by external contamination with alcohol hair products. If a hair sample is also positive for EtG (cutoff of 30 pg/mg hair), this indicates excessive alcohol use during the tested time frame, and the potential influence of hair care products is eliminated.[29]

BIOMARKERS FOR DRUGS OF ABUSE

Illicit substance use in women of childbearing age has increased over the past 3 decades, with a parallel increase during pregnancy.[5] Drug use during pregnancy is a risk factor for both maternal and fetal complications.[31] As well, children exposed to drug use in their environment are susceptible to many adverse outcomes associated with drug use affecting their physical and mental health, as well as their social well-being.[32] The overall increased use of drugs of abuse has necessitated the development of biomarkers of drug use, obviating the shortcomings of maternal reports, providing clinicians with tools that can detect exposure to or use of these illicit compounds. Biomarkers for individual drugs or xenobiotics, each with unique impacts on the health of the child, are discussed.

Cocaine

Prenatal cocaine exposure is associated with low birth weight, prematurity, spontaneous abortions, stillbirths, and microcephaly. In addition, placenta complications have been described, including placental abruption and increased risk of diminished blood flow to the fetus.[33] Exposure to cocaine during childhood can increase the risk for hypertension, ventricular arrhythmia, seizures, and intracranial bleeding.[34] Behavioral problems also present themselves during development to both prenatally and postnatally exposed children. Infants exposed in utero are found to have attention deficits with an increased incidence of attention-deficit/hyperactivity disorder.[32]

Because of the short elimination half-life of cocaine (50 minutes), detection in blood or urine matrices is limited to a few days after use.[34] Because cocaine and its metabolites readily accumulate in both hair and meconium, these matrices can provide information on in utero exposure for infants as well as environmental exposure in older children.

Cocaine crosses the placenta via passive diffusion and is almost always found with at least 1 of its metabolites in meconium samples.[15] The site of metabolite production, either fetal or maternal, is undetermined. The most common cocaine metabolite tested and found in biologic matrices is benzoylecgonine. This metabolite is formed through hydrolysis.[15] Other metabolites, including norcocaine and cocaethylene, are also used in sample analysis for cocaine.

Using all 4 of these biomarkers allows clinicians to obtain an accurate picture of cocaine exposure and make a correct clinical interpretation. The latter is important because environmental cocaine exposure occurs in different ways, including inhalation of crack cocaine smoke, exposure to cocaine residues on surfaces, and through direct contact with a cocaine-using caregiver. The presence of cocaine in a child without the metabolites that are produced systemically indicates environmental exposure, with low risk of systemic exposure. If benzoylecgonine is also detected at concentrations at least 10% of cocaine hair levels, it is a strong indication of systemic exposure by the child. The presence of norcocaine indicates higher levels of exposure, because this metabolite is not so readily detected, as is benzoylecgonine.

Cocaethylene is an emerging biomarker that can provide additional information regarding exposure. This metabolite is formed when cocaine and ethanol are present concurrently.[35] By using cocaethylene as a biomarker, alcohol use can be detected without assessing alcohol-specific biomarkers. This strategy has great advantages for detecting a risk of fetal alcohol syndrome in neonates who are positive for this metabolite.

Opioids

Opioid use has been reported in 1% to 21% of pregnant women.[5] With increasing rates of opioid use and dependency, the incidence of neonatal abstinence syndrome (NAS) has doubled in the past 5 years in Ontario, Canada.[36] Because most infants born to opioid-dependent mothers suffer from NAS, this has become a real public health issue.[37] NAS is characterized by the presence of central nervous system hyperirritability, gastrointestinal dysfunction, and metabolic, vasomotor, and respiratory disturbances.[36] The treatment required for these symptoms increases the hospital stay to an average of 30 to 40 days for infants, primarily in a neonatal intensive care unit.[36] The recent introduction of buprenorphine has resulted in a decreased hospital stay and shorter duration of treatment of infants.[36] Testing women suspected of using opioids could allow for early treatment of the baby and mother. Although the methadone-treated mother is commonly known to the medical system and social services, expecting mothers addicted to other opioids may go undetected, and use of meconium or hair biomarkers may be the first clue to the poor neonatal adaptation shown by the neonate.

Heroin use during pregnancy may be involved in a cycle of overdose and withdrawal and is associated with complications, including spontaneous abortion, antepartum hemorrhage, and stillbirth.[38,39] Heroin is rapidly deacetylated to the active metabolite 6-monoacetylmorphine (6-MAM), readily crosses the placenta, and is incorporated into fetal tissues within 1 hour of administration.[5] Because 6-MAM persists in the system for a longer period than heroin, it is used as a biomarker to detect heroin use. Along with heroin metabolism to 6-MAM, detectable levels of morphine can also be produced.[40] In addition, illicit heroin usually contains acetylcodeine, and users commonly top up their heroin with codeine before injection.[40] This practice may complicate the interpretation of test results, because the source of codeine and morphine may be unknown in 6-MAM–positive samples.

Codeine and morphine are commonly tested together because morphine is a metabolite of codeine through CYP2D6 metabolism.[41] Morphine is widely distributed in fetal tissues and its level in meconium has been found to correlate with maternal dose, time, and duration of gestational exposure.[15] Similar to codeine and morphine testing, oxycodone and its metabolite oxymorphone are commonly tested together. Hydrocodone is tested with one of its metabolites, hydromorphone, which is also available as a separate analgesic. It is best to determine which drug was prescribed before interpreting the results, because each of the metabolites is also a prescription drug. Because opioids are not contraindicated during pregnancy and can be used during labor, it is necessary to try to identify all medications administered to the mother to properly assess opioid levels.

Amphetamines

This group of drugs of abuse includes methamphetamine (commonly called crystal meth), amphetamine (commonly called speed, also Adderall or Dexedrine), and

MDMA (3,4-methylenedioxy-N-methylamphetamine) (commonly called ecstasy). Case reports have reported congenital abnormalities, including heart defects and cleft palate, in infants exposed to amphetamines during the first trimester.[5] All of these compounds have been associated with similar impacts on behavior and cognition of exposed children, including lower IQ scores, difficulties with advancement in school, and physical fitness activities.[32] In addition, children of addicted mothers have been found to show more behavioral problems.[32] Each compound in this group has its own method of detection, and results are used in conjunction to provide a more accurate interpretation.

Methamphetamine is able to cross the placenta at a rapid rate and even at lower levels on the fetal side; it persists because of slower elimination, resulting in prolonged fetal exposure.[15,42] The fetal elimination rate of amphetamine is also reduced, but to a greater extent than that of methamphetamine.[42] The prolonged elimination of both methamphetamine and amphetamine can cause accumulation of both compounds on the fetal side if the mother is using these compounds on a consistent basis. Environmental exposure is also a concern for children, especially if methamphetamine is smoked in the household.

Each one of these amphetamine derivatives can be tested for in meconium and hair samples to assess exposure in children. Interpretation of samples positive for amphetamines can become complex depending on which compounds are detected. If either methamphetamine or amphetamine is detected alone, this indicates exposure or use of this compound. Samples positive for both methamphetamine and amphetamine can be interpreted in 3 ways. First, the amphetamine could be a product of methamphetamine metabolism, indicating methamphetamine use or exposure. Second, seized illicit methamphetamine contains amphetamine as well, indicating methamphetamine use and, unknowingly, amphetamine exposure. Third, it can suggest both methamphetamine and amphetamine were used during the tested time frame. It is necessary to test for all amphetamine compounds if exposure is suspected, because the interpretation of amphetamines can be complex.

Cannabinoids

No clear increase in pregnancy complications for users of marijuana is known. However, some studies have associated marijuana use during pregnancy with lower birth weights and longer gestations.[5] Users of marijuana have been documented to use other illicit drugs, which increases the risk of complications. In addition, it was recently found that children exposed to marijuana had lower performance on standardized tests, indicating that long-term behavioral and neurodevelopmental issues may occur in these children.[43]

Cannabis sativa, marijuana, produces the group of cannabinoids, with more than 50 unique compounds. Δ9-tetrahydrocannabinol (THC) is the primary compound of the cannabinoids and is metabolized to the active compound 11-hydroxy-Δ9-tetrahydrocannabinol and subsequently 11-nor-Δ9-tetrahydrocannabinol-9-carboxylic acid (THC-COOH).[15] Analysis of samples for cannabinoid content is primarily conducted using enzyme-linked immunosorbent assay (ELISA) techniques and yields a qualitative result of positive or negative depending on the cutoff value set for the method. Because of the commonality of infrequent cannabis users and their chance of increasing false-negative results, the sensitivity of the immunoassay analysis can vary depending on the tested population.[15] Confirmation of ELISA results can be conducted using gas chromatography-mass spectrometry, but because of the nature of THC and the extraction methods used, which alter the ratio between THC-COOH and total cannabinoids, lower rates of confirmation have been found.[15] Positive ELISA results for cannabinoids indicate use or high exposure, because THC and its metabolites are not readily incorporated into matrices. Implementing liquid chromatography-mass spectrometry analysis is a potential method for THC analysis, because it is able to detect lower levels of compounds.

BIOMARKERS OF ENVIRONMENTAL EXPOSURES

Although there are numerous biomarkers for a multitude of environmental chemical exposures, we use 1 powerful example of environmental exposure through diet primarily to show the importance of biomarkers in this field.

Methylmercury

Methylmercury is a known neurotoxin produced from inorganic mercury by anaerobic organisms that live in aquatic environments.[44] Because methylmercury strongly binds to cysteine-containing proteins, it is not readily eliminated from the body; its elimination half-life is approximately 60 days, and it can also accumulate in the environment.[45] Fish consumption is the main source of methylmercury ingestion, with a dose-response relationship between the amount of fish consumed and the total systemic mercury burden, which can be measured in hair and blood.[44] Methylmercury readily crosses the placenta and because the blood-brain barrier does not fully develop until 6 months after birth, prenatal exposure can result in adverse neurodevelopmental effects.[45] These adverse neurodevelopment effects can include deficits in the functional domains of language, memory, and attention.[45] Adverse effects of high prenatal exposure to methylmercury have been well documented because of 2 serious poisoning events in Japan and Iraq.[45] In addition, neurologic damage can also occur in children and adults who consume fish containing high mercury levels on a regular basis. This damage is often characterized by ataxia, sensory disturbances, and mental state changes.[45]

Total mercury levels are commonly tested in hair samples, both maternal and fetal. Data show that methylmercury makes up 80% of the total mercury detected in hair, with the remaining 20% being inorganic mercury.[45] With respect to maternal hair, levels as low as 10 μg/g hair have been associated with severe adverse effects to the fetus.[44] In a recent meta-analysis, the lower observable adverse effect level of mercury for adverse fetal outcome was defined at 0.3 μg/g maternal hair.[46] Analysis of hair of women who consume more than 340g (12oz) of fish per week could be a useful tool to assess whether this consumption is associated with increased mercury levels. If so, these women may wish to modify their diet before becoming pregnant, decreasing the body's burden of mercury and ensuring minimal fetal exposure to methylmercury.[44]

IMPORTANCE OF BIOMARKERS

Substance abuse, prenatal or not, is an ongoing public health concern, affecting not only the user themselves but also their families, and the health system economically. Beyond being biomarkers for physical and neurologic well-being of exposed children, hair and meconium measures identify women who continue to use drugs of abuse or alcohol despite being aware of their pregnancy. Children raised by an addicted mother have increased risk for neglect and abuse.[8] Behavioral problems associated with exposure to drugs of abuse can commence in utero, but the quality of the postnatal environment can also modify the child's behavior and development.[32] Hence, these biomarkers constitute strong predictors of environmental risk for the child, and a need for close follow-up of the well-being of the child. Identifying abuse is critical to allow social workers and children's aid societies to implement the necessary interventions and provide the best environment possible for the child.

Polydrug use is commonly reported in those who tested positive for certain drugs. In terms of opioid-dependent women, benzodiazepines, cocaine, and marijuana are the most common concomitantly used drugs.[36] This finding was confirmed by showing that meconium samples positive for opioids were likely to also be positive for cocaine, benzodiazepines, methadone, and FAEEs in a previous study.[37] As well, stimulant use of amphetamines and cocaine by the mother was a potential risk factor of alcohol use and subsequently fetal alcohol exposure.[19] Knowing which drugs are often used concomitantly can allow clinicians to potentially diagnose drug exposures in children that otherwise would have gone undetected.

Environmental exposures to chemicals are increasingly becoming more publicly acknowledged. Developing biomarkers for specific environmental toxicants can help clinicians detect both high-level and low-level exposures in humans. Detection can then lead to a decrease in exposure to these toxicants, and possibly discontinuing public use of compounds causing major adverse effects on health.

SUMMARY

The impact that drug and alcohol use or abuse during pregnancy can have on neonates and infants is serious. Because mothers may grossly underreport use because of fears and embarrassment, identification of biomarkers in newborns that point to such use has become a major research focus and is becoming more commonly accepted and used in clinical practice. Using such biomarkers provides clinicians with an opportunity to appropriately diagnose and, where possible, treat newborn conditions associated with prenatal alcohol or drug abuse. It also provides social workers with the opportunity to implement necessary interventions to provide a safer environment for the child. Similarly, the development of effective biomarkers to detect environmental chemical exposures allows the health care team to implement, where available, mitigating interventions to minimize their adverse effects.

REFERENCES

1. Biomarkers Definitions Working Group. Biomarkers and surrogate endpoints: preferred definitions and conceptual framework. Clin Pharmacol Ther 2001;69: 89–95.
2. Goodsaid FM, Frueh FW, Mattes W. Strategic paths for biomarker qualification. Toxicology 2008;245:219–23.
3. Timbrell JA. Biomarkers in toxicology. Toxicology 1998;129:1–12.
4. Goel N, Beasley D, Rajkumar V, et al. Perinatal outcome of illicit substance use in pregnancy–comparative and contemporary socio-clinical profile in the UK. Eur J Pediatr 2011;170:199–205.
5. Keegan J, Parva M, Finnegan M, et al. Addiction in pregnancy. J Addict Dis 2010; 29:175–91.
6. Zelner I, Shor S, Gareri J, et al. Universal screening for prenatal alcohol exposure: a progress report of a pilot study in the region of Grey Bruce, Ontario. Ther Drug Monit 2010;32:305–10.
7. Klein J, Karaskov T, Koren G. Clinical applications of hair testing for drugs of abuse–the Canadian experience. Forensic Sci Int 2000;107:281–8.
8. Koren G, Hutson J, Gareri J. Novel methods for the detection of drug and alcohol exposure during pregnancy: implications for maternal and child health. Clin Pharmacol Ther 2008;83:631–4.

9. Gareri J, Koren G. Prenatal hair development: implications for drug exposure determination. Forensic Sci Int 2010;196:27–31.

10. Kulaga V, Velazquez-Armenta Y, Aleksa K, et al. The effect of hair pigment on the incorporation of fatty acid ethyl esters (FAEE). Alcohol Alcohol 2009;44:287–92.

11. Harkey MR. Anatomy and physiology of hair. Forensic Sci Int 1993;63:9–18.

12. Henderson GL. Mechanisms of drug incorporation into hair. Forensic Sci Int 1993; 63:19–29.

13. Jurado C, Kintz P, Menendez M, et al. Influence of the cosmetic treatment of hair on drug testing. Int J Legal Med 1997;110:159–63.

14. Moller M, Koren G. Unsuspected prenatal opioid exposure: long-term detection by alternative matrices. Ther Drug Monit 2010;32:1–2.

15. Gareri J, Klein J, Koren G. Drugs of abuse testing in meconium. Clin Chim Acta 2006;366:101–11.

16. Szeto HH. Kinetics of drug transfer to the fetus. Clin Obstet Gynecol 1993;36:246–54.

17. Gareri J, Lynn H, Handley M, et al. Prevalence of fetal ethanol exposure in a regional population-based sample by meconium analysis of fatty acid ethyl esters. Ther Drug Monit 2008;30:239–45.

18. Chan D, Caprara D, Blanchette P, et al. Recent developments in meconium and hair testing methods for the confirmation of gestational exposures to alcohol and tobacco smoke. Clin Biochem 2004;37:429–38.

19. Kulaga V, Shor S, Koren G. Correlation between drugs of abuse and alcohol by hair analysis: parents at risk for having children with fetal alcohol spectrum disorder. Alcohol 2010;44:615–21.

20. Hutson JR, Rao C, Fulga N, et al. An improved method for rapidly quantifying fatty acid ethyl esters in meconium suitable for prenatal alcohol screening. Alcohol 2011;45:193–9.

21. Zelner I, Shor S, Lynn H, et al. Clinical use of meconium fatty acid ethyl esters for identifying children at risk for alcohol-related disabilities: the first reported case. J Popul Ther Clin Pharmacol 2012;19:e26–31.

22. Brien JF, Chan D, Green C, et al. Chronic prenatal ethanol exposure and increased concentration of fatty acid ethyl esters in meconium of term fetal guinea pig. Ther Drug Monit 2006;28:345–50.

23. Caprara DL, Klein J, Koren G. Diagnosis of fetal alcohol spectrum disorder (FASD): fatty acid ethyl esters and neonatal hair analysis. Ann Ist Super Sanita 2006;42:39–45.

24. Chan D, Klein J, Karaskov T, et al. Fetal exposure to alcohol as evidenced by fatty acid ethyl esters in meconium in the absence of maternal drinking history in pregnancy. Ther Drug Monit 2004;26:474–81.

25. Chan D, Bar-Oz B, Pellerin B, et al. Population baseline of meconium fatty acid ethyl esters among infants of nondrinking women in Jerusalem and Toronto. Ther Drug Monit 2003;25:271–8.

26. Caprara DL, Klein J, Koren G. Baseline measures of fatty acid ethyl esters in hair of neonates born to abstaining or mild social drinking mothers. Ther Drug Monit 2005;27:811–5.

27. Chan D, Klein J, Koren G. Validation of meconium fatty acid ethyl esters as biomarkers for prenatal alcohol exposure. J Pediatr 2004;144:692.

28. Zelner I, Hutson JR, Kapur BM, et al. False-positive meconium test results for fatty acid ethyl esters secondary to delayed sample collection. Alcohol Clin Exp Res 2012. [Epub ahead of print].

29. Gareri J, Appenzeller B, Walasek P, et al. Impact of hair-care products on FAEE hair concentrations in substance abuse monitoring. Anal Bioanal Chem 2011; 400:183–8.

30. Kulaga V, Pragst F, Fulga N, et al. Hair analysis of fatty acid ethyl esters in the detection of excessive drinking in the context of fetal alcohol spectrum disorders. Ther Drug Monit 2009;31:261–6.
31. Bandstra ES, Morrow CE, Mansoor E, et al. Prenatal drug exposure: infant and toddler outcomes. J Addict Dis 2010;29:245–58.
32. Lester BM, Lagasse LL. Children of addicted women. J Addict Dis 2010;29:259–76.
33. Joya X, Gomez-Culebras M, Callejon A, et al. Cocaine use during pregnancy assessed by hair analysis in a Canary Islands cohort. BMC Pregnancy Childbirth 2012;12:2.
34. Taguchi N, Mian M, Shouldice M, et al. Chronic cocaine exposure in a toddler revealed by hair test. Clin Pediatr (Phila) 2007;46:272–5.
35. Natekar A, Koren G. Interpretation of combined hair fatty acid ethyl esters, cocaine and cocaethylene. Ther Drug Monit 2011;33:284.
36. Abrahams R, Chase C, Desmoulin J, et al. The opioid dependent mother and newborn–an update. The 6th Annual Ivey Symposium. J Popul Ther Clin Pharmacol 2012;19:e73–7.
37. Moller M, Karaskov T, Koren G. Opioid detection in maternal and neonatal hair and meconium: characterization of an at-risk population and implications to fetal toxicology. Ther Drug Monit 2010;32:318–23.
38. Su PH, Chang YZ, Yang C, et al. Perinatal effects of combined use of heroin, methadone, and amphetamine during pregnancy and quantitative measurement of metabolites in hair. Pediatr Neonatol 2012;53:112–7.
39. Mactier H. The management of heroin misuse in pregnancy: time for a rethink? Arch Dis Child Fetal Neonatal Ed 2011;96:F457–60.
40. Lee S, Cordero R, Paterson S. Distribution of 6-monoacetylmorphine and morphine in head and pubic hair from heroin-related deaths. Forensic Sci Int 2009;183:74–7.
41. Kirchheiner J, Schmidt H, Tzvetkov M, et al. Pharmacokinetics of codeine and its metabolite morphine in ultra-rapid metabolizers due to CYP2D6 duplication. Pharmacogenomics J 2007;7:257–65.
42. White S, Laurenzana E, Hendrickson H, et al. Gestation time-dependent pharmacokinetics of intravenous (+)-methamphetamine in rats. Drug Metab Dispos 2011;39:1718–26.
43. Goldschmidt L, Richardson GA, Willford JA, et al. School achievement in 14-year-old youths prenatally exposed to marijuana. Neurotoxicol Teratol 2012;34:161–7.
44. Koren G, Bend JR. Fish consumption in pregnancy and fetal risks of methylmercury toxicity. Can Fam Physician 2010;56:1001–2.
45. Schoeman K, Bend JR, Koren G. Hair methylmercury: a new indication for therapeutic monitoring. Ther Drug Monit 2010;32:289–93.
46. Schoeman K, Bend JR, Hill J, et al. Defining a lowest observable adverse effect hair concentrations of mercury for neurodevelopmental effects of prenatal methylmercury exposure through maternal fish consumption: a systematic review. Ther Drug Monit 2009;31:670–82.

New Ways to Detect Adverse Drug Reactions in Pediatrics

Michael Rieder, MD, PhD, FRCPC, FRCP (Glasgow)[a,b,c,*]

KEYWORDS

- Adverse drug reactions • Children • Safety assessment • Immunopharmacology
- Pharmacogenomics

KEY POINTS

- It is clear that adverse drug reactions (ADRs) are a major problem in the care of children, and that the approach to these is primarily clinical.
- Recent developments in the characterization assessment and therapy of common and serious ADRs are likely to change the approach to ADRs in children, notably for special populations such as premature neonates and children with cancer.
- These developments should bring child health care practitioners closer to the shared goal of safe and effective drug therapy for children.

ADVERSE DRUG REACTIONS—THE NATURE AND SCOPE OF THE PROBLEM

For most of recorded history, medical treatment was conducted using therapies that would today be considered complementary or alternative medicine.[1] Medications were typically prepared—frequently by compounding—largely from botanic or other natural sources, and there was little standardization or regulation. Occasionally this approach resulted in the development of a specific therapy, of which the most notable example would be the development of digoxin for the treatment of cardiac disease by William Withering in the 18th century.[2] In this case, a series of unique circumstances led to this discovery. Withering, who in addition to being a physician was a trained botanist, was interested in understanding how an herbal mixture used by a folk healer in Shorpshire, in the West Midlands region of England, improved dropsy (edema usually associated with heart failure) among patients who did not respond to the best medical therapy of the day. In this case, Withering's botanic knowledge enabled him to determine that, among the 20 herbs in the mixture, only one, *Digitalis purpurea*

[a] Department of Paediatrics, Schulich School of Medicine & Dentistry, Western University, London, Ontario, Canada; [b] Departments of Physiology & Pharmacology, Schulich School of Medicine & Dentistry, Western University, London, Ontario, Canada; [c] Department of Medicine, Schulich School of Medicine & Dentistry, Western University, London, Ontario, Canada
* Department of Paediatrics, Children's Hospital, London Health Sciences Centre, 800 Commissioner's Road East, London, Ontario N6C 2V5, Canada.
E-mail address: mrieder@uwo.ca

Pediatr Clin N Am 59 (2012) 1071–1092
http://dx.doi.org/10.1016/j.pcl.2012.07.010
0031-3955/12/$ – see front matter © 2012 Elsevier Inc. All rights reserved.
pediatric.theclinics.com

or Foxglove, was likely to have biologic activity. Withering then conducted a series of clinical studies to determine what would be the most effective and safe dose of Foxglove to treat dropsy. His landmark publication in 1785, "An Account of the Foxglove and Some of Its Medical Uses; With Practical Remarks on Dropsy and Other Diseases," is remarkable not only in the detail of the clinical investigations undertaken, but also in Withering's candor in acknowledging that his studies had included treating patients with doses that produced toxicity.[2] This early description of the potential for hazards associated with therapy was, unfortunately, largely unheeded.

The contemporary era of specific therapy has been most frequently attributed to the discovery of the antimicrobial activity of sulfanilamide.[1,3] In 1935 Gerhard Domagk, a physician working for the pharmaceutical division of the German conglomerate IG Farbenindustrie (which previously and later was the Bayer Company) published his key paper describing the results of his work over the previous 3 years, which demonstrated that Prontosil, a compound derived from azo dyes, was able to treat streptococcal infection in mice.[4] Subsequently it was discovered that the pharmacologically active molecule was sulfanilamide. While Sir Alexander Fleming had demonstrated the antibacterial effects of penicillin in 1929, his work had been conducted entirely in vivo and was framed in the context of using penicillin as a tool for isolation of certain bacteria.[5] In contrast, by 1937 sulfanilamide was being routinely used clinically, with penicillin not being commonly available until the pressures of World War II led the British and American governments and industrial sectors to push the evaluation and manufacture of penicillin in industrial quantities.[6]

The impact of introducing specific drug therapy cannot be overestimated. Infection was among the most common causes of death for patients of all ages, and the impact of effective antibiotic therapy was, in the words of Louis Thomas, "as if we could cure cancer".[1] However, while the ability to cure infections produced a paradigm change in medical care, this was not without cost. In fact, soon after sulfanilamide entered into routine clinical practice, rash and fever were described as associated with sulfanilamide therapy.[7] It is likely that this was an early example of drug hypersensitivity. Crystalluria, the most notorious adverse event associated with sulfanilamide therapy, however, was toxicity produced by a solvent used in drug preparation. The early sulphonamides were very water-insoluble, and indeed crystalluria was a problem associated with sulphonamide therapy.[7] The problem for children using sulphonamide treatment was compounded by the need to develop an alternative to the large sulphonamide tablets used at that time. An elixir of sulfanilamide was prepared using diethylene glycol as a solvent.[8] Diethylene glycol is an excellent solvent, and a potent nephrotoxin. Elixir of sulfanilamide was responsible for more than 100 deaths, and the ensuing public outrage resulted in, among other things, the creation of the US Food and Drug Administration (FDA) and led to developments that produced today's drug regulatory process.[7,9]

These 2 adverse events—rash and fever associated with drug therapy and unexpected nephrotoxicity of a component in a drug formulation—provide examples of the diversity of effects manifested as ADRs. An ADR has been defined as "a response to a drug which is noxious and unintended and which occurs at doses normally used in man for prophylaxis, diagnosis, or therapy of disease, or for the modification of physiologic function".[10] This broad definition includes a wide range of possible complications of therapy, but does not include errors seen related to incorrect drug administration such as giving a drug by the wrong route or in a toxic dose. The latter events are referred to as adverse drug events.[11,12]

It is now appreciated that ADRs are both common and important complications of therapy.[13] While the rate of ADRs varies depending on a number of variables including the drug, disease being treated, and the circumstances of the individual patient, it appears that for most drugs the minimal rate of ADRs that can be expected during therapy is approximately 5%, with many drugs being associated with substantially higher rates of ADRs.[7,14,15] Consequently, ADRs are associated with substantial morbidity and mortality. In fact, ADRs have been estimated to be between the 4th and 6th most common causes of death in the United States and Canada and have been associated with health care costs in the billions of dollars.[14,16]

ADVERSE DRUG REACTIONS—IMPLICATIONS FOR CHILD HEALTH

There are several myths that enjoy widespread circulation as to the degree and range to which drug therapies, and as a consequence ADRs, are used in children, as well as to relative risks of ADRs in children versus adults. These myths have led to complacency, which has not fostered a culture of patient safety in child health care.

The first of these myths has to do with drug utilization. It is commonly believed that children rarely receive drug therapy and when they do it is primarily in the form of antibiotics. This issue has actually been studied. All prescriptions dispensed to a cohort of 1 million Canadian children, roughly 15% of all children in Canada, in 1999 were retrieved.[17] Over this 1-year period, the 1,031,731 Canadian children (<18 years) received 4,028,502 prescriptions, roughly 4 prescriptions per child per year.[17] Of the drugs prescribed, antibiotics were indeed the most commonly prescribed drugs. However, they accounted for less than half of all drugs prescribed. There was a wide range—indeed more than 1300 distinct pharmacologic entities—that accounted for the remainder of the drugs prescribed (**Table 1**). As well, the overall numbers require some context to understand actual drug use among children. Despite the large number of prescriptions, most children are well and need few if any prescription drugs. As shown in **Fig. 1**, the largest amount of drug utilization—in fact, more than 70— occurs among roughly 25% of children. Thus, there are 2 distinct populations of children, children who are otherwise well and need perhaps one prescription a year, often an antibiotic or a respiratory drug, and a group of children with chronic health issues who require multiple prescriptions from a wide range of therapeutic classes.

Table 1
Drug utilization of 1 million Canadian children with respect to drug classes—data on selected drug classes derived

Drug Class	Percentage of All Prescriptions
Antibiotics	43%
Respiratory drugs	18%
Acne drugs	6%
Contraceptives	5%
Stimulants	4%
Analgesics (prescription)	3%
Antidepressants	2%
Anticonvulsants	1%
Gastrointestinal drugs (prescription)	1%
Antidiabetic drugs	1%

Data from Khaled LA, Ahmad F, Brogan T, et al. Prescription drug use by one million Canadian children. Paediatr Child Health 2003;8(Suppl A):6A–56A.

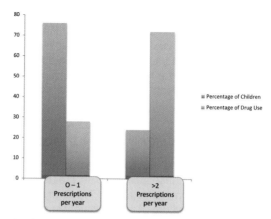

Fig. 1. Drug utilization by Canadian children, 1999. Most children have zero to 2 prescriptions per year, but approximately a quarter of children account for 70% of drug utilization. (*Data from* Khaled LA, Ahmad F, Brogan T, et al. Prescription drug use by one million Canadian children. Paediatr Child Health 2003;8(Suppl A):6A–56A.)

The second myth is that children are at a relatively reduced risk for ADRs compared with adults. While it has been accepted for some time that the preterm neonate is a distinct exception to this, a combination of faith in the general good health of children and unique cultural issues germane to certain specialty practices has fueled this myth. In fact, children are typically at either the same risk for ADRs as adults or even more; for example, it could be argued that essentially every child treated for leukemia experiences a series of ADRs, which are a regrettably but currently necessary part of life-saving therapy.

The fact that children are at an appreciable risk for ADRs, in some cases at higher risk than adults, is not surprising when one considers the 7 generally accepted risks for ADRs. These include: (1) previous adverse reaction to another drug, (2) polypharmacy, (3) female gender, (4) extremes of age, (5) reduction in capacity of the organs of excretion (liver, kidney), (6) larger drug dose, and (7) certain genetic polymorphisms.

These risk factors often operate in synergy (eg, patients at the extremes of age — the very premature infant or the very elderly senior) often have (for different reasons) reduced liver and kidney capacity, and often (again for different reasons) are prescribed multiple drugs.[18] As well, although the developmentally related reductions in drug clearance are well known in the case of the premature infant, the fact that the liver is the largest relative percentage of body mass at any time during life during the toddler years (with consequent implications for activation-induced adverse drug events such as valporic acid-induced hepatotoxicity, lamotrigine-induced serious skin rash, ifosfamide-induced nephrotoxicity and cefaclor-induced serum sickness-like reactions) is much less well appreciated.[19–22] Children are also at special risk for adverse drug events such as 10-fold errors in medication administration.[23] This phenonemon—almost unknown in adults—occurs in children due to a combination of drugs with child-unfriendly dosing formulations and mathematical problems on the part of some health care personnel.[24–26]

Thus, there are clear and compelling reasons that suggest that children are likely to be at a substantial risk for ADRs, and in certain circumstances may be at an even higher risk than adults.[27–29] Indeed, as noted previously, there are certain populations of children (eg, the premature neonate and children with cancer) for whom ADRs are essentially universal and are accepted as an undesired but currently necessary cost associated with therapy.[30,31] Given the increasing variety and complexity of therapies for children, the ability of clinicians to be able to appreciate, evaluate, treat, and ultimately prevent ADRs constitutes a core clinical skill for child health care practitioners in the upcoming decades.[32] Regrettably, despite the importance of ADRs in child health care, this is an area that is poorly taught in most pediatric residency programs.

THE CONTEMPORARY APPROACH TO ADRS

The current dealing with ADRs is primarily clinical, and can best be remembered as 5 As: appreciation, assessment, analysis, assistance, and aftermath.

This approach starts with clinicians appreciating the possible risk of an ADR. Succinctly put, the diagnosis of an ADR necessitates the consideration that it is a possibility. While this seems intuitive, assessment of ADR risk and the communication of this risk to patients and families are often less than optimal, even in settings in which ADR risk is clear and virtually certain. Some pediatric specialities (eg, pediatric oncologists) have developed widely adopted standard operating procedures prior to starting therapy that go to considerable lengths to ensure that patients and families understand the risks associated with chemotherapy.[33] However, such an approach has not been as well developed for many other child health disciplines. This is compounded by the complexity of therapies administered to chronically ill children as noted previously. Children who require drug therapy often require complex combinations. Given that there are over 3500 distinct therapeutic agents on the American market, it is a real challenge for health care providers to be aware of what are common and important ADRs, notably for new drugs or for drugs with which they are unfamiliar. Another layer of challenge is caused by the fact that the care of sick children is often multidisciplinary, requiring clear communication between members of the team, most notably in the area of therapeutics. In many hospitals, clinical pharmacists have indeed become essential to optimize the ability of providing safe and effective therapy.

When an adverse event occurs in the context of therapy, a distinction needs to be made as to whether the event is disease- or medication-related. While somewhat of a generalization, it is common for patients and families to associate the adverse event with therapy, while health care providers, especially those who prescribe therapy, quite commonly tend to associate the adverse event with the disorder being treated. This dichotomy serves as a useful starting point for the key diagnostic question: is the adverse event described drug-related or not.[34]

This brings one to assessment, the second step after appreciation. To make an adequate assessment it is crucial to have a clear and complete understanding of the events that led to the suspicion of an ADR. This includes both a comprehensive history as well as a relevant physical examination. Key elements in history include the rationale for therapy, the timing and dose of the drug(s) in question, the timing and nature of the symptoms and signs of concern, any interventions used with respect to the symptoms and signs of concern, and any potential confounders. As an example, it would be distinctly inappropriate to attribute a rash to a drug if the rash had been present before the drug was given. While somewhat an extreme example, much information can be obtained from a careful temporal analysis of the course of the disorder being treated, the course of therapy, and the course of the symptoms or signs of interest. Similarly, the physical examination may be extremely helpful. As an illustration, while an urticarial rash may be strongly suggestive of drug allergy, a nonpruritic, nonurticarial erythematous rash—of the type often called maculopapular—may be more suggestive of nondrug etiologies. While a thorough history and physical examination can be of great help in assessing ADRs, laboratory and other tests are usually less helpful. Laboratory tests can indeed identify worrisome findings, but often cannot tell whether the abnormality is drug-induced or not. For example, the presence of elevated serum transaminases can signal drug-induced hepatoxicity, but the results cannot differentiate drug-induced causes from infectious (viral hepatitis) ones. The main role of laboratory tests at the present time is to identify potential nondrug-induced causes (eg, viral hepatitis) and thus exclude drug-related causes, rather than to confirm the role of drugs in the sign or symptom of interest.[35] Testing can also confirm a clinical impression (eg, the demonstration of leukoclastic vasculitis can support the diagnosis of drug eruption). However, as will be noted, this may well change over the next decade.

There are several drugs for which laboratory testing in fact may be helpful. These include ADRs resulting from the use of penicillins as well as local anesthetics. Pencillin allergy is perhaps the most commonly stated drug allergy. While penicillin can cause ADRs mediated by a variety of mechanisms, including Gell and Coombs class 1 to 4 hypersensitivity, type 1 hypersensitivity (ie, immunoglobulin E [IgE]-mediated allergy) is the most common and most serious ADR associated with penicillin.[28,36] This is 1 case of an ADR where the pathophysiological mechanism is known in reasonably complete detail and in fact has been used to develop testing to predict ADR risk. Assessment can be done in vivo using penicillin skin testing, which is predictive of the risk for penicillin allergy and can provide a reliable risk for the likelihood of a serious allergic reaction with future penicillin therapy.[36,37] As well, in vitro assessment of risk can be done by determining if the patient has pencillin-specific IgE using a radioaller-gosorbent test (RAST).[36,37] The use of in vitro assessments for penicillin allergy is less specific than skin testing but is reasonably sensitive, notably when combined with a rechallenge following a negative in vitro test. Positive results are highly significant (ie, they are associated with a significant risk for a serious ADR with future therapy), but negative in vitro results are not a guarantee of safety; thus rechallenge is important if future therapy is planned on the basis of a negative in vitro test. Assessment for penicillin allergy is of importance given both the frequency with which penicillin can induce allergy and the regrettable fact that, although penicillin allergy is common, it is not nearly as common as it is reported. When patients are asked as to which drugs they are allergic, to up to 10% will mention a penicillin allergy; however, it has been demonstrated that most patients who present with a history of penicillin allergy are in fact not allergic to penicillin. Interestingly, many parents whose children have a history of a possible ADR to penicillin remain reluctant to treat their children with penicillin despite negative testing.[38]

In addition to assessment of the risk of penicillin allergy, in vivo testing can be useful in the evaluation of allergy to local anesthetics.[39] In this case, testing is not to confirm or refute the association of a local anesthetic with an adverse event but rather to determine safety for future therapy. As most ADRs to local anesthetics are class-specific, typically the approach is to undertake skin testing with an agent of another class (eg, if the patient is believed to have an allergic reaction to an amide local anesthetic, then it would be appropriate to conduct skin testing using an ester local anesthetic).[39,40] Patch testing has been used for the assessment of a number of compounds, but patch testing requires special expertise and is not widely available.[41] Finally, in vitro testing can be very useful for the evaluation of possible pseudocholinesterase deficiency in patients who have had prolonged duration of effect from paralyzing agents such as succinylcholine.[42]

Analysis follows appreciation and assessment. Analysis essentially is putting together a differential diagnosis guided by the information gathered during assessment. It is often difficult for clinicians to reach a conclusion when assessing the potential role of a drug in an adverse event, and thus several algorithms have been developed to help guide the process of determining causation.[43] However, consistency between these algorithms is often poor; moreover, many algorithms do not take key confounders into account.[43,44] The algorithm that is used most commonly is the Naranjo score, a score derived from an algorithm developed by Naranjo and colleagues[45] for the assessment of possible ADRs in adult patients treated with neurotropic drugs. Decisions as to whether an adverse event is an unlikely, possible, probable, or definite ADR is made by adding up the score assigned to a number of variables, including timing of drug exposure, likelihood of other causes, and whether the response changed in response to changes in drug dose or use of a placebo (**Table 2**).[45] This algorithm was extremely useful when it was developed, but changes in medical practice and differences in approach between adults and children have made this algorithm less useful in pediatrics.

The next step is assistance, which for most ADRs is relief of symptoms and to decide whether to continue therapy. In the case of serious ADRs—notably those mediated, even in part, by the immune system—it is usually necessary to stop the offending drug. If the ADR is acute or life-threatening, such as anaphylaxis, then additional timely and acute intervention is often needed to prevent serious injury or death.[46,47] As an example, there is emerging evidence that immune modulation may alter the course of serious drug hypersensitvities such as Stevens Johnson syndrome or toxic epidermal necrolysis.[28,48] However, for most ADRs, the best therapy is symptom management. Part of assistance is also the evaluation as to whether the drug used needs to be replaced, if the disorder that led to the drug prescription persists, or whether the drug can be permanently discontinued as the disorder has resolved. Occasionally, treating through ADRs is indicated. This approach has merit when the symptoms are troublesome but expected to diminish in severity or even disappear over time. An example is the fine hand tremor associated with aerosol albuterol (salbutamol) therapy. This ADR relates to stimulation of the beta receptors on skeletal

Table 2
The Naranjo scale. Possible scores range from >9 (definite ADR), 5–8 (probable ADR), 1–4 (possible ADR) or 0 or below (doubtful ADR)

Question	Yes	No	Do Not Know
Are there previous conclusive reports on this reaction?	1	0	0
Did the adverse event appear after the drug was given?	2	−1	0
Did the adverse event improve after the drug was stopped or a specific antagonist was given?	1	0	0
Did the adverse event appear when the drug was readministered?	2	−1	0
Are there alternate causes that could have caused the adverse event?	−1	2	0
Did the reaction reappear when a placebo was given?	−1	1	0
Was the drug detected in any body fluid in toxic concentrations?	1	0	0
Was the reaction more severe when the dose was increased or less severe when the dose was decreased?	1	0	0
Did the patient have a similar reaction to the same or similar drugs in a previous exposure?	1	0	0
Was the adverse event confirmed by any objective evidence?	1	0	0

Data from Naranjo CA, Busto U, Sellers EM, et al. A method for estimating the probability of adverse drug reactions. Clin Pharmacol Ther 1981;30:239–45.

muscle. It is common when therapy for reactive airways disease or asthma is started but typically goes away with continued therapy.[34]

The final step in managing an ADR is aftermath. There are several consequences of having had an ADR, some predictable and some not. While patients will often return to their usual state of health after resolution of an ADR, some ADRs have significant long-term consequences in terms of organ impairment. As an example, some patients with ifosfamide-induced nephrotoxicity will have long-term kidney dysfunction, which in rare cases can even progress to the point of requiring a renal transplant.[30,49] Similar considerations apply to cisplatin-induced ototoxicity and anthracycline-induced cardiotoxicity.[30,50,51] Thus, additional interventions may be needed.

Communication is an important part of the aftermath of an ADR that is often underappreciated. First, it is crucial that the patient and family understand what has happened and what the implications are. It is also important to ensure clear communication with other health care practitioners who are involved in managing the patient and his or her family. Finally, and especially for new drugs, it is important that the respective drug regulatory authorities (eg, the FDA) are made aware of ADRs, most notably unexpected ones. This is obviously less important for older drugs (eg, the FDA is very aware that amoxicillin therapy can result in penicillin allergy) than it is for new drugs. The cold hard reality is that drugs enter the market being tested in relatively few people, and thus serious ADRs that are occurring in a frequency of 1 case per 1000 population or less are very unikely to be detected prior to drug approval. It is worthwhile to remember that every serious drug hypersensitivity described has occurred after the drug was marketed, often as a result of a report by an astute clinician.

This, then, is the current approach to adverse events associated with drug therapy in children. This approach has been less than satisfactory in informing safe drug therapy, especially in the area of ADR prevention, and new approaches are clearly needed. What is exciting is that there are several developments underway that offer great promise in enhancing safe and effective drug therapy in children.

SYSTEMS APPROACHES TO DRUG ERROR

As noted previously, there are certain patterns of ADRs that are much more common in children than adults. These include 10-fold errors.[23–25] While medication dosing errors can be attributed to individual errors, many have their origin in system weaknesses. Improving health care systems seems to have had a favorable impact on medication errors, whether it is the use of clinical pharmacists to review orders and intervene when appropriate or the use of continuous critical incident monitoring to develop prevention strategies.[52,53] The introduction of the electronic health record has brought additional opportunities, and challenges, to safer drug therapy for children.

CAUSALITY EVALUATION

One of the major challenges in the assessment of adverse events associated with drug therapy is the likelihood of whether the event was caused by the drug in question. While there have been causality algorithms used since the 1970s, some are quite complex, and some are quite focused.[42] As an example, Kramer and colleagues[54,55] have developed an algorithm that appears to be valid but involves 6 flow sheets, while the algorithm developed by Maria and Victorina is specific to drug-induced liver injury. As noted earlier, the most commonly used causality algorithm, the Naranjo score, was designed for adult psychiatric patients.[45] When used in the evaluation of children, it is rarely possible to rank an event as definitive.

This problem has been appreciated for some time. Over the last several years, research has been on-going to develop tools that are better suited for a pediatric population. Wei Du and a group of pediatric clinical pharmacologists from across North America have recently created a novel tool specifically designed for the assessment of possible ADRs in neonates.[56] This instrument was developed using data extracted from a review of ADRs in their neonatal intensive care units (NICUs), from which key questions were derived. Cases were then evaluated by 5 experienced pediatric clinical pharmacologists using these questions; an evaluation using a defined subset of questions was then further refined and validated on a series of 50 cases from the NICUs. When the results of this validation were compared with Naranjo scores derived from the same cases, this new instrument was demonstrated to be significantly more valid and reliable than the Naranjo scale.[56] While this instrument needs further validation in a larger cohort and in a series of different NICUs, this new tool is very promising for use in the neonatal population.

Similarly, the Adverse Drug Reactions In Children (ADRIC) group at Alder Hey in Liverpool (United kingdom) has been developing an instrument for the assessment of ADRs in children with a broader age range, not just neonates.[57] This instrument, the Liverpool Causality Assessment Tool, uses a stepwise algorithm to determine the likelihood that an adverse event is drug-related or not (**Fig. 2**). This approach uses a flow chart format that is intended to be more user-friendly than the use of scales. The Liverpool Causality Assessment Tool appears to be able to evaluate a number of possibilities with better inter-rater reliability than the Naranjo scale when used to assess over 80 case reports as well as 37 published ADR cases.[57] This instrument is potentially quite useful but needs evaluation in other clinical settings.

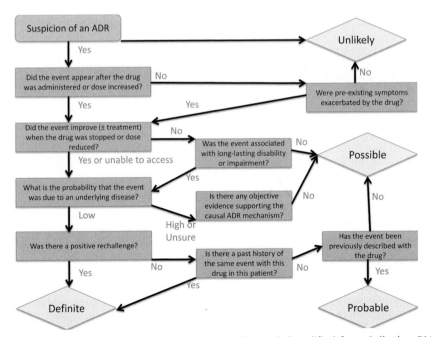

Fig. 2. The Liverpool adverse drug reaction causality tool. (*Modified from* Gallagher RM, Kirkham JJ, Mason JR, et al. Development and inter-rater reliability of the Liverpool adverse drug reaction causality assessment tool. PloS One 2011;6:e28096; with permission.)

TESTING FOR ASSESSMENT OF POTENTIAL ADRS

Currently there are limited tests available for the diagnosis of ADRs. There are, however, several assays used for research that have potential for clinical use. Most of these in vitro tests focus on immune-mediated ADRs.[58] Immune-mediated ADRs are not the most common ADRs, but they account for a disproportionately large number of serious and life-threatening ADRs (**Fig. 3**). In order to appreciate the potential utility of this testing, it would be helpful to appreciate which immune mechanisms mediate various ADRs (**Table 3**). The pathophysiology of ADRs mediated by type 1 hypersensitivity—classical IgE mediated allergy—is reasonably well understood, and thus there are both in vivo and in vitro tests that are routinely used clinically to evaluate ADRs mediated by IgE.[36–40] In sharp contrast, ADRs that are T cell-mediated are much less well understood.

The pathogenesis of drug hypersentivity has become more clear over the past decade, but there remains controversy as to the mechanistic details. There is clear consensus that the clinical signs and symptoms of delayed drug hypersensitivity, such as Stevens Johnson syndrome, are caused by a T cell-driven immune response.[28,59] However, the exact mechanism leading to this response remains unclear and somewhat controversial. The hapten hypothesis, initially advanced by Park and colleagues,[60] remains the oldest and most widely accepted theory as to how delayed drug hypersensitivity evolves. This hypothesis argues that bioactivation of a drug to

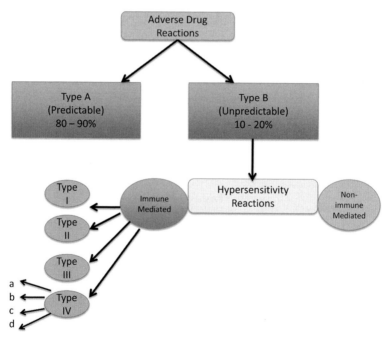

Fig. 3. Overview of ADRs. The overall classification is based on the system of Rawlins and Thompson, while the classification of immune-mediated ADRs is based on recommendations of the Nomenclature Review Committee of the World Allergy Organization. (*Data from* Gell PGH, Coombs RRA, editors. Clinical aspects of immunology. 1st edition. Oxford (England): Blackwell; 1963; Rajan TV. The Gell-Coombs classification of hypersensitivity reactions: a reinterpretation. Trends Immunol 2003;24:376–9; and Davies DM, editor. Textbook of adverse drug reactions. Oxford (United Kingdom): Oxford University Press; 1977.)

Table 3
Immune-mediated ADRs and immune mechanisms involved

Adverse Drug Reaction	Presumed Immune Mechanism
Anaphylaxis	IgE
Urticaria	IgE
Bronchospasm	IgE
Stevens Johnson syndrome	T cells/danger signals
Toxic epidermal necrolysis	T cells/danger signals

a reactive intermediate that haptenates protein, and the subsequent immune processing of the haptenated drug-protein complex, leads to an immune response manifested clinically as drug hypersensitivity (see **Fig. 3**).[28,60] More recently, Pischler and colleagues have advanced an alternate theory, the pharmacologic interference concept, which argues that low-affinity association of drugs with key immune receptors, notably with drugs that would not be capable of covalent binding, can produce immune responses leading to clinical expression such as drug hypersensitivity (**Fig. 4**).[28,61–63] In addition, the danger hypothesis, which suggests that danger signals from injured or dying cells may be important in initiating the immune response,[63] may play a role in idiosyncratic drug reactions including drug hypersensitivity.

The selection of a test to evaluate immune-mediated ADRs is highly dependent on the immune mediation of the event. As noted, measurement of IgE either in vitro or by

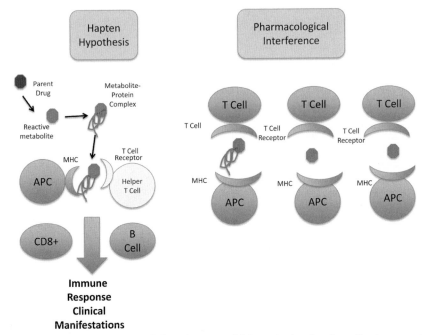

Fig. 4. Putative pathogenesis of drug hypersensitivity—the hapten hypothesis versus the pharmacologic interference concept. Abbreviations: APC, antigen presenting cell; MHC, major histocompatability complex. For the pharmacologic interference concept part of the figure, the 3 conditions represent (*left to right*) hapten, nickel, and pharmacologic interference. (*Modified from* Rieder MJ. Immune mediation of hypersensitivity adverse drug reactions: implications for therapy. Expert Opin Drug Saf 2009;8:331–43; with permission.)

in vivo demonstration of sensitivity can be done for several drugs.[36–40] An alternate approach is the basophil activation test, which assesses the release of histamine and other markers of basophil activation in response to stimulation with specific drugs as an indicator of allergy to these drugs.[64] In this context, assessment of basophil activation is used as a marker for immediate hypersensitivity. While this approach historically has been seen as less promising due to low sensitivity, coupling this assay with fluorescent antibodies for surface markers of basophil activation such as CD-63 has markedly improved the sensitivity of the assay.[65] The basophil activation test has been used for the assessment of immediate hypersensitivity to nonsteroidal anti-inflammatory drugs, muscle relaxants, β-lactam antibiotics, and pyrazolones. While this is a promising approach, this assay continues to be problematic due to relatively low sensitivity and the fact that it is only applicable to a limited number of drugs.[64,66–68]

The assessment of delayed hypersensitivity is much more problematic (**Fig. 5**). There have been several approaches developed to determine risk for drug hypersensitivity, one being the lymphocyte transformation test (LTT).[69] The basis of this test is the differential proliferation of lymphocytes from patients with drug hypersensitivity in response to the drug in question. This proliferation typically is measured by incorporation of tritiated thymidine and assessed by the comparison of vehicle- and drug-exposed lymphocytes as well as by comparison of the lymphocytes of patients and controls.[70] The LTT has been an extremely useful test for research into the pathophysiology of drug hypersensitivity.[69] However, utilization of this test for clinical purposes has been limited by several issues. First, the test is technically somewhat complicated and lacks standardization.[69] Additionally, timing is a key issue with the LTT. There appear to be 3 time windows for the LTT. During the first 4 weeks after a hypersensitive ADR, the patient's lymphocytes are highly reactive, so much so that they will not

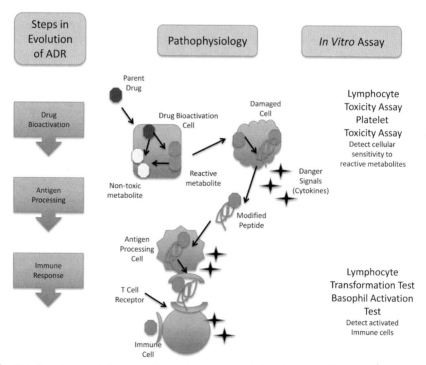

Fig. 5. Laboratory tests to assess the various stages of drug hypersensitivity.

respond to additional in vitro stimulation.[71] This is followed by a long period, usually years, during which drug-specific T cells can be detected in the peripheral blood. These cells respond well to in vitro stimulation.[72] Finally, during the last stage, no drug-specific T cells can be detected in the peripheral blood.[70] However, despite the absence of detectable drug-specific T cells, patients can develop a severe ADR if re-exposed to the drug in question. The LTT is highly mechanism-specific, and as a result is of great use for some drugs but may have no use in other types of drug hypersensitivity.[73,74] There are a number of promising developments to refine the assay, such as using flow cytometry for evaluation and the use of different targets such as expression of key markers like interleukin (IL)-5, IL-10, and CD69 or proinflammatory proteins as granulysin; these may make the LTT more suitable for adaption to the clinical setting.[75-78]

An alternate assay used to analyze drug hypersensitivity is the lymphocyte toxicity assay (LTA).[58,79-86] The basis of this assay is differential cellular sensitivity to reactive drug metabolites between the cells of patients who have developed drug hypersensitivity and the cells of patients who have not.[58,81,83] The test is performed using the peripheral mononuclear cells of patients and controls, largely T lymphocytes. After the white cells are isolated, they are incubated with the drug in question, a vehicle control, and either a reactive metabolite or the parent drug plus an activation system.[58,69] The purpose of the activation system is to generate reactive metabolites, which given their nature are often quite unstable and difficult to synthesize in quantities suitable for conducting assays.[69] The activation system has classically used microsomes, typically murine, but can also use chemical-based systems.[21,58] After incubation, the viability of the cells is determined to identify differences in sensitivity to reactive drug metabolites between patients who are drug tolerant and those who have developed drug hypersensitivity. While the earlier assays used visual scoring systems such as tryphan blue dye exclusion, refinements to the LTA have included the use of semiautomated viability assessments such as tetrazolium dye conversion or flow cytometry.[58,80-83]

The LTA has, as the LTT, been a useful tool for research into the pathophysiology of drug hypersensitivity.[58] In addition, there has been some experience with the use of this assay for the clinical assessment of adverse events that were possibly drug hypersensitive in nature.[87] In a study evaluating the use of the LTA, the author found that overall the assay had a sensitivity of 40% and a specificity of 90%, but the results were dependent on the drug evaluated; for the ß-lactam antibiotics, specificity and especially sensitivity were low, while for the sulfonamide antibiotics, both specificity and sensitivity were much higher, and the positive predictive value of the test was 100%.[87] This assay can also be used to analyze samples send to a laboratory (eg, the author has used the LTA in the laboratory to evaluate samples sent from the United States).[58,86] While the LTA has been a very useful assay for studying mechanisms of drug hypersensitivity, the problem of defining the optimal activation system and determining sensitivity and specificity limits its clinical applicability. As an illustration, the studies described previously using the ß-lactam antibiotics relied on a murine microsomal activating system, while for the sulfonamide antibiotic assays, the author used the chemically synthesized hydroxylamine derivative of sulfamethoxazole.[87,88] It would not be surprising to find more reproducible and robust toxicology data given the greater ability to control concentrations of reactive derivatives using this approach as opposed to relying on production of the metabolite by microsomal oxidation.

In addition to the issues cited previously, both the LTT and LTA have a problem unique to children; the blood sample size required to obtain the requisite number of cells is relatively large.

As part of research investigating new approaches to the study of drug hypersensitivity, the author has developed new assays to evaluate drug and metabolite toxicity.[58] Most recently, the author and colleagues have developed a toxicity assay using a new target, the platelet.[89,90] Platelets are metabolically active non-nucleated cells that have a pivotal role in hemostatis.[89] It is also now increasingly appreciated that platelets have an important role in immunity, inflammation, allergy, and hypersensitivity reactions.[91–93] The in vitro platelet toxicity assay (iPTA) is conducted by isolating platelets from patients with drug hypersensitivity and controls who are incubated with the drug in question, a vehicle control, and either a chemically synthesized reactive derivative or a microsomal activating system. After incubation, viability is determined using a semiautomated assay.[94] In a small case series, the author found that the iPTA appears to be equivalently specific and more sensitive than the LTA, while the small size and low density of platelets facilitate sample processing using differential centrifugation.[94] This is 1 approach to make testing more child-friendly and address the issue of sample volume and cell numbers.

Thus, while there are relatively few tests currently available for the diagnosis of ADRs, there are several possible approaches being developed that may be useful elements in the evaluation of adverse events associated with drug therapy.

GENE-BASED APPROACHES TO DRUG SAFETY

One of the most promising approaches to the evaluation—and notably prevention—of ADRs is with the focused use of pharmacogenomics. Personalized therapy for children is not novel; indeed, pediatricians and other specialists who care for children are accustomed to altering drug doses based on age, weight, and comorbidity.[95] Interestingly, while this same group of health care providers clearly is aware of the importance of genetically determined disease, genetics has not been a factor used in determining drug therapy.[96] However, the potential importance of genetics in both response and adverse events for therapy in children has been appreciated for some time, with the pioneering work of Weinshilbaum and colleagues demonstrating that polymorphisms in thiopurine S-methyltransferase were important determinants of drug toxicity in the context of chemotherapy for cancer.[97–99] While there has been consensus on the importance of these variations in the homozygous state, controversy as to the extent to which this applies to heterozygotes and whether this is a cost-effective approach has somewhat limited the consistent use of this genetic information in clinical practice.[100]

Over the past 2 decades, there has been a significant increase in both fundamental and applied knowledge of genetics and pharmacogenomics.[101] With this knowledge, assessment of the genetic contribution to drug toxicity has entered into routine clinical practice for certain conditions. The routine screening of people living with human immunodeficiency virus for HLA-B*5701, for example, has reduced the rate of serious hypersensitivity reactions to the antiviral agent abacavir from around 6% to essentially zero.[102] Similarly, the use of an algorithm combining clinical data with the assessment of genetic variations in cytochrome P450 2C9 (CYP29) and vitamin K epoxide reductase complex 1 (VKORC1) has improved the ability to obtain therapeutic warfarin levels in a timely manner in adult patients with atrial fibrillation.[103] In addition, the cost and time required for genetic studies have fallen sharply, enabling results to be available in real time and hence relevant to guide clinicians in their decision-making.[101,103,104] Finally, the development of research networks has enabled markedly more rapid and robust data collection. Linking networks in active surveillance for serious ADRs with pharmacogenomic and pharmacologic studies has, as exemplified by the Canadian Pharmacogenomic Network for Drug Safety (CPNDS), allowed investigators to develop novel and innovative approaches to defining the genetic contribution to serious ADRs.[105]

As noted (see **Fig. 1**), a relatively small percentage of children accounts for a relatively large percentage of total drug use, clearly reflecting populations of children with chronic and serious diseases such as cancer and epilepsy. Based on this, one can expect to see pharmacogenomic-guided therapies for children to have its first, and likely most profound, impact in these pediatric patient populations, most notably pediatric oncology.[106] As an example, the CPNDS group has studied serious ADRs associated with cisplatin and the anthracyclines, commonly used drugs in pediatric oncology.[107,108] Cisplatin is a highly effective chemotherapeutic agent associated with a significant risk for hearing loss, especially when used in children.[50,109] In a Canada-wide study, the CPNDS identified that functional variants in thiopurine S-methyltransferase and catechol O-methyltransferase are strongly correlated with risk for cisplatin-induced hearing loss.[107] Mechanistically, this is a fascinating finding, as neither enzyme is involved directly in the clearance of cisplatin. However, alterations in the activity of these enzymes may have a significant impact on the oxidative environment in the inner ear.[107,110] Aside from the clear benefits to individual patients, modeling the potential economic impact of pharmacogenomic testing to guide cisplatin therapy has suggested that the routine use of this testing would save over $19 million per year in Canada.[111]

Anthracyclines are used for many childhood cancers but are associated with a significant risk for cardiac toxicity, a risk that is greater among younger children.[112] Using similar methodology as described previously, the CPNDS has demonstrated an association between anthracycline-induced cardiotoxicity and functional variants of the SLC28A3 gene, as well as SLC28A1 and the adenosine triphosphate-binding cassette transporters ABCB1, ABCB4, and ABCC1, for a total of 4 risk and 5 protective variants.[108] When used in a multimarker model, patients in the high-risk group had a 38% chance of manifesting cardiac toxicity in the first year of treatment and an 80% chance of developing cardiac toxicity over time, whereas in the low risk group, the lifetime risk was less than 10% (**Fig. 6**).

The value of pharmacogenomics has also been demonstrated clearly when analyzing ADRs to codeine, in which common variants of CYP2D6 and UDP-glucuronosyltransferase can result in fatal toxicity in breast-fed infants as well as in children after tonsillectomy.[113–115] These data have generated considerable interest and have changed both clinical practice and public policy.[116]

While it is likely that there will be an important and growing role for pharmacogenomic testing as part of strategies to diagnose, and hopefully prevent, serious ADRs, it remains unclear presently who should be tested for what, how to deal with the information obtained, and how to best use these findings as part of public policy and clinical practice. This shows the need for clear and evidence-based guidelines for health care practitioners, many of whom are not currently adequately trained in the interpretation and use of pharmacogenomic testing.[101,117]

THERAPY FOR SERIOUS ADRS

While therapy for ADRs is primarily supportive in nature, there is emerging evidence that immunomodulation may be a useful strategy to reduce the severity of drug hypersensitivity.[28] With little evidence to guide clinicians as to the type and intensity of immunomodulation, emerging networks and collaborations, often international, have begun to define what might constitute safe and effective interventions for drug hypersensitivity.[48,118,119]

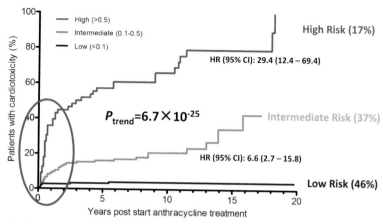

Fig. 6. Kaplan-Meier curve for the risk of anthracycline-induced cardiac toxicity among high-, intermediate-, and low-risk groups; risk groups were defined by a multimarker model with 4 risk and 5 protective genes; risk is maximal in the first year but progressively rises thereafter. (*Data from* Visscher H, Ross CJ, Rassekh SR, et al. Pharmacogenomic prediction of anthracycline-induced cardiotoxicity in children. J Clin Onc 2012;30:1422–8.)

THE UNDISCOVERED COUNTRY

Shakespeare defined the future as the undiscovered country, and in the case of ADRs in children, there remains much to be discovered. It is clear that ADRs are a major problem in the care of children, and that the approach to these is primarily clinical. Recent developments in the characterization assessment and therapy of common and serious ADRs are likely to change the approach to ADRs in children, notably for special populations such as premature neonates and children with cancer. These developments should bring child health care practitioners closer to the shared goal of safe and effective drug therapy for children.

REFERENCES

1. Thomas L. The youngest science: notes of a medicine-watcher. New York: Viking Press; 1983.
2. Aronson JK. An account of the foxglove and its medical uses 1785-1985. New York: Oxford University Press; 1986.
3. Weinshilboum RM. The therapeutic revolution. Clin Pharmacol Ther 1987;42: 481–4.
4. Domagk GJ. Ein Beitrag zur Chemotherapie der bakteriellen infektionen. Dtsch Med Wochenschr 1935;61:250–3 [in German].
5. Fleming A. On the antibacterial action of cultures of a penicillium, with special reference to their use in the isolation of B. influenzae. Br J Exp Pathol 1929; 10:3–13.
6. Zaffiri L, Gardner J, Toledo-Pereyra LH. History of antibiotics. From salvarsan to cephalosporins. J Invest Surg 2012;25:67–77.
7. Choonara I, Rieder MJ. Drug toxicity and adverse drug reactions in children— a brief historical review. Paed Perinatal Drug Therapy 2002;5:12–8.
8. Rieder MJ. If children ruled the pharmaceutical industry. Drug News Perspect 2010;23:1–8.

9. Wax PM. Elixirs, diluents, and the passage of the 1938 Federal Food, Drug and Cosmetic Act. Ann Intern Med 1995;122:456–61.
10. Nebeker JR, Barach P, Samore MH. Clarifying adverse drug events: a clinician's guide toterminology, documentation, and reporting. Ann Intern Med 2004;140: 795–801.
11. Bates DW, Leape LL, Petrycki S. Incidence and preventability of adverse drug events in hospitalized adults. J Gen Intern Med 1993;8:289–94.
12. Kaushal R, Bates DW, Landrigan C, et al. Medication errors and adverse drug events in pediatric inpatients. JAMA 2001;285:2114–20.
13. Edwards IR, Aronson JK. Adverse drug reactions: definitions, diagnosis, and management. Lancet 2000;356:1255–9.
14. Lazarou J, Pomeranz BH, Corey PN. Incidence of adverse drug reactions in hospitalized patients: a meta-analysis of prospective studies. JAMA 1998;279:1200–5.
15. Impicciatore P, Choonara I, Clarkson A, et al. Incidence of adverse drug reactions in paediatric in/out-patients: a systematic review and meta-analysis of prospective studies. Br J Clin Pharmacol 2001;52:77–83.
16. White TJ, Arakelian A, Rho JP. Counting the costs of drug-related adverse events. Pharmacoeconomics 1999;15:445–58.
17. Khaled LA, Ahmad F, Brogan T, et al. Prescription drug use by one million Canadian children. Paediatr Child Health 2003;8(Suppl A):6A–56A.
18. Kearns GL, Abdel-Rahman SM, Alander SW, et al. Developmental pharmacology–drug disposition, action, and therapy in infants and children. N Engl J Med 2003;349:1157–67.
19. Chitturi S, George J. Hepatotoxicity of commonly used drugs: nonsteroidal anti-inflammatory drugs, antihypertensives, antidiabetic agents, anticonvulsants, lipid-lowering agents, psychotropic drugs. Semin Liver Dis 2002;22:169–83.
20. Hirsch LJ, Weintraub DB, Buchsbaum R, et al. Predictors of Lamotrigine-associated rash. Epilepsia 2006;47:318–22.
21. Kearns GL, Wheeler JG, Rieder MJ, et al. Serum sickness-like reaction to cefaclor: lack of in vitro cross-reactivity with loracarbef. Clin Pharmacol Ther 1998; 63:686–93.
22. Chen N, Aleksa K, Woodland C, et al. Ontogeny of drug elimination by the human kidney. Pediatr Nephrol 2006;21:160–8.
23. Ligi I, Arnaud F, Jouve E, et al. Iatrogenic events in admitted neonates: a prospective cohort study. Lancet 2008;371:404–10.
24. Glover ML, Sussmane JB. Assessing pediatrics residents' mathematical skills for prescribing medication: a need for improved training. Acad Med 2002;77: 1007–10.
25. Koren G, Haslam RH. Pediatric medication errors: predicting and preventing tenfold disasters. J Clin Pharmacol 1994;34:1043–5.
26. Kozer E, Scolnik D, Jarvis AD, et al. The effect of detection approaches on the reported incidence of tenfold errors. Drug Saf 2006;29:169–74.
27. Clavenna A, Bonatti M. Adverse drug reactions in childhood: a review of prospective Studies and safety alerts. Arch Dis Child 2009;94:724–8.
28. Rieder MJ. Immune mediation of hypersensitivity adverse drug reactions: implications for therapy. Expert Opin Drug Saf 2009;8:331–43.
29. Aagaard L, Christensen A, Hansen EH. Information about adverse drug reactions reported in children: a qualitative review of empirical studies. Br J Clin Pharmacol 2010;70:481–91.
30. Rosoff PM. The two-edged sword of curing childhood cancer. N Engl J Med 2006;355:1522–3.

31. Agarwal S, Classen D, Larsen G, et al. Prevalence of adverse events in pediatric ICUs in the United States. Pediatr Crit Care Med 2010;11:568–78.

32. Rieder M. If children ruled the pharmaceutical industry: the need for pediatric formulations. Drug News Perspect 2010;23:458–64.

33. Paolucci P, Jones KP, del Carmen Cano Garcinuno M, et al. Challenges in prescribing drugs for children with cancer. Lancet Oncol 2008;9:176–83.

34. Rieder MJ, Carleton B. Mechanisms of adverse drug reactions in children. In: Yaffe SJ, Aranda JV, editors. Neonatal and pediatric pharmacology. 4th edition. Philadelphia: Lippincott Williams & Wilkins; 2010. p. 896–904.

35. Grant LM, Rockey DC. Drug-induced liver injury. Curr Opin Gastroenterol 2012; 28:198–202.

36. Chang C, Mahmood MM, Teuber SS, et al. Overview of penicillin allergy. Clin Rev Allergy Immunol 2011. [Epub ahead of print].

37. Lagace-Wiens P, Rubinstein E. Adverse reactions to beta-lactam antibiotics. Expert Opin Drug Saf 2012;11:381–99.

38. Paradia PM, Nguyen M, Begin P, et al. Outpatient penicillin use after negative skin testing and drug challenge in a pediatric population. Allergy Asthma Proc 2012;33(2):160–4.

39. Thyssen JP, Menne T, Elberling J, et al. Hypersensitivity to local anaesthetics—update and proposal of evaluation algorithm. Contact Derm 2008;59:69–78.

40. Warrington R, Silviu-Dan F. Drug allergy. Allergy Asthma Clin Immunol 2011; 10:S10.

41. Elzagallaai AA, Knowles SR, Rieder MJ, et al. Patch testing for the diagnosis of anticonvulsant hypersensitivity syndrome: a systematic review. Drug Saf 2009; 35:391–408.

42. Soliday FK, Conley YP, Henker R. Pseudocholinesterase deficiency: a comprehensive review of genetic, acquired and drug influences. AANA J 2010;78: 313–20.

43. Macedo AF, Marques FB, Ribeiro CF, et al. Causality assessment of adverse drug reactions: comparison of the results obtained from published decisional algorithms and from the evaluations of an expert panel. Pharmacoepidemiol Drug Saf 2005;14:885–90.

44. Arimone Y, Begaud B, Miremont-Salame G, et al. Agreement of expert judgment in causality assessment of adverse drug reactions. Eur J Clin Pharmacol 2005; 61:169–73.

45. Naranjo CA, Busto U, Sellers EM, et al. A method for estimating the probability of adverse drug reactions. Clin Pharmacol Ther 1981;30:239–45.

46. Buchmiller BL, Khan DA. Evaluation and management of pediatric drug allergy reactions. Curr Allergy Asthma Rep 2007;7:402–9.

47. Sheikh A, Shehata YA, Brown SG, et al. Adrenaline (epinephrine) for the treatment of anaphylaxis with and without shock. Cochrane Database Syst Rev 2008;(8):CD006312.

48. Del Pozzo-Magana B, Lazo-Langner A, Carleton B, et al. A systematic review of treatment of drug-induced Stevens-Johnson syndrome and toxic epidermal necrolysis in children. J Popul Ther Clin Pharmacol 2011;18:e121–33.

49. Loebstein R, Koren G. Ifosfamide-induced nephrotoxicity in children: critical review of predictive risk factors. Pediatrician 1998;101:E8.

50. Coradini PP, Cigana L, Selistre SG, et al. Ototoxicityfrom cisplatin therapy in childhood cancer. J Pediatr Hematol Oncol 2007;29:355–60.

51. Lipshultz SE, Alvarez JA, Scully RE. Anthracycline associated cardiotoxicity in survivors of childhood cancer. Heart 2008;94:525–33.

52. Fernandez-Llamazares CM, Calleja-Hernández MA, Manrique-Rodríguez S, et al. Prescribing errors intercepted by clinical pharmacists in paediatrics and obstetrics in a tertiary hospital in Spain. Eur J Clin Pharmacol 2012. [Epub ahead of print].

53. Ligi I, Millet V, Sartor C, et al. Iatrogenic events in neonates: beneficial effects of prevention strategies and continuous monitoring. Pediatrician 2010;126(6): e1461–8.

54. Kramer MS, Leventhal JM, Hutchinson TA, et al. An algorithm for the operational assessment of adverse drug reactions. I. Background, description, and instructions for use. JAMA 1979;242:623–32.

55. Maria VA, Victorino RM. Development and validation of a clinical scale for the diagnosis of drug-induced hepatitis. Hepatology 1997;26:664–9.

56. Du W, Tutag Lehr V, Lieh-Lai M, et al. An algorithm to detect adverse drug reactions in the neonatal intensive care unit: a new approach. J Clin Pharmacol 2012. Available at: http://jcp.sagepub.com/content/early/2012/01/17/0091270011433327.

57. Gallagher RM, Kirkham JJ, Mason JR, et al. Development and inter-rater reliability of the liverpool adverse drug reaction causality assessment tool. PLoS One 2011;6:e28096.

58. Elzagallaai AA, Koren G, Bend JR, et al. In vitro testing for hypersensitivity-mediated adverse drug reactions: challenges and future directions. Clin Pharmacol Ther 2011;90:455–60.

59. Uetrecht J. Idiosyncratic drug reactions: current understanding. Annu Rev Pharmacol Toxicol 2007;47:513–39.

60. Park BK, Coleman JW, Kitteringham NR. Drug disposition and drug hypersensitivity. Biochem Pharmacol 1987;36:581–90.

61. Posadas SJ, Pichler WJ. Delayed drug hypersensitivity reactions – new concepts. Clin Exp Allergy 2007;37:989–99.

62. Pichler W, Beeler A, Keeller M, et al. Pharmacological interaction of drugs with immune receptors with immune receptors: the p-i concept. Allergol Int 2006; 55(1):17–25.

63. Zhang X, Liu F, Chen X, et al. Involvement of the immune system in idiosyncratic drug reactions. Drug Metab Pharmacokinet 2011;26:47–59.

64. Mayorga C, Sanz ML, Gamboa PM, et al. In vitro diagnosis of immediate allergic reactions to drugs: an update. J Investig Allergol Clin Immunol 2010;20:103–9.

65. Sanz ML, Gamboa P, de Weck AL. A new combined test with flow cytometric basophil activation and determination of sulfidoleukotrienes is useful for in vitro diagnosis of hypersensitivity to aspirin and other nonsteroidal anti-inflammatory drugs. Int Arch Allergy Immunol 2005;136(1):58–72.

66. De Weck AL, Sanz ML, Gamboa PM, et al. Nonsteroidal anti-inflammatory drug hypersensitivity syndrome. A multicenter study. I. Clinical findings and in vitro diagnosis. J Investig Allergol Clin Immunol 2009;19:355–69.

67. Abuaf N, Rajoely B, Ghazouani E, et al. Validation of a flow cytometric assay detecting in vitro basophil activation for the diagnosis of muscle relaxant allergy. J Allergy Clin Immunol 1999;104(2 Pt 1):411–8.

68. Torres MJ, Padial A, Mayorga C, et al. The diagnostic interpretation of basophil activation test in immediate allergic reactions to beta lactams. Clin Exp Allergy 2004;34:1768–75.

69. Elzagallaai AA, Knowles SR, Rieder MJ, et al. In vitro testing for the diagnosis of anticonvulsant hypersensitivity syndrome: a systematic review. Mol Diagn Ther 2009;13:313–30.

70. Pichler WJ, Tilch J. The lymphocyte transformation test in the diagnosis of drug hypersensitivity. Allergy 2004;59:809–20.

71. Kano Y, Hirahara K, Mitsuyama Y, et al. Utility of the lymphocyte transformation test in the diagnosis of drug sensitivity: dependence on its timing and the type of drug eruption. Allergy 2007;62:1439–44.

72. Beeler A, Engler O, Gerber BO, et al. Long-lasting reactivity and high frequency of drug specific T cells after severe systemic drug hypersensitivity reactions. J Allergy Clin Immunol 2006;117:45–62.

73. Matsuno O, Okubo T, Hiroshige S, et al. Drug-induced lymphocyte stimulation test is not useful for the diagnosis of drug-induced pneumonia. Tohoku J Exp Med 2007;212:49–53.

74. Mantani N, Kogure T, Tamura J, et al. Lymphocyte transformation test for medicinal herbs yields false-positive results for first-visit patients. Clin Diagn Lab Immunol 2003;10:479–80.

75. Sachs B, Erdmann S, Al-Masaoudi T, et al. In vitro drug allergy detection system incorporating human liver microsomes in chlorazepate-induced skin rash: drug-specific proliferation associated with interleukin-5 secretion. Br J Dermatol 2001; 114:316–20.

76. Merk MF. Diagnosis of drug hypersensitivity: lymphocyte transformation test and cytokines. Toxicology 2005;209:217–20.

77. Abe R, Shimizu T, Shibaki A, et al. Toxic epidermal necrolysis and Stevens-Johnson syndrome are induced by soluble Fas ligand. Am J Pathol 2003;162: 1515–20.

78. Chung WH, Hung SI, Yang JY, et al. Granulysin is a key mediator for disseminated keratinocyte death in Stevens-Johnson syndrome and toxic epidermal necrolysis. Nat Med 2008;14:1343.

79. Shear NH, Spielberg SP. Anticonvulsant hypersensitivity syndrome. In vitro assessment of risk. J Clin Invest 1988;82(6):1826–32.

80. Spielberg SP, Gordon GB, Blake DA, et al. Predisposition to phenytoin hepatotoxicity assessed in vitro. N Engl J Med 1981;305:722–7.

81. Rieder MJ, Uetrecht J, Shear NH, et al. Diagnosis of sulfonamide hypersensitivity reactions by in-vitro "rechallenge" with hydroxylamine metabolites. Ann Intern Med 1989;110:286–9.

82. Rieder MJ, Krause R, Bird IA, et al. Toxicity of sulfonamide-reactive metabolites in HIV-infected, HTLV-infected and noninfected cells. J Acquir Immune Defic Syndr Hum Retrovirol 1995;8:134–40.

83. Tschen A, Rieder MJ, Oyewumi K, et al. The cytotoxicity of clozapine metabolites: implications for predicting clozapine-induced agranulocytosis. Clin Pharmacol Ther 1999;65:526–32.

84. Manchanda T, Hess D, Dale L, et al. Haptenation of sulfonamide reactive metabolites to cellular proteins. Mol Pharmacol 2002;62:1011–26.

85. Arp J, Rieder MJ, Urquhart B, et al. Hypersensitivity of HIV-1 infected cells to reactive sulfonamide metabolites correlated to expression of the HIV-1 viral protein tat. J Pharmacol Exp Ther 2005;314:1218–25.

86. Elzagallaai B, Garcia-Bournissen F, Finkelstein Y, et al. Severe bullous hypersensitivity reactions after exposure to carbamazepine in a Han Chinese child with a positive HLA-B*1502 and a negative lymphocyte toxicity assay: evidence for different pathophysiological mechanisms. J Popul Ther Clin Pharmacol 2011;18(1):e1–9.

87. Elzagallaai AA, Jahedmotlagh Z, Del Pozzo-Magana BR, et al. Predictive value of the lymphocyte toxicity assay in the diagnosis of drug hypersensitivity syndrome. Mol Diagn Ther 2010;14:317–22.

88. Rieder MJ, Uetrecht J, Shear NH, et al. Synthesis and in vitro toxicity of hydroxylamine metabolites of sulphonamides. J Pharmacol Exp Ther 1988;244:724–8.

89. White J. Platelet structure. In: Michelson A, editor. Platelets. Burlington (MA): AcademicPress; 2007. p. 45–74.

90. McNicol A. Platelet preparation and estimation of functional responses. In: Watson S, Authi K, editors. Platelets. Oxford (United Kingdom): Oxford University Press; 1996. p. 1–26.

91. Capron A, Joseph M, Ameisen JC, et al. Platelets as effectors in immune and hypersensitivity reactions. Int Arch Allergy Appl Immunol 1987;82:307–12.

92. Pitchford SC. Defining a role for platelets in allergic inflammation. Biochem Soc Trans 2007;35:1104–8.

93. Pitchford SC, Yano H, Lever R, et al. Platelets are essential for leukocyte recruitment in allergic inflammation. J Allergy Clin Immunol 2003;112:109–18.

94. Elzagallaai A, Rieder M, Koren G. In vitro platelet toxicity assay (iPTA): a novel diagnostic test for drug hypersensitivity syndrome. J Clin Pharmacol 2011;51: 428–35.

95. Anderson BJ. My child is unique; the pharmacokinetics are universal. Paediatr Anaesth 2012;10.

96. Becker ML, Leeder JS. Identifying genomic and developmental causes of adverse drug reactions in children. Pharmacogenomics 2010;11:1591–602.

97. Lennard L, Lilleyman JS, Van LJ, et al. Genetic variation in response to 6-mercaptopurine for childhood acute lymphoblastic leukaemia. Lancet 1990; 336:225–9.

98. Cheok MH, Evans WE. Acute lymphoblastic leukaemia: a model for the pharmacogenomics of cancer therapy. Nat Rev Cancer 2006;6:117–29.

99. Ujiie S, Sasaki T, Mizugaki M, et al. Functional characterization of 23 allelic variants of thiopurine S-methyltransferase gene (TPMT*2–*24). Pharmacogenet Genomics 2008;18:887–93.

100. Donnan JR, Unger WH, Mathews M, et al. A cost effectiveness analysis of thiopurine methyltransferase testing for guiding 6-mercaptopurine dosing in children with acute lymphoblastic leukemia. Pediatr Blood Cancer 2011;57: 231–9.

101. Russo R, Capasso M, Paolucci P, et al. Pediatric pharmacogenetic and pharmacogenomic studies: the current state and future perspectives. Eur J Clin Pharmacol 2011;67(Suppl 1):17–27.

102. Martin MA, Klein TE, Dong BJ, et al. Clinical pharmacogenetics implementation consortium guidelines for HLA-B genotype and abacavir dosing. Clin Pharmacol Ther 2012;91:734–8.

103. Gong IY, Tirona RG, Schwarz UI, et al. Prospective evaluation of a pharmacogenetics-guided warfarin loading and maintenance dose regimen for initiation of therapy. Blood 2011;118:3163–71.

104. VanderVaart S, Berger H, Sistonen J, et al. CYP2D6 polymorphisms and codeine analgesia in postpartum pain management: a pilot study. Ther Drug Monit 2011;33:425–32.

105. Loo TT, Ross CJ, Sistonen J, et al. Pharmacogenomics and active surveillance for serious adverse drug reactions in children. Pharmacogenomics 2010;11: 1269–85.

106. Ross CJ, Visscher H, Rassekh SR, et al. Pharmacogenomics of serious adverse drug reactions in pediatric oncology. J Popul Ther Clin Pharmacol 2011;18: e134–51.

107. Ross C, Katzov-Eckert H, Dube MP, et al. TPMT and COMT genetic variants are predictive for severe hearing loss in children receiving cisplatin chemotherapy. Nat Genet 2009;41:1345–9.

108. Visscher H, Ross CJ, Rassekh SR, et al. Genetic determinants of anthracycline cardiotoxicity in children. J Clin Oncol 2012;30:1422–8.

109. Li Y, Womer RB, Silber JH. Predicting cisplatin ototoxicity in children: the influence of age and the cumulative dose. Eur J Cancer 2004;40:2445–51.

110. Rybak LP, Whitworth CA, Mukherjea D, et al. Mechanisms of cisplatin-induced ototoxicity and prevention. Hear Res 2007;226:157–67.

111. Dionne F, Mitton C, Rassekh R, et al. Economic impact of a genetic test for cisplatin induced ototoxicity. Pharmacogenomics J 2011;12(4):1–9.

112. Kremer LC, van Dalen EC, Offringa M, et al. Frequency and risk factors of anthracycline induced clinical heart failure in children: a systematic review. Ann Oncol 2002;13(4):503–12.

113. Koren G, Cairns J, Chitayat D, et al. Pharmacogenetics of morphine poisoning in a breastfed neonate of a codeine-prescribed mother. Lancet 2006;368:704.

114. Sistonen J, Madadi P, Ross CJ, et al. Prediction of codeine toxicity in infants and their mothers using a novel combination of maternal genetic markers. Clin Pharmacol Ther 2012;91:692–9.

115. Kelly LE, Rieder M, van den Anker J, et al. More codeine fatalities in North American children. Pediatrics 2012;129(5):e1343–7.

116. Pat Clarke, FDA's Center for Drug Evaluation and Research, Codeine Side-Effects in Nursing Infants. Available at: http://www.fda.gov/Drugs/DrugSafety/PostmarketDrugSafetyInformationforPatientsandProviders/ucm124889.htm. Accessed August 9, 2012.

117. Amstutz U, Carleton BC. Pharmacogenetic testing: time for clinical practice guidelines. Clin Pharmacol Ther 2011;89:924–7.

118. Romano A, Torres MJ, Castells M, et al. Diagnosis and management of drug hypersensitivity reactions. J Allergy Clin Immunol 2011;127(Suppl 3):S67–73.

119. Hanly LN, Chen N, Aleksa K, et al. N-acetylcysteine as a novel prophylactic treatment for ifosfamide-induced nephrotoxicity in children: translational pharmacokinetics. J Clin Pharmacol 2012;52(1):55–64.

Pharmacotherapy of Pediatric HIV Infection

Natella Rakhmanina, MD, PhD, AAHIVS[a,b,]*,
B. Ryan Phelps, MD, MPH, AAHIVS[a,c]

KEYWORDS

- HIV • AIDS • Antiretroviral drugs • Children • Adolescents

KEY POINTS

- Human immunodeficiency virus (HIV) infection represents one of the most serious pediatric morbidities in the world, with an estimated 3.4 million children infected with HIV globally.
- Important etiologic, physiologic, psychological, and social differences between children and adults create unique consideration for antiretroviral therapy in pediatric patients.
- Antiretroviral therapy significantly decreases HIV-associated morbidity and mortality, assures normal growth and development, and improves survival and quality of life in children and adolescents.
- Limited data on the long-term effects of antiretroviral drugs exposure in utero, infancy, and throughout childhood warrants further investigation.
- With only 23% of children infected with HIV having access to antiretroviral therapy, the development and delivery of pediatric antiretroviral formulations needs to continue.

INTRODUCTION

Human immunodeficiency virus (HIV) infection represents one of the most serious pediatric diseases globally, with an estimated 3.4 million children living with HIV on our planet.[1] The majority of HIV infection among children are acquired through mother-to-child transmission (MTCT) of the virus from women with HIV during pregnancy, delivery, and breastfeeding. In 1990, the landmark Pediatric AIDS Clinical Trials

The views and opinions expressed in the article are solely those of the authors and do not necessarily reflect those of the US Agency for International Development nor those of the US Government.

[a] Division of Infectious Diseases, Children's National Medical Center, Washington, DC, USA;
[b] Department of Pediatrics, The George Washington University School of Medicine and Health Sciences, Washington, DC, USA; [c] USAID Office of HIV/AIDS, Washington, DC, USA
* Corresponding author. Special Immunology Program, Children's National Medical Center, 3.5 West, 111 Michigan Avenue Northwest, Washington, DC 20010.
E-mail address: nrakhman@cnmc.org

Pediatr Clin N Am 59 (2012) 1093–1115
http://dx.doi.org/10.1016/j.pcl.2012.07.009
0031-3955/12/$ – see front matter © 2012 Elsevier Inc. All rights reserved.

Group 076 study demonstrated that the antiretroviral (ARV) drug zidovudine (AZT) administered to the mother and infant around delivery significantly reduced MTCT.[2] Since then, the use of antiretroviral therapy (ART) during pregnancy, delivery, and postpartum has become the widespread method of the prevention of MTCT (PMTCT). Such unique and unprecedented pharmacologic intervention has been shown to be highly efficient by decreasing the natural rates of MTCT from 30% to 40% to less than 2%.[3,4]

Currently available ART uses 5 major classes of ARV drugs: nucleoside/nucleotide analogue reverse transcriptase inhibitors (NRTIs/NtRTIs), non-nucleoside reverse transcriptase inhibitors (NNRTIs), protease inhibitors (PIs), entry and fusion inhibitors, and integrase inhibitors. The combination ART, also defined as highly active ART, is comprised of 3 ARV drugs from at least 2 major classes to achieve maximal suppression of HIV replication and preservation of immune function affected by HIV disease.[5] Another major benefit of ART is its capacity to reduce the transmission of the virus from one person to another, including the prevention of vertical transmission of HIV from the infected mother to her fetus, newborn child, and infant.[5,6]

In the countries with guaranteed access to ARV drugs, the number of perinatally acquired pediatric HIV infections is very low and is limited to cases of missed opportunities for the timely identification of HIV, lack of prenatal care, and poor adherence to ARV prophylaxis.[7] In resource-limited settings, which are most heavily affected by the HIV epidemic, the major barriers to effective PMTCT are the lack of adequate prenatal care, lack of HIV testing, limited access to ART, and the need for continued breastfeeding to assure infant's survival. Despite ongoing efforts to guarantee universal access to PMTCT in the world, the World Health Organization (WHO) reports that approximately half (48% [44%–54%]) of pregnant women living with HIV currently receive ARV prophylaxis for MTCT.[8] Because of the limited access to universal diagnostics and PMTCT, the WHO estimates that 1000 children continue to be infected with HIV each day, with most new cases (97%) occurring in middle- and low-income countries.[1,9] In addition to perinatally infected children, approximately 2520 new HIV infections per day occur through horizontal transmission in adolescents who are 15 to 24 years of age, with almost half (48%) of the cases among adolescent girls, creating the potential for continued MTCT.[10]

With the ongoing epidemic of pediatric HIV infection in the world, the delivery of efficient ART to children and adolescents is crucial to saving and improving the lives of millions of children worldwide. Per WHO estimates, without therapeutic intervention approximately one-third of the infected infants will die by 1 year of age and about half will die by 2 years of age.[3] ART has been demonstrated to significantly decrease HIV-associated morbidity and mortality, assure normal growth and development, and improve survival and quality of life in children and adolescents.[11–13]

Following the adult ART development, the treatment of pediatric HIV infection has evolved from monotherapy with AZT to dual therapy with NRTIs and subsequently to multi-drug therapy involving a combination of 3 or more ARV drugs.[14] The pathogenesis and the general virologic and immunologic principles of HIV generates an infectious inflammatory process that is similar in adults and children infected with HIV. However, the important etiologic, physiologic, psychological, and social differences between children and adults create a unique consideration for ART in pediatric patients.

Early initiation of ART in children allows achieving maximal suppression of HIV replication, to preserve immunologic function, and to prevent disease progression while allowing for normal growth and development. The immunologic outcome (activation and suppression of the CD4+ cell count) of HIV infection is closely related to the child's development and creates age-specific parameters for the evaluation of therapeutic response to ART in pediatric HIV disease. In addition to the changes in immunologic response to the HIV infection, the development and maturation of organ systems involved in drug absorption, distribution, metabolism, and elimination determine significant changes in the pharmacokinetics (PK) of ARV drugs throughout childhood. As a child grows and matures, ART transforms from the administration of small amounts of liquid preparations to tablet formulations of coformulated ARV drugs. In this article, the authors review the evolution of ART throughout childhood from early infancy into adolescence.

PERINATAL EXPOSURE TO ART
ART During Pregnancy and Delivery

ART during pregnancy can be used for the purpose of maternal therapy and/or PMTCT. When a woman infected with HIV meets the standard treatment initiation criteria for her disease, ART is used for both maternal therapeutic and neonatal prophylactic purposes. When there are no indications for treatment initiation, ART in pregnancy is used solely for the purpose of PMTCT. The use of ART during delivery is based solely on the purpose of PMTCT.

To achieve a high level of PMTCT in utero, ARV drugs need to cross the placenta and produce adequate systemic drug levels in unborn infants. Pregnancy affects the disposition of ART through physiologic changes affecting absorption, biotransformation, and elimination of ARV drugs.[15–19] In addition, placental transport, compartmentalization, biotransformation, and elimination of ARV drugs in the embryo, fetus, and placenta can all affect the PK of ARV drugs in the mother and child.

Current data indicate that despite some changes in the PK parameters of the NRTIs and NNRTIs during pregnancy, overall exposure to these classes of medications is similar between pregnant and non-pregnant women, and a dose change is not warranted for these ARV drugs. The effect of pregnancy on the already highly variable PK parameters of the PIs appears to be more significant. Reports of decreased PIs exposure during the third trimester of pregnancy when compared with non-pregnancy stage warrants dose adjustment (increase) considerations during the last trimester of pregnancy for lopinavir (LPV) and atazanavir (ATV) in combination with a standard dose of boosting ritonavir (RTV).[6,20]

In developed countries, 3-drug ART throughout pregnancy followed by intrapartum intravenous AZT is considered the standard of care for PMTCT. In case a woman does not require ART for her HIV disease, delayed initiation of ART at the end of the first trimester of the pregnancy can be recommended, although earlier initiation can be considered. Maintaining adequate levels of ARV exposure in infants becomes more important during delivery when infants come in close contact with the maternal genital tract virus during the birth process. With chronic ART use during pregnancy, the exposure to ARV drugs is at a steady state at the time of delivery. If initial ARV doses are administered during labor, several PK parameters (clearance, plasma elimination half-life) are increased, whereas the area under the time versus concentration curve and peak concentration are decreased.[21] The choice of intravenous AZT is based on the ability to achieve high plasma, cord blood, and genital fluid concentrations of the ARV drug during delivery.[22]

Because of the cost and storage requirement considerations, a full schedule of prenatal PMTCT (prenatal ART starting at the end of the first trimester plus intravenous AZT during delivery) is largely limited to developed-world settings. More practical (eg, oral drugs only), less intensive, less expensive, and shorter-duration ART regimens have been designed for the PMTCT in resource-limited settings and include the following schemes:

- Mono or dual ART with AZT and lamivudine (3TC) starting at 28 to 36 weeks gestation, triple ART with AZT/3TC plus abacavir (ABC), nevirapine (NVP), nelfinavir (NFV), or LPV/RTV starting at 26 to 34 weeks gestation
- Single-dose NVP (sdNVP) intrapartum in combination with an antepartum course of AZT plus 3TC
- sdNVP plus oral AZT plus oral 3TC intrapartum
- sdNVP intrapartum without additional ART (no longer considered the most optimal approach for PMTCT)

The choice of sdNVP administered to the mother during labor is based on the rapid absorption and distribution of NVP in adults, high penetration of the drug to the umbilical cord blood (80%), prolonged NVP elimination half-life, affordable costs, and high heat resistance.[23–25]

Multiple studies with these ARV regimens conducted through international networks in diverse settings around the globe have clearly shown that the combination ART is more efficient in assuring higher levels of PMTCT than mono and dual ARV drug combinations.[6,26] Equally, the 3-component ART (antepartum, intrapartum, and postpartum in neonates) has been shown to be superior to alternative regimens which choice has been primarily dictated by cost and availability considerations in resource-limited settings.

Monitoring of Perinatal ARV Exposure

As with any pharmacologic exposure in utero, there is a concern for the short- and long-term consequences of transplacental and vaginal ARV drug exposure. Despite more than 20 years of using ART for PMTCT, data on the effect of ART on the fetus remain limited.

Long-term controversy surrounds the potential harmful effect of in utero NRTIs exposure on the mitochondrial function in neonates and children. Through the process of binding to the mitochondrial gamma DNA polymerase, NRTIs (particularly didanosine [ddI] and stavudine [d4T]) are capable of interfering with mitochondrial replication resulting in mitochondrial DNA depletion and dysfunction.[27] Clinical symptoms of mitochondrial toxicity in newborns associated with in utero NRTIs exposure, including severe (rarely fatal) neurologic, muscular, and cardiac disease and hyperlactatemia, were reported in a large cohort of French children.[28,29] The observation of several other large prospective cohorts of perinatally NRTIs-exposed children from the United States and Europe did not find a similar association.[30–32] A potential effect of genetic predisposition has been suggested to play a role in the cause of mitochondrial toxicity following exposure to NRTIs in utero. A thorough evaluation for mitochondrial toxicity is recommended for any newborn and infant with an unclear cause of neurologic, cardiac, and systemic disorders.[6]

Animal teratogenic data and case reports of central nervous system abnormalities have raised concerns for using the first-generation NNRTI efavirenz (EFV) during pregnancy (particularly during the first trimester).[33] Although recent data in humans have reported no increased risk of birth defects in children born with in utero EFV exposure, the drug remains classified as Food and Drug Administration (FDA) pregnancy category D; the use of alternative regimens, when possible, is recommended.[6] However, when potential benefits are considered to outweigh potential risks, as in the case of the resource-limited settings without widespread access to the PIs, the use of the category D drugs (such as EFV) in pregnant women is considered permissible. Because of possible risks of ART exposure in pregnancy, the most recent version of the US perinatal treatment and prophylaxis guidelines recommend repeat (second trimester) ultrasound evaluation of fetal abnormality to women with a history of ART use (particularly to EFV) during the first trimester.[6]

In the United States and Europe, the most commonly used ART during pregnancy is comprised of 2 NRTIs in combination with an RTV-boosted PI, such as ATV and LPV. A small increase in the risk of prematurity has been reported in women infected with HIV on PI-based ART during pregnancy. However, the benefits of PMTCT and the clinical usefulness of a PI-based ART (lack of hepatotoxicity and CD4+ cell count considerations associated with NVP) currently seem to outweigh the risks of prematurity. Among other considerations of PIs exposure, there is also a recent report from France linking in utero and postnatal LPV/RTV exposure to transient neonatal adrenal dysfunction.[34]

The accumulation of data on the use of newer classes of ARV drugs in pregnancy, such as entry and fusion inhibitors, may make the pendulum swing toward the preferred choice of such agents as raltegravir (RAL) and maraviroc (MVC) for future considerations of ART in the prenatal period.

To collect human data on the potential risks of ART exposure in infants and their mothers, a collaborative epidemiologic project (Antiretroviral Pregnancy Registry available at http://www.APRegistry.com) was created in collaboration with pharmaceutical manufactures with advisory committees of pediatricians and obstetricians. This anonymous, observational database is open for the reporting of any nonexperimental adverse events of perinatal ARV exposure by health providers providing care to women infected with HIV and their children. Close long-term follow-up throughout all stages of growth and development is recommended for children with a history of in utero ART exposure.

NEONATAL ARV PROPHYLAXIS AND THERAPY
Neonatal ARV Prophylaxis

In addition to complete elimination of breastfeeding, 6 weeks of neonatal AZT prophylaxis started immediately (within 6–12 hours) postpartum is recommended for PMTCT by the perinatal ART guidelines in the United States.[6] The ability of AZT to induce transient macrocytic anemia, which can become clinically significant, particularly in premature infants, has raised concerns for the length of the AZT exposure. As a result of these considerations following comparative pediatric studies, a 4-week postpartum neonatal AZT prophylaxis with complete elimination of breastfeeding is now recommended for infants with a history of adequate prenatal and intrapartum ART in Europe and the United Kingdom.[35,36]

As with maternal prophylaxis of MTCT, the use of combination postpartum ART is considered to be more efficient in PMTCT than monotherapy, particularly in high-risk scenarios, such as a lack or inconsistent use of prenatal and/or intrapartum ART, unsuppressed maternal viral load at delivery, and a history of maternal HIV resistance. Although in practice the use of different combinations of ARV drugs in newborns postpartum is widely used for the described scenarios, few studies have prospectively evaluated the use of combination ART in neonates. Most of the studies published to date evaluated the following combinations of ARV drugs in newborns[6,26]:

- AZT plus 3TC
- AZT plus NVP
- AZT plus 3TC plus NVP
- AZT plus 3TC plus NFV

Recent data from a large international trial have shown higher rates of neutropenia and anemia associated with dual (AZT plus 3TC) and triple (AZT plus 3TC plus NFV) ART when compared with AZT monotherapy.[37] In addition, high variability of NFV exposure with the potential for subtherapeutic exposure in newborns has been reported.[37,38] As a result of this study, NFV and 3TC are no longer recommended in the neonatal period in the United States and a dual ART prophylaxis with an addition of 3 doses of NVP (birth to 48 hours, 48 hours, 96 hours postpartum) in the first week of life has been recommended to be considered in cases with a high risk for MTCT.[6] Monotherapy with NVP remains an equitable alternative to AZT neonatal prophylaxis in WHO guidelines.[8]

As described earlier, postnatal ARV prophylaxis is discontinued after 4 to 6 weeks in exclusively formula fed children. Breastfed infants, who represent most newborn children in HIV-epidemic areas in the world, remain at risk for MTCT for the duration of breastfeeding. Because of the multiple economical and logistical obstacles, most importantly the lack of clean water and high infant morbidity and mortality associated with formula feeding, complete elimination of breastfeeding and substitution with exclusive formula feeding has not proven to be a safe or feasible alternative in resource-limited settings.[8,26] With continued breastfeeding, the ongoing need for PMTCT generates consideration for ART in breastfeeding women and their nursing infants.

For resource-limited settings, the WHO recommends daily NVP in infants from birth until 1 week after cessation of all breastfeeding as option A.[26] Under the same option, 4 to 6 weeks of daily NVP is recommended for infants without breastfeeding or those breastfed by women on ART.[8] As option B (including B+), daily AZT or NVP therapy for 4 to 6 weeks is recommended for neonates independent of infant feeding (breastfed or formula fed), whereas triple maternal ART is recommended until 1 week after cessation of all breastfeeding.[8] Because of the availability and cost considerations, an ART regimen with 2 NRTIs (AZT, 3TC, tenofovir disoproxil fumarate [TDF]) in combination with one NNRTI (EFV, NVP) or coformulated boosted PIs (LPV/RTV) are most frequently considered for maternal ART during breastfeeding.[8]

During breastfeeding, maternal ART continues playing a dual role of treating maternal HIV disease and preventing MTCT. The goal of treatment is to maximally suppress the maternal HIV viral load and to significantly diminish the risk of the viral passage through the breast milk. ARV drugs ingested by the infant during breastfeeding may equally provide some protection against HIV acquisition. Because of the low breast milk/plasma ratio and rapid renal elimination, breastfed infants exposed to maternal AZT do not have detectable plasma AZT concentrations. NRTIs (3TC, TDF), NNRTIs (NVP, EFV), and PIs (NFV, indinavir [IDV]), however, have all been detected in breast milk at different ratios with maternal plasma concentrations of lactating women on ART.[39–43] With low penetration of some of these ARV drugs into the breast milk (TDF, EFV, NFV), subtherapeutic infant plasma ARV concentrations may generate the development of viral resistance in infants infected with HIV.[42]

Pharmacokinetics of ARV Drugs in Infants

Compared with older children, neonates and young infants had delayed absorption, reduced liver metabolism, and renal elimination of drugs.[44–48] Rapid changes in renal function occur in the first days of life, making the dosing of ARV in neonates a challenging task. Despite the wide use of ART in noninfected and HIV-infected neonates, the PK data on neonatal ARV exposure and the dosing guidelines are limited to the handful of ARV drugs used for PMTCT: AZT, ddI, d4T, and 3TC for NRTIs, NVP for NNRTIs, and NFV and LPV/RTV for PIs (**Table 1**). For premature infants, AZT is the only drug with available PK and dosing data.[49]

Table 1
Available pediatric dosing and formulations of ARV drugs

Drug (Abbreviation)	FDA Licensed in Children	Age Restriction	Formulations Available	Dosing Regimen in Children and Adolescents Younger than 18 Years Old
NRTIs				
Zidovudine (AZT)	Yes	No	Tablets: 60 mg, 300 mg Capsules: 100 mg, 250 mg Liquid: 10 mg/mL	Twice daily
Stavudine (d4T)	Yes	No	Capsules: 15 mg, 20 mg, 30 mg Liquid: 1 mg/mL	Twice daily
Abacavir (ABC)	Yes	≥3 months	Tablets: 60 mg, 300 mg Liquid: 20 mg/mL	Twice daily[a]
Lamivudine (3TC)	Yes	No	Tablet: 150 mg Liquid: 10 mg/mL	Twice daily[a]
Didanosine (ddI)	Yes	≥2 wk	Chewable tablets: 25 mg, 50 mg, 100 mg, 200 mg Capsules (delayed release): 125 mg, 200 mg, 250 mg, 400 mg Liquid: 10 mg/mL	Twice daily Once-daily delayed-release capsules with weight ≥20 kg
Emcitritabine (FTC)	Yes	No[b]	Capsule: 200 mg Liquid: 10 mg/mL	Twice daily[a]
Tenofovir Disoproxil Fumarate (TDF)	Yes	≥2 y	Tablets: 150 mg, 200 mg, 250 mg, 300 mg Powder: 40 mg/gm	Once daily

(continued on next page)

Table 1
(continued)

Drug (Abbreviation)	FDA Licensed in Children	Age Restriction	Formulations Available	Dosing Regimen in Children and Adolescents Younger than 18 Years Old
NNRTIs				
Efavirenz (EFV)	Yes	≥3 y[c]	Tablets: 200 mg, 600 mg Capsules: 50 mg, 100 mg, 200 mg Liquid: 30 mg/mL	Once daily
Nevirapine (NVP)	Yes	>2 weeks old	Tablets: 50 mg, 100 mg, 200 mg Liquid: 10 mg/mL	Twice daily 400 mg extended-release NVP currently not approved in children
Etravirine (ETV)	Yes	≥6 y and ≥16 kg	Tablets: 25 mg, 100 mg	Twice daily
Protease Inhibitors (PIs)				
Atazanavir (ATV)	Yes	≥6 y[d]	Capsules: 100 mg, 150 mg, 200 mg, 300 mg	Once daily RTV boosting preferred[e]
Darunavir (DRV)	Yes	≥3 y and ≥10 kg	Tablets: 75 mg, 150 mg, 400 mg, 600 mg Liquid: 100 mg/mL	Twice daily Should be boosted with RTV Once-daily dose can be used if therapy naïve and >12 y
Fosamprenavir (FPV)	Yes	≥2 y if therapy naïve and ≥6 y if therapy experienced	Tablet: 700 mg Liquid: 50 mg/mL	Twice daily Should be boosted with RTV if therapy experienced and may be boosted with RTV if therapy naïve[e]
Indinavir (IDV)	No	N/A	Capsules: 100 mg, 200 mg, 400 mg	N/A
Nelfinavir (NFV)	Yes	≥2 y	Tablets: 250 mg, 625 mg Oral powder: 50 mg/gm (50 mg/scoop)	Twice daily

Lopinavir/ritonavir (LPV/r)	Yes	>42 wk gestation and >14 d old	Coformulated tablets with RTV: 100 mg LPV+25 mg RTV 200 mg LPV+50 mg RTV Coformulated capsule with RTV: 133 mg LPV+33 mg RTV Liquid: 80 mg LPV/ml + 20 mg RTV/ml	Twice daily
Ritonavir (RTV)	Yes	No	Coformulated with LPV (see lopinavir) Tablet: 100 mg Liquid: 80 mg/mL	Used to boost other PIs
Saquinavir (SQV)	No	N/A	Tablets: 500 mg Hard gel capsule: 200 mg	N/A
Tipranavir (TPV)	Yes	≥2 y	Capsule: 250 mg Liquid: 100 mg/mL	Twice daily Should be boosted with RTV
Fusion and Entry Inhibitors				
Raltegravir (RAL)	Yes	≥2 y and ≥10 kg	Chewable tablet: 25 mg Tablet: 400 mg	Twice daily
Maraviroc (MVC)	No	N/A	Tablets: 150 mg, 300 mg	N/A
Enfuvirtide (ENF)	Yes	≥6 y	Lyophilized powder for subcutaneous injection: 108 mg/vial (90 mg/mL when reconstituted with water)	Twice daily

Abbreviation: N/A, non applicable.

Information on the drug formulation, dosing, and approval were obtained from the FDA, HHS, and WHO pediatric guidelines.[4,26,107]

a Once-daily dosing not approved, but PK data encouraging.

b Limited PK data in children younger than 3 months old.

c Limited PK data for children younger than 3 years or weighing less than 10 kg.

d Limited PK data available for children aged 3 months to 6 years.

e Specifics on RTV boosting outlined in 2012 labeling revision (Available at: http://www.accessdata.fda.gov).

The immaturity of the glucuronide conjugation and glomerular filtration in the early neonatal period affects the elimination and clearance of NRTIs. The elimination of orally administered AZT in infants increases rapidly during the first days of life and reaches adult levels by 4 to 8 weeks of life.[50,51] The clearance of AZT is even more decreased in premature infants requiring a significant increase in the dosing interval to avoid potentially toxic exposure.[49,52,53] Similar to AZT, 3TC clearance is prolonged immediately after birth, requiring a 50% dose reduction in younger (<1 month) infants; for ddl, the recommended dose in newborns is 50 mg/m^2 compared with 90 to 150 mg/m^2/dose in older infants and children.[4,54–56] A similar dose reduction is required for d4T, with 50% of a pediatric dose in the first 13 days of life compared with the full pediatric dosing starting at 14 days postpartum.[57]

Among all ARV drugs used in the neonatal period, NVP has the longest elimination half-life ($t_{1/2}$).[21] Following the administration of an sdNVP to infants at 48 to 72 hours after birth, the median $t_{1/2}$ is 43.6 hours (range: 23.6–81.6 hours). Because NVP is a substrate and inducer of hepatic metabolism by enzymes of the CYP450 family (primarily CYP3A4 and CYP2B6), chronic (not single dose) maternal NVP use before delivery may produce in utero induction of NVP metabolism and accelerate NVP elimination in the infant after birth.[58] Additional NVP doses postpartum (48 and 96 hours) should allow, however, maintaining adequate NVP concentrations in infants born to mothers with chronic NVP therapy, especially when used secondary to unsuppressed viral load and inconsistent use of NVP.[6]

Similar mechanism of the increased CYP450 metabolism in newborns might be responsible for the lower PIs exposure in the neonatal period. Although NFV is no longer recommended for use in neonatal prophylaxis, its PK has been known to be significantly lower in the neonatal period.[59] PK studies of LPV/RTV in neonates suggest that higher (300 mg/m^2/dose) than the pediatric (230 mg/m^2/dose) dose is required in younger infants, and frequent dose adjustments are necessary to assure adequate LPV exposure throughout the first 12 months of life.[60] The liquid formulation of the LPV/RTV, however, contains high amounts of ethanol and propylene glycol, which may be potentially toxic to preterm and very young infants. Recent reports of the LPV-associated neonatal cardiac (atrioventricular block, bradycardia, cardiomyopathy), metabolic (lactic acidosis), renal (renal failure), and central nervous system (depression) toxicity have led the FDA's and the Department of Health and Human Service's (HHS) US guidelines to limit the use of LPV/RTV to term (>42 weeks' gestation) and older (postnatal age ≥14 days) neonates.[6,61]

TREATMENT OF HIV INFECTION IN CHILDREN
Pediatric ARV Drugs

The development and maturation of the organ systems involved in the absorption, metabolism, and elimination of ARV drugs produce significant changes in the PK and pharmacodynamics (PD) of ART throughout childhood. Faster clearance of ARV drugs by children compared with adults requires significantly higher per weight or body surface area dosing of ARV drugs in younger children to achieve similar systemic ARV exposures.

In addition to the developmental changes in the PK of ARV drugs, multiple factors, such as nutritional status and comorbidities, have the potential to influence the PK and PD of ART in children. In resource-limited settings, significant anemia, decreased weight, and delayed growth among children infected with HIV represent common challenges to ART.[62–64] Concomitant illnesses, such as hepatitis, malabsorption, and diarrhea, have the potential to alter the absorption of ARV drugs. Metabolic and endocrine abnormalities associated with malnutrition have the potential to influence the volume of distribution and the total body clearance of lipophilic ARV drugs, such as PIs.[65] Moreover, therapeutic interventions for comorbidities, such as tuberculosis, with a significant potential for drug-drug interactions further complicate the choice of ART in children.

Although an important success has been achieved in the development of the pediatric ART dosing guidelines, the data on the developmental changes in the ARV PK/PD are still limited in children. Therapeutic drug monitoring of ARV drugs needs to be considered in pediatric patients with drug-drug interactions and ART failure, particularly in scenarios when adherence failure has not been established.[66] The use of the PK data in combination with viral resistance may provide grounds for a successful individualized dosing of ARV drugs in children and adolescents.[67]

Currently, out of 22 FDA-approved marketed ARV drugs for treating adults and adolescents infected with HIV, 19 drugs are approved for use in children and 16 are available in pediatric formulations (see **Table 1**).[68] In addition to the single-drug ARV preparations, following a successful development and use of the fixed-dose coformulations (FDCs) of ARV drugs in adults, five 2-in-1 and four 3-in-1 pediatric FDCs have been developed and received quality certification by the WHO and the FDA (**Table 2**).[69] A recent increase in the certification and pooled purchasing of high-quality generic drugs produced in Brazil, India, South Africa, and Thailand has increased the availability of pediatric ART in resource-limited settings.[69] Despite significant global progress in scaling up the access to ART among children and adolescents in recent years, children continue to have limited access to ART than adults, with only 23% of children (20%–25%) receiving ART in 2010.[10,70]

Even with the availability of the pediatric formulations of the ARV drugs, serious challenges to an efficient pediatric ART remain across the countries and continents. Among those are specific pediatric adherence barriers, such as palatability and high dosing volumes of the liquid ARV formulations; pill-swallowing capacity of the child; dispensability of the pediatric ARV preparations; bioavailability of the FDC ARV components; parental and child behavior-modification skills; disclosure of HIV status; handling and delivery of pediatric ART to the caregivers; and, most importantly, the caregiver's experience and capacity to administer ART to younger patients and to serve as a supplier of ART, encouragement, and support for older children.[71–82]

Current Approach to Pediatric ART

Following the introduction of new ARV drugs in adults and the accumulation of new data on the PK and PD of ARV drugs in children, the pediatric HIV treatment guidelines have significantly evolved throughout the years. The most recent WHO and US (HHS) pediatric guideline updates were released in the summers of 2010 and 2011, respectively.[3,4] The updated version of the pediatric US guidelines is due for release in 2012. European (Pediatric European Network for Treatment of AIDS [PENTA]) pediatric guidelines were updated in the fall of 2009 and had a letter with the statement position on the age of initiation of ART in children presented at the international AIDS conference in Vienna in the summer of 2010 (available at: http://www.pentatrials.org).[83]

Both US and European guidelines recommend universal treatment of all children infected with HIV younger than 12 months of age.[4,83] The 2010 WHO pediatric guidelines have increased the age of universal initiation ART to 24 months, with an obligatory recommendation for infants younger than 12 months and conditional recommendation for children older than12 months and younger than 24 months of age.[3] The increase of the threshold for universal ART from 12 months to 24 months of age in WHO guidelines is based on the statistics of the higher infant and young children mortality from HIV in resource-limited settings (particularly in sub-Saharan Africa) when compared with

Table 2		
Selected FDA-approved FDCs of ARV drugs for children[a]		
Drugs (Abbreviations)	**FDCs Available**	**Dosing Frequency**
2-in-1 FDCs		
Stavudine/lamivudine/(d4T/3TC)	Pedi tabs: d4T 6 mg + 3TC 30 mg d4T 12 mg + 3TC 60 mg Adult tabs: d4T 30 mg + 3TC 150 mg	Twice daily
Zidovudine/lamivudine (3TC/AZT)	Pedi tabs: AZT 60 mg + 3TC 30 mg Adult tabs: AZT 300 mg + 3TC 150 mg	Twice daily
Abacavir/lamivudine (ABC/3TC)	Pedi tabs: ABC 60 mg + 3TC 30 mg Adult tabs: ABC 600 mg + 3TC 300 mg	Twice daily
Tenofovir/emtricitabine (TDF/FTC)	Pedi tabs: N/A[b] Adult tabs: TDF 300 mg + FTC 200 mg	Once daily[b]
3-in-1 FDCs		
Zidovudine/lamivudine/nevirapine (AZT/3TC/NVP)	Pedi tabs: AZT 60 mg + 3TC 30 mg + NVP 50 mg Adult tabs: AZT 300 mg + 3TC 150 mg + NVP 200 mg	Twice daily
Stavudine/lamivudine/nevirapine (d4T/3TC/NVP)	Pedi tabs: d4T 6 mg + 3TC 30 mg + NVP 50 mg d4T 12 mg + 3TC 60 mg + NVP 100 mg Adult tabs: d4T 30 mg + 3TC 150 mg + NVP 200 mg	Twice daily
Abacavir/zidovudine/lamivudine (ABC/AZT/3TC)	Pedi tabs: ABC 60 mg + AZT 60 mg + 3TC 30 mg Adult tabs: ABC 300 mg + AZT 300 mg + 3TC 150 mg	Twice daily

Abbreviations: Pedi, Pediatric; tabs, Tablets.

Information on the drug formulation, dosing, and approval were obtained from the FDA, HHS, and WHO pediatric guidelines.[4,26,107]

[a] LPV is routinely coformulated with RTV and is included in **Table 1**.

[b] TDF/FTC restricted for adolescents older than 12 years and more than 35 kg.

European and American cohorts of HIV-infected peers. Moreover, the limited ability to monitor clinical CD4+ cell counts and HIV viral load progression of the disease in resource-limited settings dictates the need for ART coverage in the years when the pediatric mortality from HIV is the highest.[3]

The choice for the initiation of ART for asymptomatic children older than 12 (>24 months for WHO) months and younger than 5 years of age is guided by the age-appropriate CD4+ cell count percentage (US, WHO, Europe) and absolute CD4+ cell number (WHO, Europe) thresholds.[3,4,83] While using a similar percentage of CD4+ cell for the treatment initiation threshold in younger children (<36 months of age), European guidelines set lower CD4+ cell percentage and lower absolute CD4+ cell number in older children (>36 months and <59 months of age) as a threshold for the initiation of ART compared with the US and WHO guidelines for this age group.[3,4,83] High viral load (HIV ribonucleic acid [RNA] polymerase chain reaction [PCR] >100,000 copies/mL) is also used as a criterion for the initiation of the pediatric ART in children older than 12 months of age in the United States and Europe but is not included in the WHO guidelines because of the limited access to the HIV PCR in resource-limited settings. In children older than 5 years of age, lower CD4+ cell counts ($\leq$350 cells/mm^3 for WHO and <350 cells/mm^3 for Europe) as compared with the United States ($\leq$500 cells/mm^3) are used. Finally, the presence of the array of clinical comorbidities, including opportunistic infections and AIDS-defining conditions, or the clinical stage of the HIV infection are used to guide the initiation of ART in symptomatic children in all 3 sets of pediatric guidelines.

All 3 (WHO, European, US) pediatric ART guidelines recommend the first-line treatment of choice for children infected with HIV to be comprised of 2 NRTIs plus a third potent agent from a different class, either an NNRTI or an RTV-boosted PI (**Table 3**).[3,4,83] In European and US guidelines, 3TC and ABC are the recommended NRTIs backbone of choice with prescreening for major histocompatibility complex, class I, B (HLA-B) *5701 before the administration of ABC.[83] In the WHO guidelines, the choice of NRTI backbone starts with the combination of AZT plus 3TC, followed by 3TC plus ABC and 3TC plus d4T (see **Table 3**).[3] Among NNRTIs, in all guidelines NVP is the preferred drug in children younger than 3 years of age without previous exposure to NVP as part of maternal or neonatal PMTCT. After 3 years of age, EFV becomes a preferred NNRTI in the United States and Europe, whereas NVP and EFV remain equitable choices in the WHO guidelines.[3,4,83] LPV/RTV is the first-line choice boosted PI in the United States until 6 years of age, when ATV/RTV becomes more preferable and LPV/RTV and other boosted PIs (darunavir [DRV/RTV] and fosamprenavir [FPV/RTV]) are considered as alternatives. LPV/RTV is also listed as the preferred boosted PI in WHO guidelines for the infants born exposed to NVP as part of maternal or neonatal PMCTC (see **Table 3**).

The development of significant clinical morbidity, unsuppressed or rebound viral load, incomplete recovery, or a newly detected decline in CD4+ cell count can all serve as indicators of the first-line ART failure. A thorough investigation of the ART practices, including assessment of adherence, unidentified ARV drug toxicities, ARV drug-drug and drug-food interactions, needs to take place before considering stopping or switching ART in children. The evaluation of HIV resistance is warranted in settings where it can be obtained. Moreover, the administration of the second-line ART usually requires switching some or all of the first-line ARV drugs with an introduction of at least one new drug from a different class and requires pediatric HIV expertise in combination with enhanced adherence support.

Adherence remains one of the most important factors in the success of ART in children. Incomparable to any other pediatric morbidity, this lifelong disease universally affects one or more family members of an infected child, making most of the caregivers for children infected with HIV patients themselves. Because of the high mortality of HIV and AIDS in resource-limited settings, many perinatally infected children become orphans and are placed in remote family or institutional settings. The ability of the caregiver and the child to maintain an adequate level of adherence needs to be addressed before initiating and throughout continuation of ART in pediatric patients infected with HIV.

TREATMENT OF HIV INFECTION IN ADOLESCENTS
ART in Adolescents

HIV-infected adolescents represent a heterogeneous group of pubertal children and young adults with vertically and horizontally transmitted HIV infection and diverse

Table 3
Summary of current pediatric ART guidelines

Recommended Initial ART Regimens for Infants and Children[a]		
Source/Year	First-Line Regimen	Alternative Regimen
International (WHO)[b] 2010	<24 mo old 2 NRTIs[c] + NVP without ARV exposure[d] 2 NRTIs + LPV/RTV with ARV exposure[d] >24 mo <3 y old 2 NRTIs + NVP ≥3 y old 2 NRTIs + NNRTI (NVP or EFV)	(AZT or d4T)[e] + 3TC + ABC or if ≥3 mo old (AZT or d4T) + FTC + ABC
European (PENTA)[b] 2009	<3 y old 2 NRTIs[c] + NVP 2 NRTIs + LPV/RTV >3 y old 2 NRTIs + EFV 2 NRTIs + LPV/RTV	<3 y old[f] 3 NRTIs + NVP 3 NRTIs + LPV/RTV >40 kg 2 NRTIs + ATV/RTV 2 NRTIs + FPV/RTV 2 NRTIs + DRV/RTV 2 NRTIs + SQV/RTV
US (HHS)[b] 2011	<3 y old 2 NRTIs[c] + LPV/RTV ≥3 y old 2 NRTIs + EFV 2 NRTIs + LPV/RTV ≥6 y old 2 NRTIs + ATV/RTV 2 NRTIs + EFV 2 NRTIs + LPV/RTV	Any age 2 NRTIs + NVP ≥6 y old 2 NRTIs + DRV/RTV 2 NRTIs + FPV/RTV

[a] This table serves as a summary of recommended ART in international guidelines. Please see complete guidance for specific information at related sources.[3,4,83]

[b] WHO recommends the universal treatment of all children infected with HIV who are younger than 24 months. The PENTA and HHS guidelines recommend universal initiation of ART in all infants infected with HIV who are younger than 12 months.

[c] The most preferred combination of NRTIs across all guidelines include
- ABC plus 3TC or (FTC) (if ≥3 months old).
- AZT plus 3TC or (FTC) (if ≥3 months old).
- TDF (if ≥12 years and Tanner stage 3) plus 3TC or FTC.
- 3TC plus d4T (alternative in the United States and one of the preferred choices in WHO guidelines).

[d] ARV exposure in younger infants (<12 months) includes exposure to maternal PMTC (including sdNVP).

[e] AZT and d4T are both thymidine analogues and cannot be coadministered.

[f] Some clinicians consider using 3 NRTIs (AZT+3TC+ABC) in combination with NVP.
   Data from Refs.[3,4,83]

demographic and socioeconomic status, sexual and substance abuse history, and different stages of psychosocial development.[84] With growing access to pediatric ART, an increasing number of children with perinatally acquired HIV infections are surviving into adolescence. These children are usually highly treatment experienced and might be on their second- and third-line regimen by the time they enter puberty. In addition, per WHO statistics, out of 6000 estimated new HIV infections per day among adults and adolescents older than 15 years of age, 42% of affected youth between the ages 15 and 24 years in 2010.[85]

Currently, ART during puberty is represented in both pediatric and adolescent guidelines. The choice of ARV drug dosing is usually based on the sexual maturation stages (Tanner stages I through V reflecting transition from a child to an adult body). Such an approach presumes that national and ethnic standards for sexual maturation are identical to the Tanner stages developed in Europe and that the local providers are familiar with them. For children in Tanner stages I through III, the WHO pediatric guidelines recommended using pediatric weight band dosing of ARV drugs, whereas adult dosing guidelines are used for adolescents in Tanner stages IV and V.[3] In the United States, pediatric dosing of ARV drugs is reserved for children in Tanner stages I and II and adult dosing is automatically applied for youth in Tanner stage V, whereas ARV dosing in Tanner stages II and IV is left to provider discretion.[4] Continued use of higher (weight- or surface-based) pediatric doses during adolescence can result in increased and potentially toxic drug exposure, whereas early introduction of lower adult doses can lead to suboptimal therapeutic exposure and development of drug resistance and subsequent virologic failure.[84]

Puberty produces a remarkable increase in growth velocity and changes in body composition, which vary between genders with a significant increase in lean body mass in boys and accumulation of fat in girls.[86,87] Girls are generally a year or two more advanced in pubertal maturation than boys, and the African American race has been associated with an earlier age at onset of menarche.[87,88] Limited information on the potential differences in the PK and PD of ARV drugs in adolescents is available to date, with some suggesting a potentially higher dose requirement for certain ARV drugs during puberty.[89] None of the available adolescent studies have investigated the effects of pubertal changes on the metabolism and disposition of ARV drugs, and the information on failure of ART therapy in adolescents is limited.

Compared with younger children, adolescents are more frequently exposed to antidepressants, hormonal contraceptives, anabolic steroids, alcohol, and illicit drugs. A limited number of studies is available to date on the effect of psychotropic drugs and substance abuse on drug disposition and the effect of ART in adolescence.[84] The potential drug interaction between PIs and NNRTIs with oral contraceptives has been reported in adults and needs to be addressed when prescribing ART to young female patients.[4,5]

As adolescents with perinatally acquired HIV infection approach adulthood, the attention to long-term consequences of ART exposure is renewed. Although significant knowledge has been accumulated concerning the metabolic and cardiovascular complications of ART in adults in recent years,[90,91] the data on the prevalence of pediatric ART-associated metabolic complications are just starting to emerge. The significance of childhood ART-associated lipodystrophy, dyslipidemia, insulin resistance, hyperlactatemia, renal insufficiency, and osteopenia in the development of the cardiovascular, renal, and bone disease of adulthood is not known and the management of these complications during childhood is under investigation.[92] To date, few studies have evaluated the impact of ARV drug exposure on the development of those complications.[93–96] A recent report of high rates of coronary artery abnormalities on cardiac magnetic resonance imaging in adolescents and young adults with a long-standing history of HIV exposure suggested possible early atherosclerosis in this population.[97] Although not associated with coronary artery disease in adults, coronary irregularities were seen in youth with increased cumulative exposure to TDF and 3TC.[97] Based on the potential risks of long-term associated ART toxicity and delayed onset in their clinical presentations, the accumulation of new data and the development of the biomarkers to facilitate the early identification of children at high risk for ARV associated toxicities are urgently needed.

Adherence in Adolescents

In addition to the described pediatric adherence barriers, adolescents infected with HIV face many new obstacles related to the psychological and social changes during the transition from childhood to adulthood. Among the most important adolescent adherence challenges in perinatally infected youth are the following:

- Growing independence
- Change in schedules and lifestyle
- Increased amount of time away from home
- Rebellion against parental involvement
- Increased risk-taking behavior
- Increased peer pressure
- Previous history of poor adherence
- Delay in disclosure of HIV status
- Premature transition of ART responsibility to an adolescent

For newly infected youth, denial and fear of HIV infection; lack of disclosure with the family, partners, and peers; lack of a support system; and confidentiality issues are among most challenging to address. Common for both groups are psychiatric problems (depression) and alcohol and substance abuse.[98,99] Finally, the issues of reproductive health and the potential for family planning become important considerations and need to be addressed.

A comprehensive assessment of adherence should be incorporated into the design and maintenance strategy of the ART regimen of every adolescent patient with an HIV infection.[100] Multiple interventions to improve long-term adherence in adolescents have been proposed, but little evidence-based data are available to date. A once-daily ART regimen is frequently a preferred choice by adolescents and their caregivers, particularly those who are involved in the supervision of the ARV dose intake and should be considered when possible.[4,101] Among the currently applied methods to improve adherence to ART of adolescents with HIV are:[72,102,103]

- Reminder systems (calendars, medical diaries, and text messaging and reminders via cell phones, beepers, and alarm systems)
- Pill boxes
- Directly observed therapy

Most important is the involvement of a multidisciplinary team of providers involving medical doctors; nurses; pharmacists; behavioral and mental health specialists; and other support systems, such as peer groups and the involvement of the partners. Efforts to support, evaluate, and maximize adherence should begin before the start of ART and should continue throughout the transition of the youth to adult care.

An adolescent patient who has been treated in the setting of a family centered pediatric/adolescent HIV clinic is frequently unprepared to face the busy adult individual-centered care. Transition of the perinatally infected adolescent with HIV to adult care is complicated by the high rates of viral resistance following a 10- to 15-year course of ARV drug exposure. Currently, the most treatment-experienced adolescents and young adults are residing in the areas of North America and Europe with guaranteed access to ARV drugs.[104] In a European cohort of 654 perinatally infected youth, 52% and 12% of the 166 patients have been reported to have dual- or triple-class resistance mutations, respectively.[105] The ongoing increase in ART coverage of the pediatric population in resource-limited settings certainly has the potential to generate a significant number of treatment-experienced adolescents and to lead to the global increase in ARV drug resistance among perinatally infected youth.

Multiple issues, such as insurance coverage, access to ARV drugs, different expectations from patients, and different adult-oriented support systems, are unfamiliar and can be intimidating after having a long-standing familynstyle relationship with a pediatric provider.[106] Communication between programs and medical providers and the establishment of a transition process within the participation of a multidisciplinary team of social workers, mental health providers, and nurses is crucial in assuring uninterrupted ART for many years ahead.

SUMMARY

Over the last decades, great successes have been achieved in the prevention, diagnosis, and therapy for pediatric HIV disease. Although not providing a cure, modern ART is capable of significantly reducing the MTCT, allowing the international community to generate an ambitious goal of creating an HIV-free generation. Close international collaboration involving multiple resources and continuous advocacy efforts are necessary to make this goal a reality within the next decade.

ART has dramatically decreased morbidity and mortality and provided high-quality survival to children and adolescents infected with HIV. Significant efforts have been devoted to the development, approval, and increased access to pediatric ARV drugs. Despite the obvious success of PMTCT and pediatric ARV therapy, millions of children remain affected by the disease worldwide. Children infected with HIV and their caregivers are faced with the difficult challenge of preserving long-term adherence to ART, avoiding ARV drug resistance, and ARV-associated toxicities throughout the different stages of growth and development. Multiple factors, including age-specific adherence barriers, changes in social and economical surroundings, and psychological and sexual maturation, affect the choices of ART in infants, children, and adolescents. Maintaining flexibility and focus on the therapeutic goals for this highly dynamic antiretroviral treatment process is the key to success in improving the outcome of pediatric HIV disease worldwide.

REFERENCES

1. World Health Organization Global summary of the HIV/AIDS epidemic. 2010. Available at: http://wwwwhoint/hiv/data/en/. Accessed May 17, 2012.
2. Connor E, McSherry G. Treatment of HIV infection in infancy. Clin Perinatol 1994; 21(1):163–77.
3. World Health Organization. Antiretroviral therapy of HIV Infection in infants and children: towards universal access: recommendations for a public health approach-2010 revision. Geneva (Switzerland): WHO; 2010.
4. Panel on Antiretroviral Therapy and Medical Management of HIV-Infected Children. Guidelines for the use of antiretroviral agents in pediatric HIV infection. 2011. Available at: http://aidsinfo.nih.gov/contentfiles/PediatricGuidelines.pdf. Accessed May 1, 2012.
5. Panel on Antiretroviral Guidelines for Adults and Adolescents. Guidelines for the use of antiretroviral agents in HIV-1-infected adults and adolescents. Department of Health and Human Services; 2012. Available at: http://aidsinfo.nih. gov/contentfiles/AdultandAdolescentGL.pdf. Accessed May 11, 2012.
6. Panel on Treatment of HIV-Infected Pregnant Women and Prevention of Perinatal Transmission. Recommendations for use of antiretroviral drugs in pregnant HIV-1-infected women for maternal health and interventions to reduce perinatal HIV transmission in the United States. 2011. Available at: http://aidsinfo.nih.gov/ContentFiles/PerinatalGL.pdf. Accessed May 1, 2012.

7. Peters V, Liu KL, Gill B, et al. Missed opportunities for perinatal HIV prevention among HIV-exposed infants born 1996-2000, pediatric spectrum of HIV disease cohort. Pediatrics 2004;114(3):905–6.

8. WHO. Programmatic update. Use of antiretroviral drugs for treating pregnant women and preventing HIV infection in infants. Geneva (Switzerland): WHO; 2012.

9. UNAIDS. Report on the global HIV/AIDS epidemic 2009. New York: UNAIDS; 2009.

10. WHO, UNICEF, UNAIDS progress report 2011: Global HIV/AIDS response epidemic update and health sector progress towards universal access. Available at: http://wwwwhoint/hiv/pub/progress_report2011/en/indexhtml. Accessed May 27, 2012.

11. Gortmaker SL, Hughes M, Cervia J, et al. Effect of combination therapy including protease inhibitors on mortality among children and adolescents infected with HIV-1. N Engl J Med 2001;345(21):1522–8.

12. Storm DS, Boland MG, Gortmaker SL, et al. Protease inhibitor combination therapy, severity of illness, and quality of life among children with perinatally acquired HIV-1 infection. Pediatrics 2005;115(2):e173–82.

13. Nachman SA, Lindsey JC, Moye J, et al. Growth of human immunodeficiency virus-infected children receiving highly active antiretroviral therapy. Pediatr Infect Dis J 2005;24(4):352–7.

14. Pizzo PA, Eddy J, Falloon J, et al. Effect of continuous intravenous infusion of zidovudine (AZT) in children with symptomatic HIV infection. N Engl J Med 1988;319(14):889–96.

15. Loebstein R, Lalkin A, Koren G. Pharmacokinetic changes during pregnancy and their clinical relevance. Clin Pharmacokinet 1997;33(5):328–43.

16. Morgan DJ. Drug disposition in mother and foetus. Clin Exp Pharmacol Physiol 1997;24(11):869–73.

17. Krauer B, Krauer F, Hytten FE. Drug disposition and pharmacokinetics in the maternal-placental-fetal unit. Pharmacol Ther 1980;10(2):301–28.

18. Philipson A. Pharmacokinetics of ampicillin during pregnancy. J Infect Dis 1977; 136(3):370–6.

19. Zaske DE, Cipolle RJ, Strate RG, et al. Rapid gentamicin elimination in obstetric patients. Obstet Gynecol 1980;56(5):559–64.

20. Conradie F, Zorrilla C, Josipovic D, et al. Safety and exposure of once-daily ritonavir-boosted atazanavir in HIV-infected pregnant women. HIV Med 2011; 12(9):570–9.

21. Mirochnick M, Clarke DF, Dorenbaum A. Nevirapine: pharmacokinetic considerations in children and pregnant women. Clinical Pharmacokinetic 2000;39(4): 281–93.

22. O'Sullivan MJ, Boyer PJ, Scott GB, et al. The pharmacokinetics and safety of zidovudine in the third trimester of pregnancy for women infected with human immunodeficiency virus and their infants: phase I acquired immunodeficiency syndrome clinical trials group study (protocol 082). Zidovudine Collaborative Working Group. Am J Obstet Gynecol 1993;168(5):1510–6.

23. Mirochnick M, Fenton T, Gagnier P, et al. Pharmacokinetics of nevirapine in human immunodeficiency virus type 1-infected pregnant women and their neonates. Pediatric AIDS Clinical Trials Group Protocol 250 Team. J Infect Dis 1998;178(2):368–74.

24. Musoke P, Guay LA, Bagenda D, et al. A phase I/II study of the safety and pharmacokinetics of nevirapine in HIV-1-infected pregnant Ugandan women and their neonates (HIVNET 006). AIDS 1999;13(4):479–86.

25. Mirochnick M, Siminski S, Fenton T, et al. Nevirapine pharmacokinetics in pregnant women and in their infants after in utero exposure. Pediatr Infect Dis J 2001; 20(8):803–5.

26. World Health Organization. Antiretroviral drugs for treating pregnant women and preventing HIV infection in infants: recommendations for a public health approach. – 2010 version. Geneva (Switzerland): WHO; 2010.

27. Brinkman K, ter Hofstede HJ, Burger DM, et al. Adverse effects of reverse transcriptase inhibitors: mitochondrial toxicity as common pathway. AIDS 1998; 12(14):1735–44.

28. Blanche S, Tardieu M, Rustin P, et al. Persistent mitochondrial dysfunction and perinatal exposure to antiretroviral nucleoside analogues. Lancet 1999;354(9184): 1084–9.

29. Barret B, Tardieu M, Rustin P, et al. Persistent mitochondrial dysfunction in HIV-1-exposed but uninfected infants: clinical screening in a large prospective cohort. AIDS 2003;17(12):1769–85.

30. Nucleoside exposure in the children of HIV-infected women receiving antiretroviral drugs: absence of clear evidence for mitochondrial disease in children who died before 5 years of age in five United States cohorts. J Acquir Immune Defic Syndr 2000;25(3):261–8.

31. European Collaborative Study. Exposure to antiretroviral therapy in utero or early life: the health of uninfected children born to HIV-infected women. J Acquir Immune Defic Syndr 2003;32(4):380–7.

32. Brogly SB, Ylitalo N, Mofenson LM, et al. In utero nucleoside reverse transcriptase inhibitor exposure and signs of possible mitochondrial dysfunction in HIV-uninfected children. AIDS 2007;21(8):929–38.

33. Rakhmanina NY, van den Anker JN. Efavirenz in the therapy of HIV infection. Expert Opin Drug Metab Toxicol 2010;6(1):95–103.

34. Simon A, Warszawski J, Kariyawasam D, et al. Association of prenatal and postnatal exposure to lopinavir-ritonavir and adrenal dysfunction among uninfected infants of HIV-infected mothers. JAMA 2011;306(1):70–8.

35. Ferguson W, Goode M, Walsh A, et al. Evaluation of 4 weeks' neonatal antiretroviral prophylaxis as a component of a prevention of mother-to-child transmission program in a resource-rich setting. Pediatr Infect Dis J 2011;30(5):408–12.

36. Lahoz R, Noguera A, Rovira N, et al. Antiretroviral-related hematologic short-term toxicity in healthy infants: implications of the new neonatal 4-week zidovudine regimen. Pediatr Infect Dis J 2010;29(4):376–9.

37. Nielsen-Saines K, Watts DH, Santos VV. Phase III randomized trial of the safety and efficacy of three neonatal antiretroviral regimens for preventing intrapartum HIV-1 transmission (NICHD HPTN 040/PACTG 1043). 18th Conference on Retroviruses and Opportunistic Infections. Boston, February 27-March 2, 2011.

38. Mirochnick M, Nielsen-Saines K, Pilotto JH, et al. Nelfinavir and Lamivudine pharmacokinetics during the first two weeks of life. Pediatr Infect Dis J 2011; 30(9):769–72.

39. Mirochnick M, Thomas T, Capparelli E, et al. Antiretroviral concentrations in breast-feeding infants of mothers receiving highly active antiretroviral therapy. Antimicrob Agents Chemother 2009;53(3):1170–6.

40. Shapiro RL, Holland DT, Capparelli E, et al. Antiretroviral concentrations in breast-feeding infants of women in Botswana receiving antiretroviral treatment. J Infect Dis 2005;192(5):720–7.

41. Schneider S, Peltier A, Gras A, et al. Efavirenz in human breast milk, mothers', and newborns' plasma. J Acquir Immune Defic Syndr 2008;48(4):450–4.

42. Benaboud S, Pruvost A, Coffie PA, et al. Concentrations of tenofovir and emtricitabine in breast milk of HIV-1-infected women in Abidjan, Cote d'Ivoire, in the ANRS 12109 TEmAA Study, Step 2. Antimicrob Agents Chemother 2011;55(3):1315–7.

43. Kesho Bora Study Group, de Vincenzi I. Triple antiretroviral compared with zidovudine and single-dose nevirapine prophylaxis during pregnancy and breastfeeding for prevention of mother-to-child transmission of HIV-1 (Kesho Bora study): a randomised controlled trial. Lancet Infect Dis 2011;11(3):171–80.

44. Rakhmanina NY, van den Anker JN. Pharmacological research in pediatrics: from neonates to adolescents. Adv Drug Deliv Rev 2006;58(1):4–14.

45. Arant BS Jr. Developmental patterns of renal functional maturation compared in the human neonate. J Pediatr 1978;92(5):705–12.

46. van den Anker JN, Schoemaker RC, Hop WC, et al. Ceftazidime pharmacokinetics in preterm infants: effects of renal function and gestational age. Clin Pharmacol Ther 1995;58(6):650–9.

47. Hines RN, McCarver DG. The ontogeny of human drug-metabolizing enzymes: phase I oxidative enzymes. J Pharmacol Exp Ther 2002;300(2):355–60.

48. McCarver DG, Hines RN. The ontogeny of human drug-metabolizing enzymes: phase II conjugation enzymes and regulatory mechanisms. J Pharmacol Exp Ther 2002;300(2):361–6.

49. Capparelli EV, Mirochnick M, Dankner WM, et al. Pharmacokinetics and tolerance of zidovudine in preterm infants. J Pediatr 2003;142(1):47–52.

50. Boucher FD, Modlin JF, Weller S, et al. Phase I evaluation of zidovudine administered to infants exposed at birth to the human immunodeficiency virus. J Pediatr 1993;122(1):137–44.

51. Mirochnick M, Capparelli E, Connor J. Pharmacokinetics of zidovudine in infants: a population analysis across studies. Clin Pharmacol Ther 1999;66(1):16–24.

52. Mirochnick M, Capparelli E, Dankner W, et al. Zidovudine pharmacokinetics in premature infants exposed to human immunodeficiency virus. Antimicrob Agents Chemother 1998;42(4):808–12.

53. Balis FM, Pizzo PA, Murphy RF, et al. The pharmacokinetics of zidovudine administered by continuous infusion in children. Ann Intern Med 1989;110(4):279–85.

54. Moodley D, Pillay K, Naidoo K, et al. Pharmacokinetics of zidovudine and lamivudine in neonates following coadministration of oral doses every 12 hours. J Clin Pharmacol 2001;41(7):732–41.

55. Moodley J, Moodley D, Pillay K, et al. Pharmacokinetics and antiretroviral activity of lamivudine alone or when coadministered with zidovudine in human immunodeficiency virus type 1-infected pregnant women and their offspring. J Infect Dis 1998;178(5):1327–33.

56. Mueller BU, Lewis LL, Yuen GJ, et al. Serum and cerebrospinal fluid pharmacokinetics of intravenous and oral lamivudine in human immunodeficiency virus-infected children. Antimicrob Agents Chemother 1998;42(12):3187–92.

57. Jullien V, Rais A, Urien S, et al. Age-related differences in the pharmacokinetics of stavudine in 272 children from birth to 16 years: a population analysis. Br J Clin Pharmacol 2007;64(1):105–9.

58. Mirochnick M, Dorenbaum A, Blanchard S, et al. Predose infant nevirapine concentration with the two-dose intrapartum neonatal nevirapine regimen: association with timing of maternal intrapartum nevirapine dose. J Acquir Immune Defic Syndr 2003;33(2):153–6.

59. Mirochnick M, Nielsen-Saines K, Pilotto JH, et al. NICHD/HPTN 040/PACTG 1043 Protocol Team. Nelfinavir pharmacokinetics with an increased dose during the first two weeks of life. The 15th Conference on Retroviruses and Opportunistic Infections. Boston, February 3–6, 2008.

60. Chadwick EG, Yogev R, Alvero CG, et al. Long-term outcomes for HIV-infected infants less than 6 months of age at initiation of lopinavir/ritonavir combination antiretroviral therapy. AIDS 2011;25(5):643–9.

61. Boxwell D, Cao K, Lewis L, et al. Neonatal toxicity of Kaletra oral solution: LPV, ethanol or propylene glycol? 18th Conference on Retroviruses and Opportunistic Infections (CROI). Boston, February 27–March 3, 2011.

62. Shet A, Mehta S, Rajagopalan N, et al. Anemia and growth failure among HIV-infected children in India: a retrospective analysis. BMC Pediatr 2009;9:37.

63. Naidoo R, Rennert W, Lung A, et al. The influence of nutritional status on the response to HAART in HIV-infected children in South Africa. Pediatr Infect Dis J 2010;29(6):511–3.

64. Kekitiinwa A, Lee KJ, Walker AS, et al. Differences in factors associated with initial growth, CD4, and viral load responses to ART in HIV-infected children in Kampala, Uganda, and the United Kingdom/Ireland. J Acquir Immune Defic Syndr 2008;49(4):384–92.

65. Fukushima K, Shibata M, Mizuhara K, et al. Effect of serum lipids on the pharmacokinetics of atazanavir in hyperlipidemic rats. Biomed Pharmacother 2009;63(9):635–42.

66. Rakhmanina NY, Neely MN, Capparelli EV. High dose of darunavir in treatment-experienced HIV-infected adolescent results in virologic suppression and improved CD4 cell count. Ther Drug Monit 2012;34(3):237–41.

67. Neely MN, Rakhmanina NY. Pharmacokinetic optimization of antiretroviral therapy in children and adolescents. Clin Pharmacokinet 2011;50(3):143–89.

68. Gupta RK, Gibb DM, Pillay D. Management of paediatric HIV-1 resistance. Curr Opin Infect Dis 2009;22(3):256–63.

69. Waning B, Diedrichsen E, Jambert E, et al. The global pediatric antiretroviral market: analyses of product availability and utilization reveal challenges for development of pediatric formulations and HIV/AIDS treatment in children. BMC Pediatr 2010;10(1):74.

70. WHO, UNICEF, UNAIDS. Towards universal access: scaling up priority HIV/AIDS interventions in the health sector: Progress report 2009. Geneva (Switzerland): WHO; 2009.

71. Bunupuradah T, Wannachai S, Chuamchaitrakool A, et al. Use of taste-masking product, FLAVORx, to assist Thai children to ingest generic antiretrovirals. AIDS Res Ther 2006;3:30.

72. Winnick S, Lucas DO, Hartman AL, et al. How do you improve compliance? Pediatrics 2005;115(6):e718–24.

73. Heald AE, Pieper CF, Schiffman SS. Taste and smell complaints in HIV-infected patients. AIDS 1998;12(13):1667–74.

74. Gibb DM, Goodall RL, Giacomet V, et al. Adherence to prescribed antiretroviral therapy in human immunodeficiency virus-infected children in the PENTA 5 trial. Pediatr Infect Dis J 2003;22(1):56–62.

75. Pontali E. Facilitating adherence to highly active antiretroviral therapy in children with HIV infection: what are the issues and what can be done? Paediatr Drugs 2005;7(3):137–49.

76. Chesney MA. Factors affecting adherence to antiretroviral therapy. Clin Infect Dis 2000;30(Suppl 2):S171–6.

77. Byrne M, Honig J, Jurgrau A, et al. Achieving adherence with antiretroviral medications for pediatric HIV disease. AIDS Read 2002;12(4):151–4, 161–4.
78. Gavin PJ, Yogev R. The role of protease inhibitor therapy in children with HIV infection. Paediatr Drugs 2002;4(9):581–607.
79. Van Dyke RB, Lee S, Johnson GM, et al. Reported adherence as a determinant of response to highly active antiretroviral therapy in children who have human immunodeficiency virus infection. Pediatrics 2002;109(4):e61.
80. Goode M, McMaugh A, Crisp J, et al. Adherence issues in children and adolescents receiving highly active antiretroviral therapy. AIDS Care 2003;15(3):403–8.
81. Reddington C, Cohen J, Baldillo A, et al. Adherence to medication regimens among children with human immunodeficiency virus infection. Pediatr Infect Dis J 2000;19(12):1148–53.
82. Phelps BR, Rakhmanina N. Antiretroviral drugs in pediatric HIV-infected patients: pharmacokinetic and practical challenges. Paediatr Drugs 2011;13(3):175–92.
83. Welch S, Sharland M, Lyall EG, et al. PENTA 2009 guidelines for the use of antiretroviral therapy in paediatric HIV-1 infection. HIV Med 2009;10(10):591–613.
84. Rakhmanina NY, Capparelli EV, van den Anker JN. Personalized therapeutics: HIV treatment in adolescents. Clin Pharmacol Ther 2008;84(6):734–40.
85. World Health Organization. Global report: UNAIDS report of the global AIDS epidemic 2010. Geneva (Switzerland): WHO. UNAIDS; 2010.
86. Kreipe R. Normal somatic adolescent growth and development. In: McAnarney ER, Kreipe RE, Orr DP, et al, editors. Textbook of adolescent medicine. Philadelphia: WB Saunders; 1992. p. 57.
87. Tanner J. Growth at adolescence. London: Blackwell Scientific Publications; 1962.
88. U.S. Department of Health, Education and Welfare. Public Health Service. Health Resource Administration. National Center for Health Statistics: age at menarche, US. 1973;133(11):2–3.
89. Kiser JJ, Fletcher CV, Flynn PM, et al. Pharmacokinetics of antiretroviral regimens containing tenofovir disoproxil fumarate and atazanavir-ritonavir in adolescents and young adults with human immunodeficiency virus infection. Antimicrob Agents Chemother 2008;52(2):631–7.
90. Vigano A, Cerini C, Pattarino G, et al. Metabolic complications associated with antiretroviral therapy in HIV-infected and HIV-exposed uninfected paediatric patients. Expert Opin Drug Saf 2010;9(3):431–45.
91. Miller TL, Grant YT, Almeida DN, et al. Cardiometabolic disease in human immunodeficiency virus-infected children. J Cardiometab Syndr 2008;3(2):98–105.
92. Eley B. Metabolic complications of antiretroviral therapy in HIV-infected children. Expert Opin Drug Metab Toxicol 2008;4(1):37–49.
93. Rakhmanina N, van Rongen A, van den Anker J, et al. Plasma protease inhibitor concentrations and fasting lipid profiles in HIV-infected children. 11th International Workshop on Clinical Pharmacology of HIV Therapy. Sorrento, April 7–9, 2010. Abstract 006.
94. S Kanjanavanit S, Hansudewechakul R, Kim S, et al. 2-year evolution of triglycerides and cholesterol in Thai HIV-1-infected children receiving first-line NVP- or EFV-based Regimen. 17th Conference on Retroviruses and Opportunistic Infections instead of CROI. San Francisco, February 16–19, 2010. Abstract 865.
95. Aurpibul L, Puthanakit T, Lee B, et al. Lipodystrophy and metabolic changes in HIV-infected children on non-nucleoside reverse transcriptase inhibitor-based antiretroviral therapy. Antivir Ther 2007;12(8):1247–54.

96. McComsey G, Bhumbra N, Ma JF, et al. Impact of protease inhibitor substitution with efavirenz in HIV-infected children: results of the First Pediatric Switch Study. Pediatrics 2003;111(3):e275–81.

97. Mikhail I, Purdy J, Dimock D, et al. High rate of coronary artery abnormalities in adolescents and young adults infected with HIV early in life. 17th Conference on Retroviruses and Opportunistic Infections. San Francisco, February 16–19, 2010. Abstract 864.

98. Murphy DA, Wilson CM, Durako SJ, et al. Antiretroviral medication adherence among the REACH HIV-infected adolescent cohort in the USA. AIDS Care 2001;13(1):27–40.

99. Simoni JM, Montgomery A, Martin E, et al. Adherence to antiretroviral therapy for pediatric HIV infection: a qualitative systematic review with recommendations for research and clinical management. Pediatrics 2007;119(6):e1371–83.

100. Khan M, Song X, Williams K, et al. Evaluating adherence to medication in children and adolescents with HIV. Arch Dis Child 2009;94(12):970–3.

101. Parienti JJ, Bangsberg DR, Verdon R, et al. Better adherence with once-daily antiretroviral regimens: a meta-analysis. Clin Infect Dis 2009;48(4):484–8.

102. Simoni JM, Amico KR, Pearson CR, et al. Strategies for promoting adherence to antiretroviral therapy: a review of the literature. Curr Infect Dis Rep 2008;10(6): 515–21.

103. Ford N, Nachega JB, Engel ME, et al. Directly observed antiretroviral therapy: a systematic review and meta-analysis of randomised clinical trials. Lancet 2009;374(9707):2064–71.

104. McConnell MS, Byers RH, Frederick T, et al. Trends in antiretroviral therapy use and survival rates for a large cohort of HIV-infected children and adolescents in the United States, 1989-2001. J Acquir Immune Defic Syndr 2005;38(4):488–94.

105. Foster C, Judd A, Tookey P, et al. Young people in the United Kingdom and Ireland with perinatally acquired HIV: the pediatric legacy for adult services. AIDS Patient Care STDS 2009;23(3):159–66.

106. A consensus statement on health care transitions for young adults with special health care needs. Pediatrics 2002;110(6 Pt 2):1304–6.

107. Drugs@FDA database. Available at: www.fda.gov/Drugs/InformationOnDrugs. Accessed May 11, 2012.

How to Optimize the Evaluation and Use of Antibiotics in Neonates

Evelyne Jacqz-Aigrain, MD, PhD[a,b,c,*], Florentia Kaguelidou, MD, PhD[a,b,c], John N. van den Anker, MD, PhD[d,e,f,g]

KEYWORDS

- Neonates • Sepsis • Antibiotics • Pharmacokinetics • Modeling • Simulation

KEY POINTS

- A pediatric study decision tree was designed to help researchers extrapolate existing knowledge on drugs from adult studies and ultimately avoid unnecessary trials in pediatrics.
- For antibiotics, the "bacteriologic response" is expected to be similar to that in adults. Therefore, pharmacokinetic (PK)/pharmacodynamic (PD) studies can support antibiotic administration in neonates by determining the appropriate dose required for targeted exposure.
- Extrapolating a PK/PD relationship from adults and/or children to neonates with limited PK data collected for model validation "in neonates," as well as using physiologically based PK models to link dose, concentration, and response data, should be implemented.
- Because neonatal infections present with several unique characteristics related to individual neonatal and environmental factors, the clinical response data might differ between age groups, and additional data on antibiotic response should also be collected. Randomized controlled trials and methodologies specific to the neonatal population are difficult to conduct for many reasons, but they still should be considered.

The authors have no conflict of interest.
[a] Department of Pharmacology, Université Paris Diderot, 5 rue Thomas Mann, Paris F75013, France; [b] AP-HP, Department of Pediatric Pharmacology and Pharmacogenetics, Hôpital Robert Debré, 48 boulevard Serurier, Paris F75019, France; [c] INSERM Clinical Investigation Center CIC9202, Hôpital Robert Debré, 48 boulevard Serurier, Paris F75019, France; [d] Division of Pediatric Clinical Pharmacology, Children's National Medical Center, Washington, DC, USA; [e] Department of Pediatrics, The George Washington University School of Medicine and Health Sciences, 111 Michigan Avenue, NW, Washington, DC, USA; [f] Department of Pharmacology & Physiology, The George Washington University School of Medicine and Health Sciences, 111 Michigan Avenue, NW, Washington, DC, USA; [g] Department of Pediatric Surgery, Erasmus MC-Sophia Children's Hospital, Rotterdam, The Netherlands
* Corresponding author. Department of Paediatric Pharmacology and Pharmacogenetics, Hopital Robert Debré, 48 boulevard Serurier, Paris 75019, France.
E-mail address: evelyne.jacqzaigrain@gmail.com

Pediatr Clin N Am 59 (2012) 1117–1128
http://dx.doi.org/10.1016/j.pcl.2012.07.004

INTRODUCTION

Drugs are licensed to ensure that their use is safe, effective, and of high quality. However, in pediatric medicine more than 50% of infants, children, and adolescents admitted to a hospital will receive one or more unlicensed or off-label medicines. This circumstance occurs even more in neonates, who represent a particularly vulnerable subgroup of pediatric patients, especially if born prematurely. Although they account for only a low percentage of total drug use in the pediatric age group, up to 90% of medicines in this very young population are used unlicensed or off-label, especially during their stay in a neonatal intensive care unit (NICU).[1–4] Therefore, the uncertainty about efficacy and the potential risk of adverse events with such a high incidence of unlicensed and off-label drug use is much more relevant for neonates than for older children.[5]

This review, based on the authors' experience with the FP7 TINN (Treat Infections in Neonates) project,[6] addresses the numerous challenges faced by neonatologists and pediatric clinical pharmacologists to assure safe and effective use and evaluation of antibiotics in neonates.

CHALLENGE 1: TO UNDERSTAND NEONATAL PHARMACOLOGY

Irrespective of the kind of drugs prescribed in neonates, understanding the impact of growth and development on the changes in absorption, distribution, metabolism, and excretion of drugs used during the neonatal period is essential.[7,8]

In neonates, distribution of antibiotics is affected by body composition. The relatively larger extracellular (70%–75% in neonates vs 50%–55% in adults) and total-body water compartments (40% in neonates vs 20% in adults) as well as the lower fat amount (15% in infants vs 20% in adults) affect the distribution of hydrophilic drugs, which are mainly distributed in body water, and to a lesser extent, the distribution of lipophilic drugs. Lower protein binding increases the free fraction of drugs that are highly bound in older children and adults. Drug-metabolizing enzyme activity in neonates by cytochrome P450 oxidases (phase I enzymes) and conjugating enzymes (phase II enzymes) is low, resulting in reduced metabolic clearance of drugs with a high variability between patients. The glomerular filtration rate is much lower in neonates than in older infants, children, or adults, affecting renal clearing capacity. The maturation of renal structure and function includes prolongation and maturation of renal tubules, increase in renal blood flow, and improvement of filtration efficiency, reflected by the rapid changes in the pharmacokinetics (PK) of renally excreted drugs such as amikacin.[9] The developmental differences and changes in the aforementioned physiology explain that the neonatal population is divided into groups based on gestational and postnatal age.[10]

For the majority of antibacterial agents used in the neonatal population, renal excretion is the most important and rate-limiting step in the clearance of the antibiotic or antibiotics prescribed and administered to the ill neonate. It is therefore imperative to have a useful measure of renal function in this vulnerable and rapidly developing, and therefore changing, population.

CHALLENGE 2: TO UNDERSTAND THE SPECIFIC CHARACTERISTICS OF NEONATAL SEPSIS

Neonatal sepsis, classified as early-onset and late-onset sepsis, is a major cause of mortality and morbidity, with specific pathogen distribution and infection rates in the different neonatal age groups.[11]

Sepsis in neonates during the first 48 to 72 hours after birth is defined as early neonatal sepsis. It is usually caused by vertical transmission of group B streptococcal infection.[12,13] The increased peripartal use of antibacterial agents in women colonized with group B streptococcus appears to have reduced neonatal infection.[14,15] Data on maternal risk factors for infection and effective strategies to detect maternal colonization are required before validating treatment protocols during labor and delivery.[16,17]

Sepsis in neonates after the first 2 to 3 days of life is called late-onset neonatal sepsis. It is predominantly caused by gram-positive organisms, with coagulase-negative staphylococci responsible for half the cases of sepsis. The rate of infection is inversely related to birth weight and gestational age and is associated with an increased risk of death.[18,19] Among others, previous antimicrobial exposure is an important risk factor.[20]

However, the classic separation between early-onset and late-onset infection may be questioned, as recent data in neonates suggest that extensive antibiotic use results in changes in the spectrum of organisms from predominantly gram-positive to predominantly gram-negative pathogens, with a significant increase in the incidence of *Escherichia coli*.[19,21]

Suspected infections are quite frequent in neonatal care, but microbiologically evaluable infections are rare: 1 to 2 cases per 1000 live births. Treatment is an emergency, and if treatment is delayed or ineffective, neonatal sepsis can be rapidly fatal; therefore, empiric parenteral antibiotics are always administered when this condition is suspected, mostly on clinical grounds alone.[22]

In addition to systemic bacterial infections, invasive candidiasis is also an important and often fatal pathogen in the preterm neonate of very low birth weight. Invasive candidiasis frequently results in increased morbidity, prolonged stay, death, or neurologic damage. Despite antifungal treatment, 20% of infants who develop invasive candidiasis die as a result of disease, and neurodevelopmental impairment occurs in nearly 60% of the survivors. Data from the literature and one large multicenter randomized controlled trial have shown that antifungal prophylaxis provides an effective approach to decrease the morbidity and mortality of invasive candidiasis in the premature infant, primarily in centers with a high incidence of fungal infection.[23] Although important, the use of antifungal agents is not within the scope of this review.

CHALLENGE 3: TO UNDERSTAND THE PHARMACODYNAMICS OF ANTIBIOTICS

Pharmacokinetics (PK) is the study of the time course of antimicrobial concentrations in the body, whereas pharmacodynamics (PD) defines the relationship between antimicrobial concentrations and its effect. The 3 PK parameters that are most important for evaluating antibiotic efficacy are the peak serum (plasma) concentration (C_{max}), the trough concentration (C_{min}), and the area under the serum concentration versus time curve (AUC). The primary measure of antibiotic activity is the minimum inhibitory concentration (MIC) of the pathogen, that is, the lowest concentration of an antibiotic that completely inhibits the bacterial growth in vitro. Integrating the PK parameters with the MIC has resulted in 3 PK/PD parameters: the peak/MIC ratio, the T>MIC (percentage of dose interval in which the serum level exceeds the MIC), and the 24-hour AUC/MIC ratio (determined by dividing the 24-hour AUC by the MIC). Based on these parameters, the bacterial killing activity is primarily defined as time dependent or concentration dependent.[24]

For concentration-dependent killing antibiotics with prolonged persistent effects (eg, aminoglycosides, fluoroquinolones), the 24-hour AUC/MIC ratio and the peak/MIC ratio are important predictors of antibiotic efficacy. The optimal dosing regimen should maximize concentration, because the higher the concentration, the more extensive and faster the degree of killing.

For time-dependent killing antibiotics (eg, penicillins, cephalosporins, carbapenems), the dosing regimen should maximize the duration of exposure.

For time-dependent killing antibiotics with moderate persistent killing (eg, vancomycin, azithromycin), the optimal dosing regimen maximizes the amount of drug received.

PK/PD markers, highly correlated with clinical cure, pathogen eradication, and even resistance development, have been identified for many antibacterial agents in adults. As a consequence, in neonates it is highly recommended to perform PK/PD studies instead of simple PK studies. However, as the isolation of the infective agent is infrequent, the PK/PD relationship is rarely based on the "true MIC" and the MIC distribution for wild-type pathogens, based on large epidemiologic and microbiological studies, are used.[25,26]

CHALLENGE 4: TO GET THE DOSE RIGHT

As PK parameters of drug disposition vary widely between neonates, identical dosing regimens may provide different total exposure and PK profiles.[27] Therefore, "to get the dose right" is one of the greatest challenges in neonatal drug development.[28]

Until recently, dosages were extrapolated from adult data by the use of simple allometric methods, based on empiric scaling factors such as body weight or body surface area, and PK studies were conducted a posterior in treated neonates. Pharmacokinetic studies, either classic (rich sampling) or population (sparse sampling), are now recommended although they remain difficult to perform.[29–31] Whatever the approach, in clinical practice it boils down to getting the dose right by exposing either a low number of neonates to high sampling[32] or a high number of neonates to limited sampling without knowing if the selected dose is optimal.[33–35] An intermediate proposal might be to perform an initial rich pilot study with 2 to 4 samples drawn in a limited number of infants, which consequently can be further validated by a population PK study embodied in a larger PK and/or efficacy trial. However, such a recommendation does not support the selection of the first dose to be administered in neonates.

Validation of the population PK models is required to test their predictive performance. For example, many models have been developed for vancomycin, an antibacterial agent widely used in staphylococcal infections, and an external validation has shown that, among potential other factors, the analytical techniques to measure serum creatinine as well as vancomycin concentrations had a clear impact on the prediction of vancomycin concentrations, and that dosage individualization of vancomycin in neonates should be considered.

Modeling and simulation can guide initial dosage recommendations in neonates, taking into account available information on drug characteristics, efficacy, and safety.[36] The use of physiologically based pharmacokinetic (PBPK) models are especially aiming at simulation of drug concentrations in the circulation and in tissue(s) at the individual or population level. These models can also account for age-related variability and, consequently, may be used to predict the PK of drugs in children from data in adults or from one pediatric "old" age group to a younger one.[37] Such models have already shown that they might be of great interest for use in neonates.[36] However, they will be even better performing with additional physiologic data that are still missing in preterm infants, including biological parameters.

CHALLENGE 5: TO CHOOSE THE RIGHT EMPIRIC TREATMENT AND DOSAGE SCHEDULE

Antibiotics are prescribed extensively in NICUs, as shown recently by a large cohort study over an 8-year period.[38] The major risk of such extensive use of broad-spectrum antibiotics is the induction and emergence of resistance, which is particularly true when using third-generation cephalosporins, a combination of broad-spectrum antibiotics, and/or prolonged antibacterial treatment. Major consequences of the emergence of resistant bacterial strains may include prolonged hospital stay, adverse drug reactions, and adverse neurodevelopmental outcomes associated with infection. Additional consequences include changes of the microbial flora or an increased risk of nosocomial infection.

For all these reasons and to optimize treatment, antibiotics should be selected based on the epidemiology of neonatal infections, and adapted to susceptibility patterns. For this reason, many countries have established surveillance networks to monitor changes in pathogens, and to detect changes in antibiotic sensitivity and occurrence of bacterial resistance. Moreover, data on the epidemiology of specific infections in various countries are available, such as group B streptococcus, methicillin-resistant *Staphylococcus aureus*, and fungal infections. In addition, surveys are conducted to search for modifications in clinical practices and/or drug prescriptions.

Antibiotics are usually administered intravenously either at repeated doses with a constant dosage interval or as a continuous infusion, depending on the antibiotic. For drugs with linear elimination given at a fixed dosage regimen, drug concentrations reach a steady state after 4 to 5 half-lives. In neonates, elimination is often longer than in infants or children, and a loading dose may be recommended to reach steady-state concentrations earlier.

CHALLENGE 6: TO PROMOTE ADAPTED MONITORING

Therapeutic drug monitoring (TDM) aims at measuring individual drug exposure based on validated concentrations or PK parameters that better reflect drug effect than drug dosage.[39] Optimal interpretation of the results requires a validated therapeutic range. One major limitation of TDM in neonates is that, for many medications, target concentrations are not defined in children but are only based on data obtained in adults. Indeed, for antibiotics the target range validated in adults is always used in children, including neonates, although additional data are required to validate that such bacteriologic targets are associated with efficacy in neonatal sepsis.

An important issue in neonatal TDM is the availability of bioanalytical assays validated for use of very small sample volumes. To optimize TDM, analytical methods adapted to the age of the patients, particularly for neonates, have to be developed and validated. Immunoassay techniques are widely used for TDM but, although often regarded as specific for the parent drug, the antibody may cross-react with other compounds, including metabolites of the drug. Therefore, the concentrations are often overestimated. In general, these differences do not affect significantly the clinical value of TDM, although they have an impact on the target concentration and contribute to the variability of drug concentrations reported in the literature.

Dried blood spot (DBS) sampling is an interesting option for TDM in neonates, as it is less invasive, it avoids classic venous blood sampling, it requires smaller blood volumes (less than 100 μL), its storage is simpler, and its transfer is easier at room temperature.[40–44] DBS is increasingly used for TDM of a wide spectrum of drugs including antibiotics, although assay sensitivity and specificity are still a challenge. The interpretation of drug concentrations measured during TDM should take into account all aspects and conditions of monitoring (including dose and dosage schedule, the type of biological sample, analytical techniques used, initiation of treatment, potential drug interactions, and so forth) and use of reference concentrations to make recommendations for dosage adjustments.

It is important to bear in mind that detailed information on neonatal disease and clinical conditions, biological parameters of interest, drug, dosage regimen and associated therapies, and time of sampling relative to the time of drug administration are essential to interpret TDM.[45]

CHALLENGE 7: TO PROMOTE DRUG EVALUATION IN NEONATES

Profound changes occurred over the past 10 to 20 years as the American and European regulations on the pediatric use of drugs encouraged the development of medicines for all pediatric age groups,[46,47] with the intention of having a major impact on drug evaluation in pediatric patients of all ages.[48–50]

However, there are major practical and ethical issues in evaluating medicines in preterm and term neonates. The gold standard for evaluating efficacy of antibacterial agents is a randomized controlled trial (RCT). However, for many reasons these kinds of trials are very difficult to conduct in neonates. Indeed, neonates are still less likely to be involved in an RCT.[51,52] In a recent study, the authors analyzed published RCTs conducted to evaluate antibiotics in neonates since 1995, and have shown that the number of RCTs of antimicrobial agents in neonates is small, as well as being poorly designed, conducted, and reported. Moreover, the necessity of conducting RCT trials, when antibacterial efficacy has already been established in other age groups, is questionable, and suitable methodological approaches are required to allow optimal drug evaluation. Specific guidelines, designed by experts, are available for the investigation of medicinal products in the term and preterm neonate,[53] as well as guidelines related to clinical trials in small populations, PK studies, and pharmacovigilance.[54]

As previously stated, neonatal bacterial infections are mainly suspected and are confirmed in only a limited number of cases, and antibiotic treatment protocols are designed in a probabilistic manner, according to local bacteriologic epidemiology and resistance patterns.

In these situations, evaluation of antibiotics remains a challenge,[55–57] as "new antibiotics" are introduced to the therapeutic arsenal because of their expected therapeutic benefits. Accordingly, individual clinicians are reluctant to randomize patients to an agent that they already use with highly expected benefit, which is particularly true for drug-resistant bacterial infections that require effective antibiotics, even if evaluation in neonates is limited. This fact explains why, in the absence of validated dosing regimens, major differences in dose administration and schedules may occur between countries or even between NICUs in the same country, as shown for ciprofloxacin.

In most cases, antibiotics have proven efficacy in adults and older children, and it is accepted that medicines that work in adults and older children do not always need to be tested extensively in neonates. This aspect is described as bridging and extrapolation, and is summarized in the Decision Tree of the European Medicines Agency (EMA)/Food and Drug Administration (**Fig. 1**). However, intrinsic neonatal factors such as the innate immune immaturity that may result in a broader dissemination of the infection and/or other medical factors, in addition to important limitations in diagnostic means, may influence the antibiotic's clinical efficacy; this is the reason why data on therapeutic response (clinical efficacy) must also be collected.

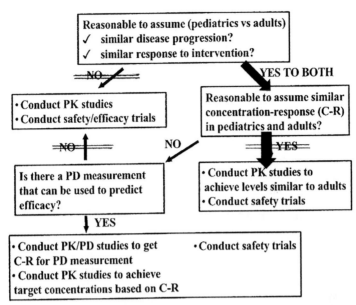

Fig. 1. Pediatric study decision tree. (*From* U.S. Department of Health and Human Services Food and Drug Administration Center for Drug Evaluation and Research (CDER) Center for Biologics Evaluation and Research (CBER). Guidance for Industry. Exposure-response relationships—study design, data analysis, and regulatory applications. Rockville, MD: U.S. Department of Health and Human Services, Food and Drug Administration, 2003. Available at: http://www.fda.gov/cber/guidelines.htm.)

As random allocation of treatment is difficult, or even impossible, for all the reasons previously discussed, effects of clinical treatment may be assessed by means of observational, nonrandomized studies. However, these studies may be hampered by several reasons for bias. When the efficacy of an antibiotic has already been demonstrated in adults, necessary data on effectiveness in neonatal use can be provided by the combination of PK/PD and clinical observational studies.[58] Indeed, observational studies generally have an important role in quantifying drug effects under the conditions of usual practice (effectiveness) whereas RCTs demonstrate drug effects under restricted conditions in terms of disease, comorbidities and concomitant treatment (efficacy). Various approaches are available such as adjustment for predefined pretreatment variables or the creation of a propensity score (ie, probability of being treated according to predefined prognostic factors).[59,60] Therefore in most cases, applications for a product license concerning antibiotics in neonates should include reliable information on the product's dosing recommendations and safety by means of trials that do not necessarily include a randomization step for treatment allocation.

CHALLENGE 8: HOW TO PREDICT TOXICITY—ROOM FOR JUVENILE ANIMAL STUDIES

When evaluating antimicrobials, the targets are pathogenic bacteria, and consequently any effects on human cells and tissues are, by definition, adverse.[27] This fact underscores the importance of safety evaluation, as the profile of adverse reactions may greatly differ between newborns and older children or adults. RCTs are often too limited in patients' sample size or too short in duration to detect any adverse events, which can be rare or may occur many years after treatment discontinuation. Indeed, most of the available information about adverse events has been derived from observational studies even in the adult population. Observational studies, either case-control or large-scale observational follow-up studies, enable adequate assessment of drug safety and have been proved to be more adequate than RCTs in evaluating safety issues.[61] Observational controlled studies should be implemented to obtain information on antibiotic safety in neonates, until 1 or 2 years of age, and should be completed by longer follow-up studies including patients who were exclusively treated with the test antibiotic until school age (6–7 years) as recommended by regulatory guidelines.[62]

Juvenile animal studies are recommended by the EMA.[63] As an example, juvenile mice studies were performed in the TINN project to evaluate the potential effects of ciprofloxacin, namely, impact on growth, neurodevelopmental toxicity, and articular toxicity. As previously stated, juvenile animal toxicity studies can be useful, although considerations on species' specificity and concerns about the physiologic comparability with humans are numerous.

CHALLENGE 9: TO DEVELOP ADAPTED FORMULATIONS

Formulations for use in neonates are required because in most cases, available age-appropriate formulations are either too concentrated, requiring multiple dilutions associated with dilution errors, or too diluted, associated with liquid overload, or even contain excessive quantities of drugs that are thrown away.[63,64] Although extensively debated and with a strong consensus among all specialists that there is a need for formulations specifically adapted to neonates, it is clear that all currently available incentives will not, in the majority of cases, result in a neonatal formulation that is commercially viable, at least in indications where the number of neonates to be treated is low.

SUMMARY

A pediatric study decision tree was designed to help researchers extrapolate existing knowledge on drugs from adult studies and ultimately avoid unnecessary trials in pediatrics.[65]

For antibiotics, the bacteriologic response is expected to be similar to that in adults. Therefore, PK/PD studies can support antibiotic administration in neonates by determining the appropriate dose required for targeted exposure. Extrapolating a PK/PD relationship from adults and/or children to neonates with limited PK data collected for model validation in neonates,[66] as well as using PBPK models to link dose, concentration, and response data, should be implemented.

Nevertheless, because neonatal infections present with several unique characteristics related to individual neonatal and environmental factors, the clinical response data might differ between age groups, and additional data on antibiotic response should also be collected. RCTs and methodologies specific to the neonatal population are very difficult to conduct for many reasons, but they still should be considered.

ACKNOWLEDGMENTS

John N van den Anker is in part supported by NIH grants (R01HD060543, K24DA027992, R01HD048689 and U54HD071601) and European Union FP7 grants TINN (223614), TINN2 (260908), NEUROSIS (223060), and GRIP (261060).

REFERENCES

1. Kumar P, Walker JK, Hurt KM, et al. Medication use in the neonatal intensive care unit: current patterns and off-label use of parenteral medications. J Pediatr 2008; 152:412–5.

2. d'Aloja E, Paribello F, Demontis R, et al. Off-label drugs prescription in neonatology: a physician's duty or a medical hazardous attitude? J Matern Fetal Neonatal Med 2011;24:99–100.
3. Nguyen KA, Claris O, Kassai B. Unlicensed and off-label drug use in a neonatal unit in France. Acta Paediatr 2011;100:615–7.
4. Conroy S, McIntyre J. The use of unlicensed and off-label medicines in the neonate. Semin Fetal Neonatal Med 2005;10:115–22.
5. Conroy S. Association between licence status and medication errors. Arch Dis Child 2011;96:305–6.
6. FP7 TINN project—Treat Infections in Neonates. Available at: www.tinn-project.org.
7. Kearns GL, Abdel-Rahman SM, Alander SW, et al. Developmental pharmacology—drug disposition, action, and therapy in infants and children. N Engl J Med 2003;349:1157–67.
8. Allegaert K, Verbesselt R, Naulaers G, et al. Developmental pharmacology: neonates are not just small adults. Acta Clin Belg 2008;63:16–24.
9. De Cock RF, Allegaert K, Schreuder MF, et al. Maturation of the glomerular filtration rate in neonates, as reflected by amikacin clearance. Clin Pharmacokinet 2012;51:105–17.
10. Noordewier B, Hook JB. Developmental aspects of renal pharmacology. Pharmacol Ther 1982;17:85–110.
11. Cohen-Wolkowiez M, Moran C, Benjamin DK, et al. Early and late onset sepsis in late preterm infants. Pediatr Infect Dis J 2009;28:1052–7.
12. Koenig JM, Keenan WJ. Group B streptococcus and early-onset sepsis in the era of maternal prophylaxis. Pediatr Clin North Am 2009;56:689.
13. Tudela CM, Stewart RD, Roberts SW, et al. Intrapartum evidence of early-onset group B streptococcus. Obstet Gynecol 2012;119:626–9.
14. Schuchat A, Zywicki SS, Dinsmoor MJ, et al. Risk factors and opportunities for prevention of early-onset neonatal sepsis: a multicenter case control study. Pediatrics 2000;105:21–6.
15. Benitz WE, Gould JB, Druzin ML. Antimicrobial prevention of early-onset group B streptococcal sepsis: estimates of risk reduction based on a critical literature review. Pediatrics 1999;103:1275.
16. Smaill FM. Intrapartum antibiotics for Group B streptococcal colonisation. Cochrane Database Syst Rev 2010;(3):CD000115.
17. Ohlsson A, Shah VS. Intrapartum antibiotics for known maternal Group B streptococcal colonization. Cochrane Database Syst Rev 2009;(3):CD007467.
18. Stoll BJ, Gordon T, Korones SB, et al. Late-onset sepsis in very low birth weight neonates: a report from the national institute of Child Health and Human Development Neonatal Research Network. J Pediatr 1996;129:63–71.
19. Stoll BJ, Hansen N, Fanaroff AA, et al. Changes in pathogens causing early-onset sepsis in very-low-birth-weight infants. N Engl J Med 2002;347:240–7.
20. Downey LC, Smith PB, Benjamin DK. Risk factors and prevention of late onset sepsis in premature infants. Early Hum Dev 2010;86:7–12.
21. Stoll BJ, Hansen NI, Higgins RD, et al. Very low birth weight preterm infants with early onset neonatal sepsis: the predominance of gram-negative infections continues in the National Institute of Child Health and Human Development Neonatal Research Network, 2002-2003. Pediatr Infect Dis J 2005;24:635–9.
22. Edmond K, Zaidi A. New approaches to preventing, diagnosing, and treating neonatal sepsis. PLoS Med 2010;7:e1000213.
23. Manzoni P, Stolfi I, Pugni L, et al, Italian Task Force for the Study, and Prevention of Neonatal Fungal Infections, Italian Society of Neonatology. A multicenter,

randomized trial of prophylactic fluconazole in preterm neonates. N Engl J Med 2007;356:2483–95.

24. Li RC, Zhu ZY. The integration of four major determinants of antibiotic action: bactericidal activity, post-antibiotic effect, susceptibility, and pharmacokinetics. J Chemother 2002;14:579–83.

25. European Committee on Antimicrobial Susceptibility Testing—EUCAST. Available at: http://www.eucast.org/.

26. Mouton JW, Brown DF, Apfalter P, et al. The role of pharmacokinetics/pharmaco-dynamics in setting clinical MIC breakpoints: the EUCAST approach. Clin Microbiol Infect 2012;18:E37–45.

27. Guideline on the evaluation of medicinal products indicated for treatment of bacterial infections. Committee for Human Medicinal Products (CHMP). Ref. EMA/CPMP/EWP/558/95/2011.

28. van den Anker J, Allegaert K. Clinical pharmacology in neonates and young infants: the benefit of a population-tailored approach. Expert Rev Clin Pharmacol 2012;5:5–8.

29. Johnson TN. Modelling approaches to dose estimation in children. Br J Clin Pharmacol 2005;59:663–9.

30. Anderson BJ, Allegaert K, Holford NH. Population clinical pharmacology of children: general principles. Eur J Pediatr 2006;165:741–6.

31. Smith PB, Cohen-Wolkowiez M, Castro LM, et al. Population pharmacokinetics of meropenem in plasma and cerebrospinal fluid of infants with suspected or complicated intra-abdominal infections. Pediatr Infect Dis J 2011;30:844–9.

32. van den Anker JN, Pokorna PP, Kinzig-Schippers M, et al. Meropenem pharmacokinetics in the newborn. Antimicrob Agents Chemother 2009;53:3871–9.

33. Guideline on reporting the results of population pharmacokinetic analysis. Committee for Human Medicinal Products (CHMP). 2006. EMEA/CHMP/EWP/147013/2004.

34. Guideline on the role of pharmacokinetics in the development of medicinal products in the paediatric population. Committee for Human Medicinal Products (CHMP). Ref. EMEA/CHMP/EWP/147013/2004.

35. Le Guellec C, Autret-Leca E, Odoul F, et al. Pharmacokinetic studies in neonatology: regulatory and methodologic problems. Therapie 2001;56:663–8.

36. Johnson TN, Rostami-Hodjegan A, Tucker GT. Prediction of the clearance of eleven drugs and associated variability in neonates, infants and children. Clin Pharmacokinet 2006;45:931–56.

37. Tod M, Jullien V, Pons G. Facilitation of drug evaluation in children by population methods and modelling. Clin Pharmacokinet 2008;47:231–43.

38. Zingg W, Pfister R, Posfay-Barbe KM, et al. Secular trends in antibiotic use among neonates: 2001-2008. Pediatr Infect Dis J 2011;30:365–70.

39. Zhao W, Jacqz-Aigrain E. Principles of therapeutic drug monitoring. Handb Exp Pharmacol 2011;205:77–90.

40. Rodvold KA. Pharmacodynamics of antiinfective therapy: taking what we know to the patient's bedside. Pharmacotherapy 2001;21:319S–30S.

41. Gunderson BW, Ross GH, Ibrahim KH, et al. What do we really know about antibiotic pharmacodynamics? Pharmacotherapy 2001;21:302S–18S.

42. Nicolau DP. Optimizing outcomes with antimicrobial therapy through pharmacodynamic profiling. J Infect Chemother 2003;9:292–6.

43. Li W, Tse FL. Dried blood spot sampling in combination with LC-MS/MS for quantitative analysis of small molecules. Biomed Chromatogr 2010;24:49–65.

44. Edelbroek PM, Heijden J, Stolk LM. Dried blood spot methods in therapeutic drug monitoring: methods, assays, and pitfalls. Ther Drug Monit 2009;31:327–36.
45. Gross AS. Best practice in therapeutic drug monitoring. Br J Clin Pharmacol 2001;52:5S–10S.
46. Dunne J. The European Regulation on medicines for paediatric use. Paediatr Respir Rev 2007;8:177–83.
47. Lehmann B. Regulation (EC) No 1901/2006 on medicinal products for paediatric use & clinical research in vulnerable populations. Child Adolesc Psychiatry Ment Health 2008;2:37.
48. Permanand G, Mossialos E, McKee M. The EU's new paediatric medicines legislation: serving children's needs? Arch Dis Child 2007;92:808–11.
49. Rocchi F, Tomasi P. The development of medicines for children. Part of a series on Pediatric Pharmacology, guest edited by Gianvincenzo Zuccotti, Emilio Clementi, and Massimo Molteni. Pharmacol Res 2011;64:169–75.
50. Olski TM, Lampus SF, Gherarducci G, et al. Three years of paediatric regulation in the European Union. Eur J Clin Pharmacol 2011;67:245–52.
51. Angoulvant F, Kaguelidou F, Dauger S, et al. Fewer infants than older patients in paediatric randomised controlled trials. Eur J Epidemiol 2010;25:593–601.
52. Cohen E, Uleryk E, Jasuja M, et al. An absence of pediatric randomized controlled trials in general medical journals, 1985–2004. J Clin Epidemiol 2007;60:118–23.
53. Guideline on the investigation of medicinal products in the term and preterm neonate. Committee for medicinal products for human use (CHMP) and paediatric committee (PDCO). 2009. Available at: http://www.emea.europa.eu.
54. International Conference of Harmonization of technical requirements for registration of pharmaceutics for human use. ICH. Harmonized tripartite guideline. Clinical investigation of medicinal products in the paediatric population. Available at: http://www.ich.org/products/guidelines/efficacy/efficacy-single/article/clinical-investigation-of-medicinal-products-in-the-pediatric-population.html.
55. Singhal N, Oberle K, Burgess E, et al. Parents' perceptions of research with newborns. J Perinatol 2002;22:57–63.
56. Singhal N, Oberle K, Darwish A, et al. Attitudes of health-care providers towards research with newborn babies. J Perinatol 2004;24:775–82.
57. Steinbrook R. Testing medications in children. N Engl J Med 2002;31(347):1462–70.
58. D'Agostino RB, d'Agostino RB. Estimating treatment effects using observational data. JAMA 2007;297:314–6.
59. Schmoor C, Caputo A, Schumacher M. Evidence from non randomized studies: a case study on the estimation of causal effects. Am J Epidemiol 2008;167:1120–9.
60. Johnston SC, Henneman T, McCulloch CE, et al. Modeling treatment effects on binary outcomes with grouped-treatment variables and individual covariates. Am J Epidemiol 2002;156:753–60.
61. Vandenbroucke JP. When are observational studies as credible as randomised trials? Lancet 2004;363:1728–31.
62. Reflection paper: formulations of choice for the paediatric population. EMEA/CHMP/PEG/194810/2005. Available at: http://www.emea.europa.eu.
63. Guideline on the need for non-clinical testing in juvenile animals of pharmaceutical for paediatric indications. 2008. Ref. EMEA/CHMP/SWP/169215/2005.
64. Wong IC, Wong LY, Cranswick NE. Minimising medication errors in children. Arch Dis Child 2009;94:161–4.
65. Guidance for Industry. Exposure-response relationships—study design, data analysis, and regulatory applications U.S. Department of Health and Human

Services Food and Drug Administration Center for Drug Evaluation and Research (CDER) Center for Biologics Evaluation and Research (CBER). 2003. Available at: http://www.fda.gov/cber/guidelines.htm.

66. Lee H, Yim DS, Zhou H, et al. Evidence of effectiveness: how much can we extrapolate from existing studies? AAPS J 2005;7:E467–74.

Pharmacotherapy for Pulmonary Hypertension

Robin H. Steinhorn, MD

KEYWORDS

- Pulmonary hypertension • Pulmonary vasculature • Vasodilator • Nitric oxide
- Phosphodiesterase • Prostacyclin • Endothelin

KEY POINTS

- Pediatric pulmonary hypertension remains a devastating illness that requires more study to appropriately adapt therapies for the unique features of the pediatric lung and its vasculature.
- Much progress has been made over the last decade, and therapies are now available that better target specific abnormalities in vascular signaling.
- Future study will likely focus on a better understanding of the signaling pathways and how they interact. For example, the combination of strategies that increase cyclic guanosine monophosphate and cyclic adenosine monophosphate together may be more effective than either treatment alone.
- It is hoped that earlier identification, combined with the development of novel and more specific therapies, will improve the life span and quality of life of these children.

NORMAL PULMONARY VASCULAR TRANSITION

During fetal life the placenta serves as the organ of gas exchange, and the fetal circulation uses a series of adaptive mechanisms to maximize delivery of oxygen to metabolically active organs such as the brain, gut, and kidney. The most highly oxygenated blood enters the fetus via the umbilical vein. To efficiently direct oxygenated blood to the systemic circulation and minimize oxygen loss, almost 90% of fetal blood flow is diverted past the lungs via anatomic shunts through the foramen ovale and the ductus arteriosus. While the lung rapidly grows its network of small pulmonary arteries during the second half of gestation,[1] blood flow in the pulmonary circulation remains highly restricted by hypoxic pulmonary vasoconstriction of small pulmonary arteries, which is reversed at birth by the sudden increase in lung oxygenation when the newborn takes his or her first breath. After birth, a rapid decrease in pulmonary vascular

Department of Pediatrics, The Ann and Robert H. Lurie Children's Hospital of Chicago, Northwestern University, 225 East Chicago Avenue, Chicago, IL 60611, USA
E-mail address: r-steinhorn@northwestern.edu

Pediatr Clin N Am 59 (2012) 1129–1146
http://dx.doi.org/10.1016/j.pcl.2012.07.011
0031-3955/12/$ – see front matter © 2012 Elsevier Inc. All rights reserved.

resistance and increase in pulmonary vascular flow occurs in response to lung expansion, increased oxygen tension, and increased pH. Pulmonary artery pressure and vascular resistance decrease more slowly, with pulmonary arterial pressure reaching its nadir approximately 2 to 3 weeks after birth. However, the responsiveness to hypoxia is retained into adulthood, and pulmonary hypertension can be easily triggered in the newborn period by hypoxic lung disease, apnea, or other causes.

DEFINITION AND CLASSIFICATION OF PEDIATRIC PULMONARY HYPERTENSION

Pulmonary hypertension is necessary to support gas exchange in the fetus, but if pulmonary arterial pressure is elevated after birth or during infancy or childhood, pulmonary hypertension becomes a serious medical problem with substantial mortality and morbidity. Pulmonary hypertension is classically defined as a mean pulmonary artery pressure of at least 25 mm Hg at rest, with a pulmonary capillary wedge pressure of 15 mm Hg or less. Numerous disease processes can produce pulmonary hypertension in both adults and children, but these 2 populations are quite different when considering classification, genetic causes and, in some cases, treatment. This difference exists largely because the exposure of the developing lung to pathologic and/or environmental insults affects lung adaptation, development, and growth, leading to far greater complexity of phenotypes.[2] The classifications of pulmonary hypertension introduced at the World Health Organization Symposium in 1998[3] and subsequently modified at the Venice and Dana Point Symposia[4,5] were primarily designed for use in adult diseases, and have been difficult to apply to pediatric populations. A new pediatric classification scheme was developed by an expert panel in Panama City in 2011 to better address the developmental underpinnings of pulmonary vascular disease in children.[2,6] For instance, while idiopathic pulmonary arterial hypertension occurs in children, pulmonary hypertension very commonly occurs in association with congenital heart disease, or other lung diseases such as lung hypoplasia or bronchopulmonary dysplasia (BPD). The latter group appears to be growing, and represents a significant proportion of patients followed by pediatric pulmonary hypertension programs. Pulmonary hypertension affects roughly one-third of infants with moderate to severe BPD,[7,8] and results in greater morbidity and mortality, poor growth and neurodevelopmental outcome, long-term mechanical ventilation support, and death due to right heart dysfunction and multiorgan failure.[9,10] Pulmonary vascular disease also contributes to the morbidity and mortality of other pediatric diseases such as sickle cell disease, interstitial lung diseases, and cystic fibrosis.[11] Relatively little is known about the epidemiology of pediatric pulmonary hypertension, and comprehensive registries to support phenotyping and clinical research are needed.[12]

Persistent pulmonary hypertension of the newborn (PPHN) is a unique and specific type of pulmonary hypertension that occurs in the neonatal period as a failure to achieve the normal drop in pulmonary vascular resistance in the early neonatal period. PPHN is a syndrome that complicates a wide range of neonatal cardiopulmonary diseases, and affects up to 10% of all preterm and term neonates that require neonatal intensive care unit (NICU) support for respiratory failure. Moderate or severe PPHN affects up to 2 to 6 per 1000 live births, and complicates the course of 10% of all infants admitted to the NICU.[13] These circulatory abnormalities are also responsible for an 8% to 10% risk of death and a 25% risk of long-term neurodevelopmental morbidity. The long-term impact of PPHN on pediatric and adult pulmonary vascular function is another important area for future research.

PHARMACOTHERAPY FOR PULMONARY HYPERTENSION

The aims of therapy for pulmonary arterial hypertension are selective pulmonary vasodilation, restoration of normal endothelial function, and reversal of remodeling of the pulmonary vasculature. All of these serve to reduce right ventricular afterload and prevent right ventricular failure. The choice of agents will often depend on the severity and acuity of illness; for instance, acute pulmonary vasodilation is needed for PPHN and acute pulmonary hypertensive crises after cardiopulmonary bypass, but long-term therapy may focus more on vascular remodeling. The main therapeutic avenues involve the nitric oxide (NO), prostacyclin, and endothelin pathways, which are summarized in excellent recent comprehensive reviews.[11,14,15] It is also of importance that the scientific understanding and therapeutic management of pulmonary hypertension are changing rapidly.

Nitric Oxide

NO is synthesized from the terminal nitrogen of L-arginine by the enzyme nitric oxide synthase (NOS). Three isoforms of NOS are present in the lung, although endothelial NOS (eNOS) is regarded as the most important regulator of NO production in the lung vasculature. NO is a gas molecule that diffuses freely from the endothelium to the vascular smooth muscle cell. The biological effects of NO in vascular smooth muscle are mediated primarily through activation of soluble guanylate cyclase, which converts guanosine triphosphate to cyclic guanosine monophosphate (cGMP) (**Fig. 1**). cGMP serves as a second messenger that relaxes vascular smooth muscle through activation of cGMP-gated ion channels and activation of cGMP-dependent protein kinase. However, recent studies indicate that alternative NO signaling pathways may also exist through reaction of NO with protein thiols to form S-nitrosothiols, which may induce vasodilation or protein modification.[16]

Lung eNOS mRNA and protein are present in the early fetus, but both increase toward the end of gestation, readying the lung to adapt to the postnatal need for pulmonary vasodilation. This increase in lung eNOS content explains the emergence of responsiveness to endothelium-dependent vasodilators, such as oxygen and acetylcholine, in late gestation.[17] Many factors associated with pulmonary hypertension have the capacity to perturb eNOS function, even if protein levels are sufficient. Presumably this is because the normal catalytic function of eNOS depends on numerous posttranslational modifications, including association with the chaperone protein Hsp90 and availability of essential substrates and cofactors including L-arginine, tetrahydrobiopterin (BH_4), nicotinamide adenine dinucleotide phosphate (reduced), and calcium/calmodulin. Depletion of Hsp90 or biopterin will reduce production or bioavailability of NO, and will also uncouple eNOS, resulting in incomplete reduction of molecular oxygen with subsequent formation of superoxide, essentially turning the enzyme into a source of oxidant stress.[18,19]

NO is currently approved by the Food and Drug Administration (FDA) only for treatment of PPHN in the neonatal period. Because eNOS is decreased or dysfunctional in PPHN, inhaled NO (iNO) is thought to provide specific replacement therapy that is inhaled directly to airspaces approximating the pulmonary vascular bed. While most commonly administered with mechanical ventilation, iNO can also be provided via continuous positive airway pressure or nasal cannula devices, although the concentration may need to be increased to account for the entrainment of room air.[20]

The safety and efficacy of iNO for PPHN have been particularly well studied through large placebo-controlled trials. iNO significantly decreases the need for extracorporeal membrane oxygenation (ECMO) support in newborns with PPHN, although mortality

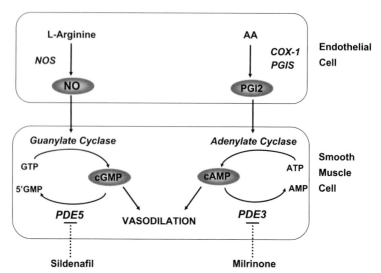

Fig. 1. Nitric oxide (NO) and prostacyclin (PGI2) signaling pathways in the regulation of pulmonary vascular tone. NO is synthesized by nitric oxide synthase (NOS) from the terminal nitrogen of L-arginine. NO stimulates soluble guanylate cyclase (sGC) to increase intracellular cyclic guanosine monophosphate (cGMP). PGI2 is an arachidonic acid (AA) metabolite formed by cyclooxygenase (COX-1) and prostacyclin synthase (PGIS) in the vascular endothelium. PGI2 stimulates adenylate cyclase in vascular smooth muscle cells, which increases intracellular cyclic adenosine monophosphate (cAMP). Both cGMP and cAMP indirectly decrease free cytosolic calcium, resulting in relaxation of smooth muscle. Specific phosphodiesterases hydrolyze cGMP and cAMP, thus regulating the intensity and duration of their vascular effects. Inhibition of these phosphodiesterases with agents such as sildenafil and milrinone may enhance pulmonary vasodilation. (*Reproduced from* Porta NF, Steinhorn RH. Pulmonary vasodilator therapy in the NICU: inhaled nitric oxide, sildenafil, and other pulmonary vasodilating agents. Clin Perinatol 2012;39:151; with permission.)

or length of hospitalization was not affected in any study. Data from the large registry maintained by the Extracorporeal Life Support Organization also indicate a 40% reduction in the number of neonates cannulated for ECMO, coincident with the FDA approval of iNO. By encompassing a range of disease severity, these studies also highlight that starting iNO for respiratory failure that is in earlier stages of evolution (for an oxygenation index of 15–25) does not decrease the incidence of ECMO and/ or death, or improve other patient outcomes.[21,22] On the other hand, delaying iNO initiation until respiratory failure is advanced (oxygenation index of >40) may increase length of time on oxygen.[23] In longer-term follow-up, iNO did not significantly alter the incidence of chronic lung disease or neurodevelopmental impairment relative to placebo.

Based on the available data, iNO should be initiated at a dose of 20 ppm, after confirming PPHN and ruling out congenital heart disease and left ventricular dysfunction. A failure to respond to 20 ppm is only rarely followed by improvement at higher doses.[24] The greatest improvement in oxygenation occurs in infants with extrapulmonary right-to-left shunting but without significant pulmonary parenchymal disease. Even if the total pulmonary vascular resistance (PVR) does not decrease, iNO can improve oxygenation through a microselective effect that reduces intrapulmonary shunting. When iNO is stopped abruptly, rebound pulmonary hypertension can develop.[25] This potentially life-threatening phenomenon can occur even if no improvement in oxygenation has been observed, and has raised questions about whether vascular cells respond to NO by upregulating vasoconstrictor pathways.[26,27] However, from a practical standpoint, the clinical problem can usually be overcome by weaning iNO to 1 ppm before discontinuation.

iNO is used to treat many other forms of pediatric and neonatal pulmonary hypertension, although its role in those settings is less well defined. For instance, randomized studies have not demonstrated a consistent improvement in oxygenation in infants with congenital diaphragmatic hernia,[28] although there appear to be benefits of stabilizing infants and preventing cardiac arrest before ECMO.[29] Up to one-third of premature infants with BPD will develop some degree of pulmonary hypertension or cor pulmonale,[7,8] and alterations in NO signaling appear to play a role in the vascular and lung injury.[30] A recent case series indicates that iNO may reduce established BPD-associated pulmonary hypertension to a greater degree than oxygen alone.[31] On the other hand, large clinical trials have shown inconsistent benefit when iNO is used to prevent BPD.[32–35]

Outside of the NICU setting, the most common clinical use of iNO is for the infant or child with congenital heart disease with associated pulmonary hypertension. Postoperatively, iNO is frequently used to prevent or treat pulmonary hypertensive crises, improve oxygenation, and increase cardiac output. Pulmonary hypertension commonly develops in infants with congenital heart lesions associated with pulmonary overcirculation, such as truncus arteriosus or atrioventricular canal. If the heart lesion is not corrected, medial and intimal thickening occur in the pulmonary vasculature over time, which eventually leads to luminal obliteration. Acute life-threatening exacerbation of pulmonary hypertension following cardiopulmonary bypass is a serious clinical problem even in very young infants. In addition, children undergoing cavopulmonary connections for single ventricle lesions require low PVR for surgical success. Several small single-center studies indicate that iNO can attenuate pulmonary hypertension in at-risk postoperative patients, reduce the number of pulmonary hypertension crises, and shorten time on mechanical ventilation.[36] In one larger randomized trial of pediatric patients, iNO (20 ppm) significantly decreased PVR and pulmonary hypertensive crises, and shortened the time to extubation readiness.[37] Responsivity to iNO has also been proposed as predictive of successful operability in patients with pulmonary hypertension associated with congenital heart disease.[38]

In clinical studies of pediatric patients with severe acute respiratory distress syndrome (ARDS), iNO produced selective pulmonary vasodilation and improved systemic oxygenation.[39] However, subsequent randomized controlled trials did not demonstrate a beneficial effect on mortality or duration of mechanical ventilation in pediatric or adult patients.[40,41] Although a transient improvement in oxygenation was observed in most of these studies, it has been speculated that because most patients dying from acute respiratory distress syndrome suffer from multiple organ systems failure, lung-selective therapy such as iNO may not improve the overall survival rate.[42] These results likely indicate that the problem of pediatric respiratory failure involves much more than vascular dysfunction, and that there is still much to be learned about the role of NO in primary lung injury.

As our understanding of NO signaling evolves, strategies will emerge that enhance function of the native NOS enzyme. For instance, sufficient synthesis of L-arginine is necessary for optimal NOS function,[43] and exogenous L-arginine supplementation enhances NOS activity in vitro. Although arginine supplementation has been less successful when attempted in vivo, L-arginine can be endogenously synthesized from L-citrulline by a recycling pathway consisting of 2 enzymes, argininosuccinate synthase and argininosuccinate lyase. Recent studies indicate that providing exogenous

L-citrulline may reverse NOS dysfunction in animal models of neonatal pulmonary hypertension.[44] In clinical studies, oral L-citrulline increased levels of both plasma citrulline and arginine in high-risk children undergoing cardiopulmonary bypass.[45] Intravenous L-citrulline has been shown to be safe and well tolerated in children undergoing cardiopulmonary bypass,[46] and clinical trials are under way.

Sildenafil

cGMP is the second messenger that regulates contractility of smooth muscle through activation of cGMP-dependent kinases, phosphodiesterases, and ion channels. In vascular smooth muscle cells, NO-mediated activation of soluble guanylate cyclase is a major source of cGMP production. Because cGMP is such a central mediator of vascular contractility, it is not surprising that its concentrations are regulated within a relatively narrow range to allow fine-tuning of vascular responses to oxygen, NO, and other stimuli.

Phosphodiesterases are a large family of enzymes that hydrolyze and inactivate cGMP and cyclic adenosine monophosphate (cAMP), thus regulating their concentrations and effects as well as facilitating cross-talk between the 2 cyclic nucleotides. Type 5 phosphodiesterase (PDE5) is especially highly expressed in the lung, and not only uses cGMP as a substrate but also contains a specific cGMP-binding domain that serves to activate its catabolic activity. As the primary enzyme responsible for regulating cGMP, PDE5 may well represent the most important regulator of NO-mediated vascular relaxation in the normal pulmonary vascular transition after birth.[47]

Fetal and neonatal lung development, along with commonly used therapies, appears to regulate PDE expression and activity. In developing lambs and rats, PDE5 is expressed according to specific developmental trajectories that result in a peak of expression during late fetal life, followed by an acute decrease around the time of birth.[48,49] This drop in PDE5 activity would be expected to amplify the effects of NO produced by birth-related stimuli such as oxygen and shear stress . By contrast, when pulmonary vessels of fetal lambs undergo remodeling by chronic intrauterine pulmonary hypertension, PDE5 activity increases relative to controls.[50,51] Even more striking is that after birth, PDE5 activity does not decrease in this lamb model of PPHN, but rather increases dramatically to levels well above those observed in spontaneously breathing or ventilated control lambs.[48,51] This abnormal increase in activity would be expected to diminish responses to both endogenous and exogenous NO, and could explain the incomplete clinical efficacy of iNO in some patients. It is also interesting that recent reports indicate that PDE5 is highly expressed in the remodeled human right ventricle, raising the possibility that sildenafil therapy may improve right ventricular function.[52]

Although sildenafil is presently only approved by the FDA for the treatment of pulmonary hypertension in adult patients, it is frequently used in children. The first clinical report of sildenafil use in children was to facilitate weaning from iNO following corrective surgery for congenital heart disease.[53] In this initial case series, enteral sildenafil increased circulating cGMP and allowed 2 of 3 infants to wean from iNO without rebound pulmonary hypertension. Subsequent case series expanded these initial observations to show that enteral sildenafil may facilitate iNO discontinuation in infants with critical illness,[54] and may also reduce duration of mechanical ventilation and length of stay in the intensive care unit.[55]

A recent large trial randomized children (approximately two-thirds of whom had pulmonary hypertension associated with cardiac disease) to low-, medium-, or high-dose sildenafil versus placebo for 16 weeks.[56] The investigators concluded that sildenafil monotherapy for 16 weeks is well tolerated for pediatric pulmonary hypertension.

The primary end point of improvement in peak oxygen consumption during exercise testing was only marginally different between sildenafil and placebo ($P = .056$), but greater effects were noted in the medium-dose and high-dose groups. Adverse events included pyrexia, upper respiratory infections, increased erections, and nausea. Patients who completed the 16-week trial were eligible to receive sildenafil for extended treatment (STARTS-2). Although there was not a placebo arm, the investigators noted that survival rates compared favorably with historical rates. The data also suggest that the overall profile favors the medium dose (roughly 0.5–1 mg/kg given 3 times daily), and there should be consideration for adjusting sildenafil to a medium dose for long-term use. The clinical use of enteral sildenafil has also been reported in infants with PPHN, including one small, randomized controlled trial with oral sildenafil that showed a dramatic improvement in oxygenation and survival.[57]

Enteral administration of sildenafil could raise concerns about gastrointestinal absorption, particularly in critically ill patients who may have compromised intestinal perfusion. An intravenous preparation of sildenafil was approved for clinical use in 2010. Two studies have reported the use of intravenous sildenafil in critically ill children. One enrolled pediatric patients with postoperative pulmonary hypertension after cardiac surgery to 1 of 3 intravenous doses of sildenafil or placebo for a minimum of 24 hours.[58] Median time to extubation and length of time in intensive care was reduced in the sildenafil arm, although the study was underpowered. An open-label pilot trial in infants with PPHN demonstrated that intravenous sildenafil, delivered as a continuous infusion, improved oxygenation.[59] Furthermore, 7 infants received sildenafil without prior use of iNO, and all experienced a significant improvement in oxygenation within 4 hours after sildenafil administration. Only 1 of these 7 infants required iNO, and the other 6 infants improved and survived to hospital discharge without requiring either iNO or ECMO.[59] A randomized controlled trial is currently under way to evaluate the efficacy of intravenous sildenafil in infants with moderate PPHN (NCT01409031).

Sildenafil is also an attractive therapeutic option for infants with chronic pulmonary hypertension caused by congenital diaphragmatic hernia or bronchopulmonary dysplasia, because it can be given orally and over longer periods of time with apparent low toxicity. In a rat model of hyperoxia-induced BPD, chronic use of sildenafil decreased medial wall thickness and right ventricular hypertrophy, and improved lung alveolarization.[60] A clinical case series examined the effect of oral sildenafil in 25 infants and children (<2 years old) with pulmonary hypertension caused by chronic lung disease (mostly BPD). Most patients showed some improvement after a median treatment interval of 40 days, and the majority of infants were able to wean off iNO.[61] Five patients died after initiation of sildenafil treatment, but none died of refractory pulmonary hypertension or right heart failure. A similar approach might benefit some infants with chronic pulmonary hypertension associated with lung hypoplasia.[62] These important pilot studies suggest that sildenafil is well tolerated in infants with pulmonary hypertension caused by chronic lung disease, and paves the way to further studies in this especially challenging population.

An interesting recent study showed that in a rat model of congenital diaphragmatic hernia, antenatal administration of sildenafil to the dam reduced PDE5 activity and increased cGMP, and produced striking reductions in the vascular findings of persistent pulmonary hypertension.[63] This finding is the first indication that pulmonary hypertension can be treated before birth, and will likely open up a productive line of investigation in antenatal diagnosis and treatment.

Tadalafil is a longer-acting selective PDE5 inhibitor recently approved by the FDA for the treatment of adult pulmonary hypertension. A recent retrospective report examined pediatric patients with pulmonary hypertension who were converted from sildenafil to tadalafil to achieve once-daily dosing at 1 mg/kg/d.[64] In addition to the ease of administration, about half of the patients exhibited significant improvements in mean pulmonary arterial pressure and PVR index measured at heart catheterization. Side-effect profiles were similar for the 2 agents. These results indicate that tadalafil may be safe for pediatric patients with pulmonary arterial hypertension, and has the advantages of only once-daily dosing.

Prostanoids

A complementary vasodilatory pathway in the fetal lung is mediated by prostacyclin (PGI_2) and cAMP (see **Fig. 1**). Prostacyclin is a metabolite of arachidonic acid that is endogenously produced by the vascular endothelium. The vascular effects of PGI_2 are mediated through its binding to a membrane IP receptor that activates adenylate cyclase and increases cAMP, which triggers relaxation of smooth muscle cells through reducing intracellular calcium concentrations. Prostacyclin production appears to increase in late gestation and early postnatal life,[65,66] indicating its importance in promoting the neonatal pulmonary vascular transition. Pulmonary hypertension in both neonates and older children is characterized by a decrease in the biosynthesis of prostacyclin accompanied by increased synthesis of the vasoconstrictor thromboxane A_2.[67] Furthermore, the PGI_2 receptor (IP) is decreased in adult and pediatric patients with pulmonary hypertension, and animal studies point to its contribution to altered vasodilation in PPHN.[68] Prostacyclin is a potent vasodilator in both the systemic and pulmonary circulations and also has antiplatelet effects.[69] Prostacyclin was one of the earliest pulmonary vasodilators used for clinical treatment of pulmonary hypertension, and was approved by the FDA in 1995 for the treatment of severe chronic pulmonary arterial hypertension.

At present, several prostanoid drug preparations are available for clinical use. Epoprostenol, delivered as a continuous intravenous infusion, remains a mainstay of therapy, and has been shown to improve pulmonary hemodynamics, quality of life, exercise capacity, and survival in adults and children with idiopathic and secondary pulmonary hypertension.[70–75] These significant long-term effects may occur even if short-term vasodilation is not observed, suggesting beneficial effects on platelet aggregation, inhibition of smooth muscle cell growth, and/or protection of right ventricular function.[76] The optimal dose of intravenous epoprostenol is not well defined, although children usually need higher doses than adults. In some children, rapid dosage escalation of infusions of PGI_2 may be necessary to promote acute pulmonary vasodilation, and tolerance can develop that requires periodic dose escalation. Adverse effects include inhibition of platelet aggregation, systemic vasodilation, and alterations in hepatic enzymes, and common side effects include diarrhea and jaw pain. Epoprostenol requires dedicated venous access, typically through a central venous line. The drug is chemically unstable at neutral pH and room temperature, and its short half-life requires continuous intravenous infusion with cold packs to maintain drug stability. Sudden interruption of the medication can lead to severe rebound pulmonary hypertension.[77]

While used commonly for chronic management, intravenous epoprostenol is less frequently used for acute pulmonary hypertension, because of the risks of ventilation-perfusion mismatch and systemic hypotension. For this reason, inhaled, oral, and subcutaneous routes of delivery have been pursued. When given as an inhaled aerosol, the vasodilator effects of PGI_2 tend to be limited to the pulmonary circulation, making this strategy appealing when acute pulmonary vasodilation is needed.[78] Reports in children have been generally positive, although to date there are few studies reporting the use of inhaled PGI_2 in neonates with PPHN.[79–81] The author's experience suggests that inhaled PGI_2 is well tolerated and may assist in recovery without ECMO in infants with severe pulmonary hypertension and inadequate response to iNO.[82] Although the optimal dosing of inhaled PGI_2 in critically ill mechanically ventilated infants is not known, short-term studies in newborn lambs with pulmonary hypertension suggest that doses up to 500 ng/kg/min produce progressive improvements in pulmonary artery pressure, PVR, and pulmonary blood flow.[83] In the author's clinical experience, doses of 50 to 100 ng/kg/min produce rapid improvement in oxygenation in infants who are refractory to iNO.[84] Concerns regarding the use of inhaled PGI_2 include airway irritation from the alkaline solution needed to maintain drug stability, rebound pulmonary hypertension if the drug is abruptly discontinued, loss of medication into the circuit owing to condensation, and alteration of characteristics of mechanical ventilation from the added gas flow needed for the nebulization. Prolonged use of continuous inhaled PGI_2 could also lead to damage of mechanical ventilator valves. Further investigations will likely focus on preparations specifically designed for inhalation, such as iloprost or treprostinil, as discussed below. An oral agent, beraprost, is a prostacyclin analogue that is less potent than epoprostenol, but chemically stable with a longer half-life of approximately 1 hour. Beraprost is currently only approved for the treatment of pulmonary hypertension in Japan and South Korea, although new oral prostanoids are currently under investigation in adult populations.

Iloprost is a chemically stable prostacyclin analogue with a half-life to 20 to 30 minutes that has been studied as an inhaled compound.[85] The advantages of an inhaled agent include improved selectivity for the pulmonary vascular bed, which is superior for patients with acute pulmonary hypertensive crisis with hemodynamic compromise and low cardiac output. This approach may improve ventilation-perfusion mismatch and oxygenation, and successful use has been reported in pediatric populations, including those with PPHN and postcardiopulmonary bypass,[85–92] and those refractory to iNO or sildenafil.[93,94] Acute bronchoconstriction is a potential adverse event, and compliance can be poor because of the need for frequent aerosol administrations, up to 8 to 12 times daily.[11]

Treprostinil is a prostacyclin analogue that is stable at room temperature and neutral pH, and with a longer half-life of about 3 hours. Treprostinil is approved by the FDA for the treatment of chronic pulmonary hypertension in adults, and can be delivered via continuous subcutaneous or intravenous infusion as well as by inhalation. Subcutaneous treprostinil produces short-term improvements in exercise tolerance and hemodynamics in some adults with pulmonary arterial hypertension, but severe local site discomfort and induration can limit its tolerance. Subcutaneous treprostinil has been used to transition some children who were chronically stable on intravenous epoprostenol,[95] and may improve the clinical course in children as an add-on therapy.[96] Placebo-controlled trials have demonstrated improved exercise tolerance, clinical symptoms, and hemodynamics in patients with pulmonary hypertension, including children.[97]

PDE3 Inhibition: Milrinone

Similar to the NO-cGMP pathway, prostacyclin-cAMP signaling is regulated by cAMP-hydrolyzing PDE isoforms such as PDE3 and PDE4. The author's group recently reported that PDE3A expression and activity in the resistance pulmonary arteries increases dramatically by 24 hours after birth.[98] These results were unexpected, as one would have predicted that PDE3 activity would decrease after birth to facilitate cAMP accumulation, similar to the patterns reported for PDE5.[47,84] It was also observed that addition of iNO dramatically increased PDE3 levels, which suggests that inhibition of PDE3 activity might enhance the vasodilatory effects of iNO/cGMP signaling in addition to its expected effects on the cAMP pathways.[68]

Milrinone is an inhibitor of PDE3 activity that is frequently used in pediatric patients to improve myocardial contractility after cardiac surgery.[99,100] Milrinone may also bypass abnormalities in endogenous PGI_2 production and/or enhance availability of cAMP, which could be useful for acute treatment of pulmonary hypertension. Recent studies have shown a potential effect on the pulmonary vascular bed as well as synergistic effects with inhaled prostanoids.[68,100,101] In animal studies, milrinone decreases pulmonary artery pressure and resistance, and acts additively with iNO.[83,102] Clinical reports indicate that milrinone may decrease rebound pulmonary hypertension after iNO is stopped,[27] and may enhance pulmonary vasodilation of infants with PPHN refractory to iNO.[103] A study to better define the pharmacokinetic profile of milrinone in infants with PPHN is ongoing (NCT01088997), and should lead to clinical trials designed to test its efficacy.

Endothelin Receptor Antagonists: Bosentan

Endothelin-1 (ET-1) is a 21-amino-acid protein formed by serial enzymatic cleavage of a larger prepropeptide to the vasoactive form, and is one of the most potent vasoconstrictors described in the pulmonary vasculature (**Fig. 2**). ET-1 is principally produced in endothelial cells in response to hypoxia, and is known to promote endothelial cell dysfunction, proliferation and remodeling of smooth muscle cells, inflammation, and fibrosis.[104] ET-1 binds to 2 receptor subtypes, ET receptors A and B, and the binding of ET-1 to the ETA receptor on smooth muscle cells produces vasoconstriction. Increased ET-1 production and altered ET-receptor activity have been consistently reported in neonatal and adult animal models of pulmonary hypertension, and lung ET-1 expression and plasma ET levels were elevated in severe pulmonary arterial hypertension in adults.[105] In several animal and human studies, plasma ET-1 concentrations are consistently increased during and following cardiopulmonary bypass, suggesting a role for ET-1 in the pathophysiology of pulmonary hypertension induced by cardiopulmonary bypass.[106–109] ET-1 is believed to play a role in the pathogenesis of

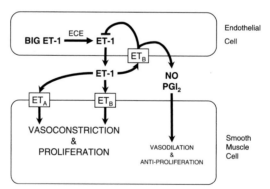

Fig. 2. Endothelin-1 (ET-1) signaling pathway in the regulation of pulmonary vascular tone. Big ET-1 is cleaved to ET-1 by endothelin-converting enzyme (ECE) in endothelial cells. ET-1 binds its specific receptors ETA and ETB with differential effects. Binding of ET-1 to ETA or ETB on smooth muscle cells leads to vasoconstrictive and proliferative effects. ETB are transiently expressed on endothelial cells after birth; binding of ET-1 to ETB on endothelial cells leads to downregulation of ECE activity and increased production of nitric oxide (NO) and prostacyclin (PGI_2), which lead to vasodilation and antiproliferation. (*Reproduced from* Porta NF, Steinhorn RH. Pulmonary vasodilator therapy in the NICU: inhaled nitric oxide, sildenafil, and other pulmonary vasodilating agents. Clin Perinatol 2012;39:151; with permission.)

neonatal pulmonary hypertension, and endothelin blockade augments pulmonary vasodilation.[104] A recent prospective examination of 40 newborns with congenital diaphragmatic hernia and poor outcome also indicated that plasma ET-1 levels were highly correlated with the severity of pulmonary hypertension.[110]

Bosentan is an oral endothelin receptor antagonist (ERA) that improves exercise capacity, pulmonary vascular resistance, and quality of life in adults[111,112] and children with pulmonary hypertension.[113,114] Bosentan lowers pulmonary artery pressure and PVR in children with diverse causes of pulmonary hypertension.[113,115] Recent case reports also suggest that bosentan may improve oxygenation in neonates with PPHN,[116,117] and a clinical trial is currently under way in that population (NCT01389856). Bosentan is generally well tolerated in children, and has also been successfully used as adjunctive treatment for children receiving long-term epoprostenol therapy.[118] Bosentan may improve functional status and survival estimates for up to 2 years,[113] although these long-term improvements may not be observed in patients with cardiac disease and systemic to pulmonary shunts.[119] Risks include hepatotoxicity (dose-dependent), teratogenicity and, possibly, male infertility.[120] Liver function should be monitored monthly, although elevated aminotransferases and drug discontinuation rates are less common in young children compared with patients aged 12 years or older.[120] A specific pediatric formulation of bosentan was recently approved for use in children by the European authorities.

Ambrisentan is a selective ETA receptor antagonist with high oral bioavailability and a long half-life.[121] This agent blocks the vasoconstrictor effect of ETA receptors while maintaining the vasodilatory and clearance effects of ETB receptors. Ambrisentan has been shown to improve exercise capacity and delay clinical worsening in patients with pulmonary arterial hypertension,[122,123] and is thought to produce less liver toxicity than bosentan, but further study is needed in children. Of note, another selective ETA receptor antagonist, sitaxentan, was recently withdrawn from the market because of concerns about severe liver toxicity.

SUMMARY

Pediatric pulmonary hypertension remains a devastating illness that requires much more study if we are to adapt therapies for the unique features of the pediatric lung and its vasculature. Still, much progress has been made over the last decade, and prognosis appears to be improving with the new therapies now available. Future study will likely focus on a better understanding of the signaling pathways and how they interact. For example, the combination of strategies that increase cGMP and cAMP together may be more effective than either treatment alone. In addition, it is hoped that earlier identification, combined with the development of novel and more specific therapies, will improve the life span and quality of life of these children.

ACKNOWLEDGMENTS

The preparation of this article was supported in part by R01HL54705 (NHLBI) and U01HL102235 (NHLBI).

REFERENCES

1. Levin DL, Rudolph AM, Heymann MA, et al. Morphological development of the pulmonary vascular bed in fetal lambs. Circulation 1976;53:144–51.

2. Cerro MJ, Abman S, Diaz G, et al. A consensus approach to the classification of pediatric pulmonary hypertensive vascular disease: report from the PVRI pediatric taskforce, panama 2011. Pulm Circ 2011;1:286–98.

3. Simonneau G, Galie N, Rubin LJ, et al. Clinical classification of pulmonary hypertension. J Am Coll Cardiol 2004;43:5S–12S.

4. Simonneau G, Robbins IM, Beghetti M, et al. Updated clinical classification of pulmonary hypertension. J Am Coll Cardiol 2009;54:S43–54.

5. Humbert M, McLaughlin VV. The 4th world symposium on pulmonary hypertension. introduction. J Am Coll Cardiol 2009;54:S1–2.

6. Lammers AE, Adatia I, Cerro MJ, et al. Functional classification of pulmonary hypertension in children: report from the PVRI pediatric taskforce, panama 2011. Pulm Circ 2011;1:280–5.

7. Slaughter JL, Pakrashi T, Jones DE, et al. Echocardiographic detection of pulmonary hypertension in extremely low birth weight infants with bronchopulmonary dysplasia requiring prolonged positive pressure ventilation. J Perinatol 2011;31:635–40.

8. An HS, Bae EJ, Kim GB, et al. Pulmonary hypertension in preterm infants with bronchopulmonary dysplasia. Korean Circ J 2010;40:131–6.

9. Farquhar M, Fitzgerald DA. Pulmonary hypertension in chronic neonatal lung disease. Paediatr Respir Rev 2010;11:149–53.

10. Khemani E, McElhinney DB, Rhein L, et al. Pulmonary artery hypertension in formerly premature infants with bronchopulmonary dysplasia: clinical features and outcomes in the surfactant era. Pediatrics 2007;120: 1260–9.

11. Abman SH, Ivy DD. Recent progress in understanding pediatric pulmonary hypertension. Curr Opin Pediatr 2011;23:298–304.

12. Robbins IM, Moore TM, Blaisdell CJ, et al. Improving outcomes for pulmonary vascular disease. Am J Respir Crit Care Med 2012;185:1015–20.

13. Walsh-Sukys MC, Tyson JE, Wright LL, et al. Persistent pulmonary hypertension of the newborn in the era before nitric oxide: practice variation and outcomes. Pediatrics 2000;105:14–20.

14. Tissot C, Ivy DD, Beghetti M. Medical therapy for pediatric pulmonary arterial hypertension. J Pediatr 2010;157:528–32.

15. Oishi P, Datar SA, Fineman JR. Advances in the management of pediatric pulmonary hypertension. Respir Care 2011;56:1314–39 [discussion: 39–40].

16. Gaston BM, Carver J, Doctor A, et al. S-nitrosylation signaling in cell biology. Mol Interv 2003;3:253–63.

17. Tiktinsky MH, Morin FC III. Increasing oxygen tension dilates fetal pulmonary circulation via endothelium-derived relaxing factor. Am J Physiol Heart Circ Physiol 1993;265:H376–80.

18. Mata-Greenwood E, Jenkins C, Farrow KN, et al. eNOS function is developmentally regulated: uncoupling of eNOS occurs postnatally. Am J Physiol Lung Cell Mol Physiol 2006;290:L232–41.

19. Farrow KN, Lakshminrusimha S, Reda WJ, et al. Superoxide dismutase restores eNOS expression and function in resistance pulmonary arteries from neonatal lambs with persistent pulmonary hypertension. Am J Physiol Lung Cell Mol Physiol 2008;295:L979–87.

20. Kinsella JP, Parker TA, Ivy DD, et al. Noninvasive delivery of inhaled nitric oxide therapy for late pulmonary hypertension in newborn infants with congenital diaphragmatic hernia. J Pediatr 2003;142:397–401.

21. Konduri GG, Solimani A, Sokol GM, et al. A randomized trial of early versus standard inhaled nitric oxide therapy in term and near-term newborn infants with hypoxic respiratory failure. Pediatrics 2004;113:559–64.

22. Konduri GG, Vohr B, Robertson C, et al. Early inhaled nitric oxide therapy for term and near-term newborn infants with hypoxic respiratory failure: neurodevelopmental follow-up. J Pediatr 2007;150:235–40, 40.e1.

23. Gonzalez A, Fabres J, D'Apremont I, et al. Randomized controlled trial of early compared with delayed use of inhaled nitric oxide in newborns with a moderate respiratory failure and pulmonary hypertension. J Perinatol 2010;30:420–4.

24. Neonatal Inhaled Nitric Oxide Study Group. Inhaled nitric oxide in full-term and nearly full-term infants with hypoxic respiratory failure. N Engl J Med 1997;336: 597–604.

25. Davidson D, Barefield ES, Kattwinkel J, et al. Safety of withdrawing inhaled nitric oxide therapy in persistent pulmonary hypertension of the newborn. Pediatrics 1999;104:231–6.

26. Black SM, Heidersbach RS, McMullan DM, et al. Inhaled nitric oxide inhibits NOS activity in lambs: potential mechanism for rebound pulmonary hypertension. Am J Physiol Heart Circ Physiol 1999;277:H1849–56.

27. Thelitz S, Oishi P, Sanchez LS, et al. Phosphodiesterase-3 inhibition prevents the increase in pulmonary vascular resistance following inhaled nitric oxide withdrawal in lambs. Pediatr Crit Care Med 2004;5:234–9.

28. Neonatal Inhaled Nitric Oxide Study Group. Inhaled nitric oxide and hypoxic respiratory failure in infants with congenital diaphragmatic hernia. Pediatrics 1997;99:838–45.

29. Fliman PJ, deRegnier RA, Kinsella JP, et al. Neonatal extracorporeal life support: impact of new therapies on survival. J Pediatr 2006;148:595–9.

30. Afshar S, Gibson LL, Yuhanna IS, et al. Pulmonary NO synthase expression is attenuated in a fetal baboon model of chronic lung disease. Am J Physiol Lung Cell Mol Physiol 2003;284:L749–58.

31. Mourani PM, Ivy DD, Gao D, et al. Pulmonary vascular effects of inhaled nitric oxide and oxygen tension in bronchopulmonary dysplasia. Am J Respir Crit Care Med 2004;170:1006–13.

32. Donohue PK, Gilmore MM, Cristofalo E, et al. Inhaled nitric oxide in preterm infants: a systematic review. Pediatrics 2011;127:e414–22.

33. Steinhorn RH, Shaul PW, deRegnier RA, et al. Inhaled nitric oxide and bronchopulmonary dysplasia. Pediatrics 2011;128:e255–6 [author reply: e6–7].

34. Ballard RA, Truog WE, Cnaan A, et al. Inhaled nitric oxide in preterm infants undergoing mechanical ventilation. N Engl J Med 2006;355:343–53.

35. Hibbs AM, Walsh MC, Martin RJ, et al. One-year respiratory outcomes of preterm infants enrolled in the nitric oxide (to prevent) chronic lung disease trial. J Pediatr 2008;153:525–9.

36. Barr FE, Macrae D. Inhaled nitric oxide and related therapies. Pediatr Crit Care Med 2010;11:S30–6.

37. Miller OI, Tang SF, Keech A, et al. Inhaled nitric oxide and prevention of pulmonary hypertension after congenital heart surgery: a randomised double-blind study. Lancet 2000;356:1464–9.

38. Atz AM, Adatia I, Lock JE, et al. Combined effects of nitric oxide and oxygen during acute pulmonary vasodilator testing. J Am Coll Cardiol 1999;33: 813–9.

39. Rossaint R, Falke KJ, Lopez F, et al. Inhaled nitric oxide for the adult respiratory distress syndrome. N Engl J Med 1993;328:399–405.

40. Dobyns EL, Cornfield DN, Anas NG, et al. Multicenter randomized controlled trial of the effects of inhaled nitric oxide therapy on gas exchange in children with acute hypoxemic respiratory failure. J Pediatr 1999;134:406–12.

41. Sokol J, Jacobs SE, Bohn D. Inhaled nitric oxide for acute hypoxemic respiratory failure in children and adults. Cochrane Database Syst Rev 2003;(1):CD002787.

42. Coggins MP, Bloch KD. Nitric oxide in the pulmonary vasculature. Arterioscler Thromb Vasc Biol 2007;27:1877–85.

43. Pearson DL, Dawling S, Walsh WF, et al. Neonatal pulmonary hypertension-urea-cycle intermediates, nitric oxide production, and carbamoyl-phosphate synthetase function. N Engl J Med 2001;344:1832–8.

44. Ananthakrishnan M, Barr FE, Summar ML, et al. L-citrulline ameliorates chronic hypoxia-induced pulmonary hypertension in newborn piglets. Am J Physiol Lung Cell Mol Physiol 2009;297:L506–11.

45. Smith HA, Canter JA, Christian KG, et al. Nitric oxide precursors and congenital heart surgery: a randomized controlled trial of oral citrulline. J Thorac Cardiovasc Surg 2006;132:56–65.

46. Barr FE, Tirona RG, Taylor MB, et al. Pharmacokinetics and safety of intravenously administered citrulline in children undergoing congenital heart surgery: potential therapy for postoperative pulmonary hypertension. J Thorac Cardiovasc Surg 2007;134:319–26.

47. Farrow KN, Steinhorn RH. Phosphodiesterases: emerging therapeutic targets for neonatal pulmonary hypertension. Handb Exp Pharmacol 2011;204: 251–77.

48. Farrow KN, Lakshminrusimha S, Czech L, et al. Superoxide dismutase and inhaled nitric oxide normalize phosphodiesterase 5 expression and activity in neonatal lambs with persistent pulmonary hypertension. Am J Physiol Lung Cell Mol Physiol 2010;299:L109–16.

49. Sanchez LS, Filippov G, Zapol WM, et al. cGMP-binding, cGMP-specific phosphodiesterase gene expression is regulated during lung development. Pediatr Res 1995;37:348A.

50. Hanson KA, Abman SH, Clarke WR. Elevation of pulmonary PDE5-specific activity in an experimental fetal ovine perinatal pulmonary hypertension model. Pediatr Res 1996;39:334A.

51. Farrow KN, Wedgwood S, Lee KJ, et al. Mitochondrial oxidant stress increases PDE5 activity in persistent pulmonary hypertension of the newborn. Respir Physiolo Neurobiol 2010;174:272–81.

52. Nagendran J, Archer SL, Soliman D, et al. Phosphodiesterase type 5 is highly expressed in the hypertrophied human right ventricle, and acute inhibition of phosphodiesterase type 5 improves contractility. Circulation 2007;116: 238–48.

53. Atz AM, Wessel DL. Sildenafil ameliorates effects of inhaled nitric oxide withdrawal. Anesthesiology 1999;91:307–10.

54. Lee JE, Hillier SC, Knoderer CA. Use of sildenafil to facilitate weaning from inhaled nitric oxide in children with pulmonary hypertension following surgery for congenital heart disease. J Intensive Care Med 2008;23:329–34.

55. Namachivayam P, Theilen U, Butt WW, et al. Sildenafil prevents rebound pulmonary hypertension after withdrawal of nitric oxide in children. Am J Respir Crit Care Med 2006;174:1042–7.

56. Barst RJ, Ivy DD, Gaitan G, et al. A randomized, double-blind, placebo-controlled, dose-ranging study of oral sildenafil citrate in treatment-naive children with pulmonary arterial hypertension. Circulation 2012;125:324–34.

57. Baquero H, Soliz A, Neira F, et al. Oral sildenafil in infants with persistent pulmonary hypertension of the newborn: a pilot randomized blinded study. Pediatrics 2006;117:1077–83.
58. Fraisse A, Butrous G, Taylor MB, et al. Intravenous sildenafil for postoperative pulmonary hypertension in children with congenital heart disease. Intensive Care Med 2011;37:502–9.
59. Steinhorn RH, Kinsella JP, Pierce C, et al. Intravenous sildenafil in the treatment of neonates with persistent pulmonary hypertension. J Pediatr 2009;155:841–7.
60. Ladha F, Bonnet S, Eaton F, et al. Sildenafil improves alveolar growth and pulmonary hypertension in hyperoxia-induced lung injury. Am J Respir Crit Care Med 2005;172:750–6.
61. Mourani PM, Sontag MK, Ivy DD, et al. Effects of long-term sildenafil treatment for pulmonary hypertension in infants with chronic lung disease. J Pediatr 2009; 154:379–84, 84 e1–2.
62. Keller RL, Moore P, Teitel D, et al. Abnormal vascular tone in infants and children with lung hypoplasia: findings from cardiac catheterization and the response to chronic therapy. Pediatr Crit Care Med 2006;7:589–94.
63. Luong C, Rey-Perra J, Vadivel A, et al. Antenatal sildenafil treatment attenuates pulmonary hypertension in experimental congenital diaphragmatic hernia. Circulation 2011;123:2120–31.
64. Takatsuki S, Calderbank M, Ivy DD. Initial experience with tadalafil in pediatric pulmonary arterial hypertension. Pediatr Cardiol 2012;33(5):683–8.
65. Brannon TS, MacRitchie AN, Jaramillo MA, et al. Ontogeny of cyclooxygenase-1 and cyclooxygenase-2 gene expression in ovine lung. Am J Phys 1998;274: L66–71.
66. Brannon TS, North AJ, Wells LB, et al. Prostacyclin synthesis in ovine pulmonary artery is developmentally regulated by changes in cyclooxygenase-1 gene expression. J Clin Invest 1994;93:2230–5.
67. Christman BW, McPherson CD, Newman JH, et al. An imbalance between the excretion of thromboxane and prostacyclin metabolites in pulmonary hypertension. N Engl J Med 1992;327:70–5.
68. Lakshminrusimha S, Porta NF, Farrow KN, et al. Milrinone enhances relaxation to prostacyclin and iloprost in pulmonary arteries isolated from lambs with persistent pulmonary hypertension of the newborn. Pediatr Crit Care Med 2009;10:106–12.
69. Jones RL, Qian Y, Wong HN, et al. Prostanoid action on the human pulmonary vascular system. Clin Exp Pharmacol Physiol 1997;24:969–72.
70. Rosenzweig EB, Kerstein D, Barst RJ. Long-term prostacyclin for pulmonary hypertension with associated congenital heart defects. Circulation 1999;99: 1858–65.
71. Barst RJ, Maislin G, Fishman AP. Vasodilator therapy for primary pulmonary hypertension in children. Circulation 1999;99:1197–208.
72. Barst RJ, Rubin LJ, Long WA, et al. A comparison of continuous intravenous epoprostenol (prostacyclin) with conventional therapy for primary pulmonary hypertension. the primary pulmonary hypertension study group. N Engl J Med 1996;334:296–302.
73. Barst RJ, Rubin LJ, McGoon MD, et al. Survival in primary pulmonary hypertension with long-term continuous intravenous prostacyclin. Ann Intern Med 1994; 121:409–15.
74. Sitbon O, Humbert M, Nunes H, et al. Long-term intravenous epoprostenol infusion in primary pulmonary hypertension: prognostic factors and survival. J Am Coll Cardiol 2002;40:780–8.

75. Yung D, Widlitz AC, Rosenzweig EB, et al. Outcomes in children with idiopathic pulmonary arterial hypertension. Circulation 2004;110:660–5.

76. D'Alonzo GE, Barst RJ, Ayres SM, et al. Survival in patients with primary pulmonary hypertension. Results from a national prospective registry. Ann Intern Med 1991;115:343–9.

77. Doran AK, Ivy DD, Barst RJ, et al. Guidelines for the prevention of central venous catheter-related blood stream infections with prostanoid therapy for pulmonary arterial hypertension. Int J Clin Pract Suppl 2008;160:5–9.

78. Zwissler B, Rank N, Jaenicke U, et al. Selective pulmonary vasodilation by inhaled prostacyclin in a newborn with congenital heart disease and cardiopulmonary bypass. Anesthesiology 1995;82:1512–6.

79. Bindl L, Fahnenstich H, Peukert U. Aerosolised prostacyclin for pulmonary hypertension in neonates. Arch Dis Child Fetal Neonatal Ed 1994;71:F214–6.

80. Soditt V, Aring C, Groneck P. Improvement of oxygenation induced by aerosolized prostacyclin in a preterm infant with persistent pulmonary hypertension of the newborn. Intensive Care Med 1997;23:1275–8.

81. Olmsted K, Oluola O, Parthiban A, et al. Can inhaled prostacyclin stimulate surfactant in ELBW infants? J Perinatol 2007;27:724–6.

82. Kelly LK, Porta NF, Goodman DM, et al. Inhaled prostacyclin for term infants with persistent pulmonary hypertension refractory to inhaled nitric oxide. J Pediatr 2002;141:830–2.

83. Kumar VH, Swartz DD, Rashid N, et al. Prostacyclin and milrinone by aerosolization improve pulmonary hemodynamics in newborn lambs with experimental pulmonary hypertension. J Appl Phys 2010;109:677–84.

84. Porta NF, Steinhorn RH. Pulmonary vasodilator therapy in the NICU: inhaled nitric oxide, sildenafil, and other pulmonary vasodilating agents. Clin Perinatol 2012;39:149–64.

85. Ewert R, Schaper C, Halank M, et al. Inhalative iloprost—pharmacology and clinical application. Expert Opin Pharmacother 2009;10:2195–207.

86. Ehlen M, Wiebe B. Iloprost in persistent pulmonary hypertension of the newborn. Cardiol Young 2003;13:361–3.

87. Eifinger F, Sreeram N, Mehler K, et al. Aerosolized iloprost in the treatment of pulmonary hypertension in extremely preterm infants: a pilot study. Klin Padiatr 2008;220:66–9.

88. Hallioglu O, Dilber E, Celiker A. Comparison of acute hemodynamic effects of aerosolized and intravenous iloprost in secondary pulmonary hypertension in children with congenital heart disease. Am J Cardiol 2003;92:1007–9.

89. Ivy DD, Doran AK, Smith KJ, et al. Short- and long-term effects of inhaled iloprost therapy in children with pulmonary arterial hypertension. J Am Coll Cardiol 2008;51:161–9.

90. Limsuwan A, Wanitkul S, Khosithset A, et al. Aerosolized iloprost for postoperative pulmonary hypertensive crisis in children with congenital heart disease. Int J Cardiol 2008;129:333–8.

91. Muller M, Scholz S, Kwapisz M, et al. Use of inhaled iloprost in a case of pulmonary hypertension during pediatric congenital heart surgery. Anesthesiology 2003;99:743–4.

92. Tissot C, Beghetti M. Review of inhaled iloprost for the control of pulmonary artery hypertension in children. Vasc Health Risk Manag 2009;5:325–31.

93. De Luca D, Zecca E, Piastra M, et al. Iloprost as 'rescue' therapy for pulmonary hypertension of the neonate. Paediatr Anaesth 2007;17:394–5.

94. Chotigeat U, Jaratwashirakul S. Inhaled iloprost for severe persistent pulmonary hypertension of the newborn. J Med Assoc Thai 2007;90:167–70.
95. Ivy DD, Claussen L, Doran A. Transition of stable pediatric patients with pulmonary arterial hypertension from intravenous epoprostenol to intravenous treprostinil. Am J Cardiol 2007;99:696–8.
96. Levy M, Celermajer DS, Bourges-Petit E, et al. Add-on therapy with subcutaneous treprostinil for refractory pediatric pulmonary hypertension. J Pediatr 2011;158:584–8.
97. Simonneau G, Barst RJ, Galie N, et al. Continuous subcutaneous infusion of treprostinil, a prostacyclin analogue, in patients with pulmonary hypertension. Am J Respir Crit Care Med 2002;165:1–5.
98. Chen B, Lakshminrusimha S, Czech L, et al. Regulation of phosphodiesterase 3 in the pulmonary arteries during the perinatal period in sheep. Pediatr Res 2009; 66:682–7.
99. Hoffman TM, Wernovsky G, Atz AM, et al. Efficacy and safety of milrinone in preventing low cardiac output syndrome in infants and children after corrective surgery for congenital heart disease. Circulation 2003;107:996–1002.
100. Chang AC, Atz AM, Wernovsky G, et al. Milrinone: systemic and pulmonary effects in neonates after cardiac surgery. Crit Care Med 1995;23:1907–14.
101. Bassler D, Choong K, McNamara P, et al. Neonatal persistent pulmonary hypertension treated with milrinone: four case reports. Biol Neonate 2006;89:1–5.
102. Deb B, Bradford K, Pearl RG. Additive effects of inhaled nitric oxide and intravenous milrinone in experimental pulmonary hypertension. Crit Care Med 2000; 28:795–9.
103. McNamara PJ, Laique F, Muang-In S, et al. Milrinone improves oxygenation in neonates with severe persistent pulmonary hypertension of the newborn. J Crit Care 2006;21:217–22.
104. Abman SH. Role of endothelin receptor antagonists in the treatment of pulmonary arterial hypertension. Annu Rev Med 2009;60:13–23.
105. Giaid A, Yanagisawa M, Lagleben D, et al. Expression of endothelin-1 in the lungs of patients with pulmonary hypertension. N Engl J Med 1993;328:1732–9.
106. Hiramatsu T, Imai Y, Takanashi Y, et al. Time course of endothelin-1 and nitrate anion levels after cardiopulmonary bypass in congenital heart defects. Ann Thorac Surg 1997;63:648–52.
107. Komai H, Adatia IT, Elliott MJ, et al. Increased plasma levels of endothelin-1 after cardiopulmonary bypass in patients with pulmonary hypertension and congenital heart disease. J Thorac Cardiovasc Surg 1993;106:473–8.
108. Reddy MV, Hendricks-Munoz KD, Rajasinghe HA, et al. Post-cardiopulmonary bypass pulmonary hypertension in lambs with increased pulmonary blood flow: a role for endothelin 1. Circulation 1997;95:1054–61.
109. Schulze-Neick I, Li J, Reader JA, et al. The endothelin antagonist BQ123 reduces pulmonary vascular resistance after surgical intervention for congenital heart disease. J Thorac Cardiovasc Surg 2002;124:435–41.
110. Keller RL, Tacy TA, Hendricks-Munoz K, et al. Congenital diaphragmatic hernia: endothelin-1, pulmonary hypertension, and disease severity. Am J Respir Crit Care Med 2010;182:555–61.
111. Rubin LJ, Badesch DB, Barst RJ, et al. Bosentan therapy for pulmonary arterial hypertension. N Engl J Med 2002;346:896–903.
112. Channick RN, Simonneau G, Sitbon O, et al. Effects of the dual endothelin-receptor antagonist bosentan in patients with pulmonary hypertension: a randomised placebo-controlled study. Lancet 2001;358:1119–23.

113. Rosenzweig EB, Ivy DD, Widlitz A, et al. Effects of long-term bosentan in children with pulmonary arterial hypertension. J Am Coll Cardiol 2005;46:697–704.
114. Maiya S, Hislop AA, Flynn Y, et al. Response to bosentan in children with pulmonary hypertension. Heart 2006;92:664–70.
115. Barst RJ, Ivy D, Dingemanse J, et al. Pharmacokinetics, safety, and efficacy of bosentan in pediatric patients with pulmonary arterial hypertension. Clin Pharmacol Ther 2003;73:372–82.
116. Nakwan N, Choksuchat D, Saksawad R, et al. Successful treatment of persistent pulmonary hypertension of the newborn with bosentan. Acta Paediatr 2009;98:1683–5.
117. Goissen C, Ghyselen L, Tourneux P, et al. Persistent pulmonary hypertension of the newborn with transposition of the great arteries: successful treatment with bosentan. Eur J Pediatr 2008;167:437–40.
118. Ivy DD, Doran A, Claussen L, et al. Weaning and discontinuation of epoprostenol in children with idiopathic pulmonary arterial hypertension receiving concomitant bosentan. Am J Cardiol 2004;93:943–6.
119. van Loon RL, Hoendermis ES, Duffels MG, et al. Long-term effect of bosentan in adults versus children with pulmonary arterial hypertension associated with systemic-to-pulmonary shunt: does the beneficial effect persist? Am Heart J 2007;154:776–82.
120. Beghetti M, Hoeper MM, Kiely DG, et al. Safety experience with bosentan in 146 children 2-11 years old with pulmonary arterial hypertension: results from the European Postmarketing Surveillance program. Pediatr Res 2008;64:200–4.
121. Channick RN, Sitbon O, Barst RJ, et al. Endothelin receptor antagonists in pulmonary arterial hypertension. J Am Coll Cardiol 2004;43:62S–7S.
122. Galie N, Badesch D, Oudiz R, et al. Ambrisentan therapy for pulmonary arterial hypertension. J Am Coll Cardiol 2005;46:529–35.
123. Galie N, Olschewski H, Oudiz RJ, et al. Ambrisentan for the treatment of pulmonary arterial hypertension: results of the ambrisentan in pulmonary arterial hypertension, randomized, double-blind, placebo-controlled, multicenter, efficacy (ARIES) study 1 and 2. Circulation 2008;117:3010–9.

Pharmacologic Management of the Opioid Neonatal Abstinence Syndrome

Walter K. Kraft, MD[a,b,c,*], John N. van den Anker, MD, PhD[d,e,f,g]

KEYWORDS

- Neonatal abstinence syndrome • Opioids • Pharmacogenetics • Withdrawal
- Phenobarbital • Clonidine

KEY POINTS

- All infants with in utero exposure to opioids demonstrate signs and symptoms of withdrawal. Two-thirds of infants require pharmacologic therapy to ensure proper feeding and development.
- Opioid replacement is the optimal primary therapy. The current standard is morphine, although there is significant heterogeneity in treatment regimens, with many centers using methadone.
- Of predictive factors, lack of polysubstance exposure, prematurity, and maternal use of buprenorphine are most strongly associated with less severe withdrawal symptoms and need for pharmacologic therapy.
- Emerging therapies include the use of buprenorphine for primary therapy, and clonidine as an adjunct.
- Pharmacogenetic profiling of infants and the use of modeling and simulation to optimize dosing are emerging, but not fully developed, technologies that may change the treatment of the neonatal abstinence syndrome.

[a] Department of Pharmacology and Experimental Therapeutics, Thomas Jefferson University, 1170 Main Building, 132 South 10th Street, Philadelphia, PA 19107, USA; [b] Department of Medicine, Thomas Jefferson University, 1170 Main Building, 132 South 10th Street, Philadelphia, PA 19107, USA; [c] Department of Surgery, Thomas Jefferson University, 1170 Main Building, 132 South 10th Street, Philadelphia, PA 19107, USA; [d] Division of Pediatric Clinical Pharmacology, Children's National Medical Center, 111 Michigan Avenue, NW, Washington, DC 20010, USA; [e] Department of Pediatrics, George Washington University School of Medicine and Health Sciences, Washington, DC, USA; [f] Department of Pharmacology & Physiology, George Washington University School of Medicine and Health Sciences, Washington, DC, USA; [g] Department of Pediatric Surgery, Intensive Care, Erasmus MC-Sophia Children's Hospital, Rotterdam, The Netherlands
* Corresponding author. Departments of Pharmacology and Experimental Therapeutics, Medicine, and Surgery, Thomas Jefferson University, 1170 Main Building, 132 South 10th Street, Philadelphia, PA 19107.
E-mail address: Walter.Kraft@jefferson.edu

Pediatr Clin N Am 59 (2012) 1147–1165
http://dx.doi.org/10.1016/j.pcl.2012.07.006
0031-3955/12/$ – see front matter © 2012 Elsevier Inc. All rights reserved.

DEFINITION OF NEONATAL ABSTINENCE SYNDROME

Neonatal withdrawal symptoms have been noted following prenatal exposure to several drugs. Examples include opioids,[1,2] benzodiazepines,[3,4] mood-stabilizing medications,[5] selective serotonin reuptake inhibitors,[6] and nicotine.[7] For all drug classes except opioids, these symptoms are usually self-limited and do not require pharmacologic treatment. Infants born to mothers with opioid abuse or receiving methadone maintenance often develop withdrawal symptoms, following the postpartum cessation of in utero exposure to opioids. This complex is known as the neonatal abstinence syndrome (NAS). The full mechanistic basis for the clinical presentation is unclear. Tolerance induced by long-term exposure to opioids is primarily mediated by receptor downregulation coupled with upregulation in the cyclic adenosine monophosphate (cAMP) pathway.[8] Other putative mechanisms include neuroimmune activation, production of anti-opioid peptides, or activation of the spinal dynorphin system. Symptoms of withdrawal are hypothesized to be due to increased adenylyl cyclase activity and an abrupt increase in norepinephrine following removal of the mu opioid ligand. NAS is characterized by signs of central nervous system (CNS) hyperirritability, gastrointestinal dysfunction, respiratory distress, and vague autonomic symptoms. Common symptoms in order of frequency includes tremor, high-pitched cry, sneezing, increased muscle tone, regurgitation and vomiting, poor sleep, loose stools, sweating, excoriation, mottling, nasal stuffiness, low-grade fever, and tachypnea. Impaired weight gain and seizures are seen with untreated NAS. All infants with prolonged in utero opioid exposure will develop signs and symptoms of withdrawal of varying severity. However, the disorder encompasses a diverse spectrum, and those with milder symptoms respond well to supportive treatments. NAS symptoms severe enough to require pharmacologic treatment occur in 55% to 94% of infants born to opioid-dependent mothers.[9]

Current use of illicit drugs occurs in 4.4% of pregnant women.[10] Heroin use during pregnancy is associated with fetal death and infant morbidity, including intrauterine growth retardation, placental insufficiency, postpartum hemorrhage, preeclampsia, and premature rupture of membranes.[11,12] In an attempt to counteract these poor outcomes, methadone maintenance in opioid-dependent pregnant women has been used for the past 35 years, and is associated with improved birth weight and improvements in multiple domains.[13–16] A more recent development is the expansion in the use and abuse of prescription opioids. Whereas the use of heroin decreased by 19% between 1998 and 2008, the abuse of prescription opioids during the same period increased by 41%.[17] In 2010, 5.1 million individuals reported nonmedical abuse of prescription pain medications within the previous month, with 71% of abused pain relievers being obtained from friends or family, and either bought or taken without permission.[10] The societal burden of NAS is difficult to assess, as is evident from the wide variations and implausible rates reported to regional authorities for hospitals in the defined geographic area with similar patient populations.[18] Such variation is due to limited self-reporting of drug abuse, and underreporting of NAS using the International Classification of Diseases.[19] In 1996, a survey by the National Institute of Drug Addiction estimated that 7000 cases occur each year, although the report conceded this is potentially an underestimation.[20] More recently, the rate of NAS in the United States has increased from 1.2 to 3.9 per 1000 live births between 2000 and 2009.[21] A similar incidence rate has been estimated in Australia.[22]

PREDICTORS OF NAS SEVERITY

The dose of maternal methadone dose as a covariate of the need for NAS treatment length has been examined extensively. Although a meta-analysis that evaluated studies by methodological quality did not identify a statistically significant difference in outcomes between high-dose and low-dose methadone, there is a suggestion of modest maternal dose dependency on outcomes.[23] However, if such an effect does exist, it is small and not relevant in terms of choosing a maternal dose or differential treatment approaches in the treatment of infants. Lower maternal methadone doses have been associated with higher rates of illicit substitution, and a consensus view is that maternal doses of methadone should not be reduced solely to reduce NAS severity. High-quality random-ized, controlled trial evidence from the MOTHER study has demonstrated that compared with methadone use, maternal buprenorphine is associated with a decreased need for morphine treatment in NAS and neonatal length of stay.[24] The maternal study population in this study has been convincingly demonstrated to be similar to the patient population at large, strongly supporting the generalizability of results.[25]

Whereas Jansson and colleagues[26] described worse NAS symptoms and pharma-cotherapy in males, severity, need for therapy, or length of therapy were not influenced by gender in a cohort study by Holbrook and Kaltenbach.[27] Similarly, there was no sex dependency in the large randomized MOTHER study, which compared use of meth-adone and buprenorphine in pregnant women.[28] Intrapartum variability or decelera-tions in fetal heart rate do not predict the need for therapy in NAS.[29] However, alternations in autonomic regulation, as measured by analysis of maternal[26] or infant[30] vagal tone, have been noted to be predictors of worse NAS symptomatology. It is postulated that infants who adapt to maternal methadone–induced autonomic changes are maladapted to more severe NAS following birth. Methadone exposure during pregnancy is associated with an approximately 2.5-fold increase in the rate of preterm birth.[31,32] Preterm infants have a well-described natural history of NAS and a need for treatment that differs from term infants. The current NAS scoring instru-ments have not been examined in this population. Need for therapy[33] and length of stay is shorter in the preterm population.[34,35] The preterm population thus appears to be categorically different in terms of in utero opioid exposure.

Polydrug abuse during pregnancy is associated with impaired fetal markers (heart rate and variability) and greater need for postpartum pharmacologic therapy.[36] A retro-spective study by Seligman and colleagues[34] demonstrated that the length of NAS treatment for all opioid only exposed infants between 2000 and 2006 was 31 days, compared with 38 days for polydrug-exposed term infants. Strikingly, a multivariate analysis of infants revealed a significant prolongation of treatment duration for NAS (31 vs 47 days, $P<.01$) of benzodiazepine versus non–benzodiazepine-exposed infants. Benzodiazepine withdrawal symptoms in adults include anxiety, tremors, anorexia, nausea, postural hypotension, and in severe cases seizures, delirium, and hyperpy-rexia. The onset of symptoms is 12 to 24 hours for short-acting agents with a peak at 72 hours, whereas longer-acting agents such as diazepam are associated with an onset of 24 to 72 hours and a peak between 5 and 8 days following the last dose.[37] Benzodiazepines cross the placenta,[38,39] but maternal confounders have made it diffi-cult to estimate adverse effects specific to in utero exposure of benzodiazepines.[40] Whereas teratogenicity is unlikely in benzodiazepine-exposed infants,[41–43] decreased birth weight and neonatal withdrawal have been noted,[3] the latter manifested by hypo-tonia and hypoventilation or tremulousness.[4] The half-life of diazepam in neonates is 31 days.[44] Thus, in contrast to that of adults, initiation of neonatal withdrawal for many benzodiazepines can be delayed with an onset at a week and effects noticeable for weeks.[45,46] There is no specific treatment for neonatal benzodiazepine withdrawal. Tobacco exposure is associated with worse NAS symptomatology.[47,48] Analysis of meconium for tobacco, methadone or its metabolites, cocaine, or opioids other than methadone, however, are not predictive of NAS outcomes.[49]

LONG-TERM AND SHORT-TERM SEQUELAE

Environmental and social factors are more important influences upon childhood development than brief periods of prepartum and peripartum exposure to drugs of abuse.[50,51] Infants exposed in utero to opioids show low birth weights, increased preterm birth, and reduced fetal growth parameters, but investigations have been hampered by the logistical difficulty of controlling for tobacco and other social factors associated with illicit drug use.[52] Studies linking in utero opioids to impaired neurodevelopment[53] have been criticized for not accounting for confounding of the child's social and environmental milieu.[54] The database for opioid exposure is less robust than that for cocaine.[55] It is possible that there are subtle neurodevelopmental effects arising from in utero opioid exposure apart from effects caused by environmental and home settings.[56] Even if this is real, however, these associations do not provide guidance about practical therapeutic decisions. For newborns, the benefits of maternal opioid therapy during pregnancy using methadone in a structured program clearly outweigh no therapy. There is evidence that untreated or undertreated women may seek street sources of opioids to treat withdrawal symptoms, which clearly has negative neonatal outcomes. Of importance, there is no evidence of long-term adverse outcomes in children treated with pharmacologic agents in comparison with infants who do not require treatment for NAS, or for treatment with different classes of agents.[57,58] Although the database of information is smaller, in human and animal studies neonatal outcomes with in utero buprenorphine exposure are generally favorable compared with methadone.[59]

CURRENT THERAPIES
Variability of Current Practice Patterns

Few studies have examined NAS prevalence and treatment patterns. Nandakumar and Sankar[60] published a survey of 17 neonatal units in the Northwest Region of the United Kingdom, revealing not only conflicting practices in scoring, identification, and management but also a deficit of reliable data to assist practitioners in determining the best regimen to treat NAS. In a survey conducted by Sarkar and Donn[61] in United States neonatal intensive care units (NICU), the focus was primarily on determining the percentage of respondents using an abstinence scoring system, those with access to formal written policies or educational programs for NAS management, and practitioners using customary pharmacologic agents for withdrawal. The 13-question survey of 102 accredited fellowship programs (which had 75 respondents) did not include questions on NAS incidence or length of hospital stay. O'Grady and colleagues[62] conducted a 15-question questionnaire of 235 neonatal units that sought to survey current NAS practices in the United Kingdom and Ireland. The survey assessed first-line and second-line agents, attitudes to breastfeeding by women on methadone, and the safety of infants discharged on medication. Crocetti and colleagues[63] assessed the number of opiate-exposed neonates identified as having NAS, as well as policies and procedures for treatment in 27 hospitals throughout Maryland. In aggregate, these surveys demonstrate significant heterogeneity in diagnosis and treatment patterns. There are clear information gaps for identification, treatment, and length of hospital stay. Moreover, there is a lack of pharmacoeconomic analyses on costs and cost-effectiveness of treatment for NAS.

Framework for Treatment

The therapeutic framework of treatment begins with the identification of infants at risk for NAS. NAS is graded using a standard checklist that identifies and stratifies severity of disease based on signs and symptoms in multiple domains. Of several scoring systems used to gauge symptom severity and titrate drug dose,[64–66] the Finnegan score (or modifications of it)[67] is the most commonly used.[61,62] A modification of the Finnegan score used in the multicenter MOTHER study of buprenorphine use for pregnant women[68,69] is the standard instrument used in other randomized NAS research trials.[70,71] The Finnegan instrument was created to assess severity of disease in those with known opioid exposure. On day 2 of life a score of 7 corresponds with the 95th percentile for nonexposed infants, meaning any score of 8 or greater is highly suggestive of in utero opioid exposure even in those denying opioid use during pregnancy.[72] Nonpharmacologic therapies should be used for all infants with in utero opioid exposure. These treatments include swaddling,[73] the use of small calorically dense formulas, rooming in, breastfeeding, and minimization of excessive external stimulation. Infants with mild symptoms should be observed in the hospital for at least 4 days. For infants with severe symptomatology manifested by seizures, poor weight gain, and elevated values in a NAS-specific scoring instrument, pharmacologic therapy is indicated. Ideal treatment uses a protocol-driven use of drug titration to control symptoms. Both symptom-driven (ie, weight-independent fixed dose titration based on severity of NAS scores) and weight-based dosing regimens have been used, with neither being identified as the standard approach.[74] Regardless of the manner of dose titration, infants who do not have control of symptoms despite high doses of the initial therapy are treated with a secondary drug. After stabilization, symptom scores are used to gradually wean the controlling drug or drugs; this occurs typically in an inpatient setting, as it allows careful observation and dose titration of infants. Some institutions stabilize an infant in an inpatient setting, with terminal weaning done as an outpatient. The use of outpatient treatment in highly selected patients is associated with shorter inpatient stays, but extended total duration of therapy.[75]

The rationale to use pharmacologic therapy is to ensure proper feeding and development, and foster the maternal infant bond. The ideal specific drug used would safely achieve these therapeutic goals, while at the same time minimizing the total duration of therapy and length of hospitalization. The most commonly used initial therapy is an opioid, while phenobarbital or clonidine are the primary adjunctive agents. Although used more commonly, phenobarbital has not been demonstrated to have improved safety or efficacy in comparison with clonidine as an adjunctive therapy. A comparison of these agents as adjuncts is currently being investigated (NCT01175668). The role of initial dual therapy of phenobarbital with an opioid has been described, but has not been compared in a large number of patients.[76] The value of this approach has not been established, but anecdotally may provide benefit in infants with polysubstance use.

Opioids

Cochrane reviews,[77,78] the American Academy of Pediatrics,[9,79] and expert reviews[80,81] identify opioid replacement as the ideal treatment for the withdrawal symptoms associated with in utero exposure to opiates. Opioid replacement as a first-line agent (1) improves weight gain but lengthens hospitalizations compared with supportive care, (2) reduces seizure rates and possibly duration of therapy compared with phenobarbital, and (3) reduces treatment failure compared with diazepam.[77] Although many of the studies cited in the Cochrane review had methodological flaws, the standard of care practice that has developed since the 1970s has generally supported this approach. There is limited evidence from which definitive recommendations can be made regarding differential safety and efficacy of specific opioids. Moreover, high-quality data on the optimal dose regimens or comparative effectiveness on use of adjunctive agents are lacking. Current practice patterns for these have been developed empirically, and remain an area that would benefit from investigations of higher quality.

Morphine

Morphine is the most commonly used opioid for replacement therapy. Paregoric, a previously commonly used morphine source, was never subject to any formal evaluation by the Food and Drug Administration, and is no longer available. Diluted, deodorized tincture of opium (DTO) has a morphine concentration of 0.4 mg/mL and an ethanol concentration of 0.19%. This agent has been largely replaced by an ethanol-free morphine solution of 0.4 mg/mL concentration. Preservative-free morphine hydrochloride solution for neonatal administration is stable at 4°C for at least 6 months.[82] Because of the relatively short half-life of morphine, best outcomes have been demonstrated when morphine doses are given no longer than 4 hours apart.[83] Accordingly, infants who are sleeping at the nominal dose time should be awakened for drug administration.

Morphine in humans is metabolized primarily to morphine-3-glucuronide (M3G) and morphine-6-glucuronide (M6G) via uridine 5′-diphosphate glucuronosyl transferase (UGT)-2B7. The ontogeny of UGT development is dynamic in the immediate postpartum period, demonstrated by reduced M6G/morphine ratio in neonates younger than 7 days as well as an associated reduced postsurgical morphine requirement in comparison with older neonates.[84] Nonlinear mixed-effects models have been used to estimate active metabolite formation as well as elimination.[85] Clearance generally correlates with glomerular filtration, with minimal fecal elimination or metabolism to normorphine. The large interpatient and intrapatient variability of intravenous morphine pharmacokinetics and pharmacodynamics in neonates is due in part to a dynamic acquisition of metabolic enzymes, renal function, and changes in fat and extracellular fluid balance.[84–86] Of note, the pharmacokinetics profile of orally administered morphine in neonates is currently unknown. An area of therapeutic need would be the characterization of the concentration-response relationship. Such a relationship, created with modeling and simulation, would be of use in designing an optimized dose regimen.

The initial dose of morphine was 0.12 to 0.6 mg/kg/d in a survey of 17 pediatric units in the United Kingdom.[60] These investigators had the opinion that a higher initial dose may be associated with better control of symptoms, but acknowledged that evidence to support this intuition was lacking. A dose of 0.24 mg/kg/d was recommended by the 1998 report of the American Academy of Pediatrics (AAP),[9] although this protocol outlined drop-unit doses that would make fine titration difficult. Neither the 2012 AAP Committee on Drugs NAS report[79] nor the Cochrane review of the topic identified a favored specific dose.[77] There is no generally accepted maximum dose of morphine used for NAS. A survey of neonatal units in the United Kingdom revealed that typical maximum doses were up to 1.3 mg/kg/d, and that one-third determined dose according to symptom control rather than a maximum predefined level.[62] Specific protocols for dose titration are based either on a weight-based increase in dose based on scores above a specific NAS score, or a weight-independent dose based on a graded severity of NAS score. **Table 1** outlines these 2 commonly used approaches.

Methadone

Methadone is a long-acting opioid commonly used for abstinence treatment. The longer half-life of methadone provides less of a flux between peak and trough levels, while also providing ease of administration at less frequent intervals. Oral bioavailability in adults is high, but variable.[87] The pharmacokinetics of methadone in the

Table 1
Morphine regimens, based on Finnegan scoring every 4 hours

Weight Based	Symptom Based	
Initial Dose:	*Initial Dose:*	
0.4 mg/kg/d in 6 divided doses	For first elevated score >8, rescore in 1 h to verify. If still elevated	
Dose Increase:		
20%/d for NAS scores >24 total on 3 measures, or a single score ≥12	Single NAS score	Dose every 4 h (mg)
	9–12	0.04
Weaning Dose:	13–16	0.08
After 48 h of clinical stability, reduce dose by 10% every 24–48 h	17–20	0.12
Reduce dose when the sum of the previous 3 scores is <18 and no single score is >8	21–24	0.16
	≥25	0.20
Cease therapy when dose is 0.15 mg/kg/d	Doses are fixed and not based on infant weight	
Rescue Dose:	Dose Increase:	
Administer additional morphine at previous dose for inadequate symptom control between scheduled dose intervals	Single NAS score	Increase Dose (mg)
	0–9	None
Adjunctive Treatment:	9–12	0.02
At dose of morphine 1.25 mg/kg/d initiate second medication[a]	13–16	0.04
	17–20	0.06
	Weaning Dose:	
	After 48 h of clinical stability, reduce dose by 0.02 mg every 24 h if scores ≤8	
	For first elevated score >8, rescore in 1 h to verify. If still elevated	
	Two NAS scores	Increase Dose (mg)
	9–12	0.01
	13–16	0.02
	17–20	0.04
	Cease therapy when dose is 0.02 mg	
	Adjunctive Treatment:	
	At dose of morphine 1.6 mg/d initiate second medication[a]	

[a] Phenobarbital loading dose of 20 mg/kg followed by 5 mg/kg/d, or clonidine.
Data from Jones HE, Kaltenbach K, Heil SH, et al. Neonatal abstinence syndrome after methadone or buprenorphine exposure. N Engl J Med 2010;363(24):2320–31; and Jansson LM, Velez M, Harrow C. The opioid-exposed newborn: assessment and pharmacologic management. J Opioid Manag 2009;5(1):47–55.

pediatric and neonatal populations has been simulated using physiologic-based pharmacokinetic modeling that suggests significant interpatient and developmental variability, but decreased systemic exposure with age.[88] This model has not been validated by rich patient-level data. There is scant published clinical trial evidence to guide its use in the neonatal population. In a single small study, outcomes with methadone were similar to those for phenobarbital or diazepam.[89] Comparisons with oral morphine are limited to a single retrospective review of 46 patients, in which there was no significant difference in length of stay between treatments.[90] A standard dose has not been established, but the protocol used by Lainwala and colleagues[90] is provided in **Box 1**. Methadone use remains relatively uncommon, ranging from fewer

---

Box 1
Methadone protocol for inpatient use

- Initial loading dose 0.1 mg/kg/dose

- Additional 0.025 mg/kg/dose given every 4 h for continuing NAS scores greater than 8 until symptoms are controlled or a maximum dose of 0.5 mg/kg/d reached

- Maintenance dose determined by calculating the total methadone dose given over previous 24 hours

- Maintenance dose administered in 2 divided doses every 12 hours

Data from Lainwala S, Brown ER, Weinschenk NP, et al. A retrospective study of length of hospital stay in infants treated for neonatal abstinence syndrome with methadone versus oral morphine preparations. Adv Neonatal Care 2005;5(5):265–72.

---

than 2% of units in the United Kingdom[62] to as many as 20% in the United States.[61] The long dosing interval has led some sites to use methadone as extended outpatient dosing. Compared with full inpatient treatment, infants discharged home on methadone have shorter hospitalizations but longer duration of therapy, though at least in one study having a similar total of methadone administered.[91] Because of the likely variability of pharmacokinetics, frequent outpatient follow-up is required to allow careful monitoring and dose titration based on symptoms.

Buprenorphine
Buprenorphine is a long-acting partial μ opioid receptor agonist that in adults is more effective for withdrawal symptoms than clonidine, and possibly methadone.[92] Use of buprenorphine in this population has gained favor, in part because of its properties of improved safety, particularly with regard to respiratory depression. Buprenorphine has compared favorably with methadone for use in pregnant women.[24] In NAS, the use of buprenorphine has been explored in 2 open-label, placebo-controlled trials.[70,93] A total of 50 infants were randomized in a 1:1 ratio to oral morphine every 4 hours or sublingual buprenorphine administered every 8 hours. The optimized initial dose was 15.9 μg/kg/d, with a maximum of 60 μg/kg/d. Doses were increased 25% until control of symptoms was obtained, and decreased by 10% until cessation of therapy when the dose was 10% of the initial dose. Doses were not adjusted for actual weight, and were instead based on the weight at initiation of therapy. Although the initial goals of this phase 1 investigation was the feasibility and safety of buprenorphine to treat NAS, an efficacy advantage over morphine was demonstrated. When the results from both cohorts were combined, treatment with buprenorphine revealed a mean length of treatment of 23 days, compared with a mean length of 34 days using standard of care oral morphine (**Fig. 1**). Following log transformation to satisfy normality assumptions, the length of treatment was on average 36% shorter (95% confidence interval [CI]: 17%–51%; $P = .001$) in the buprenorphine arm than in those administered oral morphine, and the length of stay was on average 29% shorter (95% CI: 10%–44%; $P = .006$). Caveats to these findings are an open-label study design and that, while consistent with retrospective studies at the same institution,[34] the duration of treatment and length of stay in both arms was somewhat longer than has been reported at other institutions.

Adjunctive therapy with phenobarbital was required in 6 of 25 infants in the buprenorphine group compared with 2 of 25 randomized to morphine. It is unclear whether this finding is due to a ceiling effect of buprenorphine as a partial agonist in a subset of patients with more severe disease, or if the predefined maximum dose

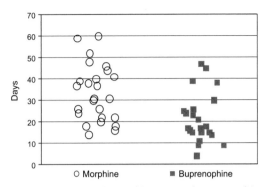

Fig. 1. Length of treatment: open-label morphine versus buprenorphine by patient.

of buprenorphine was set too low. Pharmacokinetic sampling in this trial unexpectedly revealed amelioration of withdrawal symptoms at plasma concentrations of buprenorphine below the 0.7 ng/mL threshold, estimated for relief of symptoms in adults.[94] This finding could be due to a different volume of distribution of the drug in the neonate, or a pharmacodynamic profile of withdrawal that fundamentally differs from that in adults.

Drugs for sublingual administration are formulated using buprenorphine for injection (Buprenex or equivalent generic) at a concentration of 0.075 mg/mL in a 30% ethanol solution. Buprenorphine is stable at room temperature for at least 30 days in glass vials and for at least 7 days in plastic syringes. Buprenorphine is absorbed by the sublingual route within 2 minutes in adults.[95] There was no evidence of aspiration in neonates after more than 1600 individual doses were administered in the phase 1 investigation. There were 2 serious adverse events. One infant developed cytomegalovirus in the immediate postpartum period and another had idiopathic seizure. Both events were judged to be unrelated to study treatment by the investigator, institutional review board, and data safety monitoring board.

Adjuncts

Phenobarbital

The use of phenobarbital (identified as phenobarbitone in the British nomenclature) is often used as a rescue therapy when maximum dose of opioid replacement therapy is reached without adequate resolution of symptoms, although it has also been used as an initial adjunct in combination therapy with an opioid[76] or as initial monotherapy.[96] Phenobarbital use has been examined in a Cochrane review, which concluded that opioids had a comparative advantage concerning incidence of seizures, duration of treatment, and nursery admissions, but not necessarily in the rate of treatment failure.[78] The half-life of phenobarbital in neonates decreases from 115 hours after 1 week to 67 hours after 4 weeks.[97] This prolonged half-life explains the improved outcomes through the use of a loading dose compared with dosing without a load.[98] The typical loading dose is 20 mg/kg, followed by 5 mg/kg. Phenobarbital anecdotally seems to have particular utility in those infants with polydrug exposure in utero. Phenobarbital causes increased metabolism of many drugs metabolized by the cytochrome P450 system for patients of all agents, a finding confirmed in NAS infants cotreated with phenobarbital and buprenorphine.[99] Questions raised about the potential for deleterious neurodevelopmental effects will be addressed by the ongoing PROPHENO trial (NCT01089504), scheduled to be completed in late 2014.

Clonidine

Clonidine is a centrally acting α-agonist that reduces global sympathetic tone and has been used in adult withdrawal syndromes. Clonidine is less efficacious in adults in comparison with opioids in the management of withdrawal symptoms.[92] Several small retrospective examinations had suggested clonidine as a useful adjunct therapy in NAS (**Table 2**). Agthe and colleagues[71] described a high-quality, randomized controlled trial of clonidine, 1 μg/kg every 4 hours compared with placebo as a parallel adjunct to oral morphine therapy (in the form of DTO). Clonidine solution for epidural injection (100 μg/mL) was diluted to 5 μg/mL and administered orally. The dual morphine/clonidine arm had a statistically significant shorter length of stay (11 days [95% CI: 8–15] vs 15 days [95% CI: 13–17]). In addition, the total dose of morphine was 7.7 mg with dual therapy compared with 19.2 mg with monotherapy ($P = .03$). Clonidine was generally well tolerated, with no serious hypotension or bradycardia. An episode of supraventricular tachycardia occurred in one patient 3 days after cessation of clonidine. Based on the mechanism of action of clonidine and potential for post-cessation sympathetic surge, it is plausible that this was causally related to cessation of the study drug. Three infants in the clonidine-treated group died of autopsy-verified myocarditis, sudden infant death syndrome, and homicide (methadone overdose). Each occurred at least 22 days after the cessation of the study drug and were assessed to be unrelated to the study drug.[71] Xie and colleagues[100] performed nonlinear mixed-effects modeling of clonidine pharmacokinetics and noted a rapid increase in clearance in the first month of life. A dose adjustment of 1.5 μg/kg every 4 hours starting the second week of life, based on modeling and simulation, was proposed. This dose adjustment has not been tested in a clinical trial setting.

Breastfeeding

The number of women in methadone programs who choose to breastfeed their newborns has been traditionally low, with more than half of those who start stopping after 6 days.[101] However, it is expected that this number will increase both locally and nationwide as a result of specific campaigns. In 2011, the United States Surgeon General released *A Call to Action to Support Breastfeeding*, which calls for expansion of breastfeeding for American infants. This standpoint is supported by the Department of Health and Human Services in Healthy People 2020, as well as major medical societies.[102] Methadone is passed on to neonates through breast milk, although the

Table 2 Clonidine use				
Authors,[Ref.] Year		n	Clonidine Dose (μg/kg)	Outcome in Length of Stay (LOS) or Length of Treatment (LOT)
Hoder et al,[124] 1984	Case Series	7	0.5–1.0 by mouth every 6 h	13 d LOS
Leikin et al,[125] 2009	Case Series	14	0.5–1.0 by mouth every 6 h	7 d LOT In utero exposures = 3 Iatrogenic NAS = 11
Esmaeili et al,[126] 2010	Case Series	29	0.5–3.0 h intravenous	14 d LOT 32 d LOS Chloral hydrate rescue
Agthe et al,[71] 2009	Randomized controlled trial	40	1.0 by mouth every 4 h (+morphine)	11 d LOT vs 15 for placebo

absolute amount is small (<0.2 mg/d) and does not appreciably change neonatal serum methadone concentrations.[103] However, a pharmacodynamic effect is suggested, as breastfed infants have decreased severity of NAS or need for treatment with pharmacologic agents.[104,105] Based on the small doses of drug transferred to the infant, it is not clear if this effect reflects the calming effect of the act of breastfeeding or the effect of drug.[106] For mothers maintained on usual abstinence doses, the amount of buprenorphine transferred through breast milk is 0.1 to 1.2 μg/kg/d, which represents approximately 0.02% of the maternal dose.[107–110] The bioavailability of buprenorphine transferred in breast milk is not characterized, but appears low based on measurement in neonatal blood and urine,[110] and by minimal effects in suppression of NAS symptomatology.[111–113] There are no reported safety concerns associated with breastfeeding, therefore despite the product insert that advises against breastfeeding, current national guidelines advocate breastfeeding for mothers prescribed buprenorphine.[114]

Pharmacogenetics

The interpatient variability seen in severity of withdrawal symptoms or response to therapies cannot be reduced to a monogenic etiology in either newborns or adults. However, several single-nucleotide polymorphisms (SNPs) in candidate genes have been identified that appear to determine response to opioids for pain or replacement abstinence therapy in adults, for predilection to substance abuse disorder,[115] and social hedonic capacity.[116] The μ opioid receptor (OPRM1) gene A118G SNP has been associated with differential morphine sensitivity, with decreased pain and morphine requirements with the AA genotype.[117] An exploratory examination by Wachman and colleagues[101] in 28 term infants with in utero opioid exposure revealed a significantly lower need for pharmacotherapy, lower doses, and shorter lengths of stay in patients with the AA variant compared with those with the GG variant. Catechol-O-methyltransferase (COMT), an enzyme that degrades catecholamines, was also examined. In adults, the COMT SNP (Val158Met) is associated with a lower required morphine dosage in patients with cancer,[118] although the association with addiction is much less clear.[119] Wachman and colleagues[101] reported that COMT (Val158Met) was associated with a decreased need for therapy, dose of medications, and length of stay. Variants of p-glycoprotein (MDR1) were not associated with differential NAS outcomes. These intriguing findings, if verified in a larger cohort, may have implications for identifying those most at risk for the need of therapy. Enthusiasm is tempered, however, by the example of pharmacogenetic approaches to warfarin therapy in adults, in which there is limited practitioner uptake despite evidence of efficacy and easy-to-use algorithms.

FUTURE DIRECTIONS

Future directions may include the examination of the existing scales, particularly those based on the Finnegan scale, to discern whether there it is possible to simplify the scales to include those elements most closely correlated with clinical outcomes in the management of infants with known opioid exposure. A 3-point scale consisting of hyperactive Moro reflex, mild tremors when undisturbed, and increased muscle tone has been described as discriminative between opioid-exposed and non–opioid-exposed infants, but this has not yet been validated in a large sample.[24]

Dexmedetomidine is chemically similar to clonidine, but with a greater α2-receptor specificity.[120] Dexmedetomidine has been proposed as a potential alternative for the treatment of iatrogenic pediatric opioid withdrawal syndromes, but has not been evaluated in the treatment of NAS.[121] Lofexidine and guanfacine are other α2-agonists that have been investigated for the treatment of adult withdrawal but not pediatric withdrawal, but the size and quality of studies have been limited.[122] These agents have no theoretical advantage over clonidine.

It is not clear whether a short-acting agent such as morphine, compared with longer half-life drugs such as buprenorphine or methadone, will provide better outcomes for infants who require pharmacologic therapy. Extrapolation from adult abstinence and control of withdrawal symptoms would suggest that longer-acting agents, by reducing the flux in drug concentration, would provide more uniform control of symptoms and a smoother transition to the postcessation period of therapy. However, it is also possible that morphine would provide more flexibility in titrating to a dynamic symptom complex by allowing quicker dose titration and attainment of steady state after dose adjustment. A double-blinded, double-dummy trial currently under way (NCT01452789) may provide insight into this question. The lack of published pharmacokinetic and outcomes data make methadone dosing empiric and non-evidence based.

The majority of treatment for NAS takes place in an inpatient setting, but there are institutions in which home management with phenobarbital and methadone are used. A formal comparison between these approaches would be useful. The correct location for treatment also needs to take into consideration not only the pharmacology of the replacement agent but also the dynamics of mother-infant dyad and of the social situation. In this way, any investigation should take these considerations into account in structuring a study, as well as in defining end points for examination.

Pharmacogenetics may assist in identifying infants at risk for requiring pharmacologic therapy for NAS, but will likely be only one of many covariates that would feed into a predictive disease-state model. Such a model could effectively link demographics, in utero exposures, disease severity, genetic factors, pharmacodynamic responses, pharmacokinetics, and other variables. It is likely that such a model would be actuated optimally in an electronic system that had system inputs from an electronic medical record. Modeling also will play an increasing role in the realm of quantitative methods, allowing use of the sparse data sets available in neonates. In such a fashion, pharmacometric simulations can predict dose response and help to inform the formulation of new dosing regimens or combination therapy. Using a "learn and confirm" paradigm, these models can be refined and optimized.[123]

SUMMARY

There is clearly an unmet medical need to develop improved pharmacologic treatment for infants with NAS. The mean hospital cost for an NAS admission in 2009 was $53,400.[21] Ideally such treatment would provide improved symptom control without compromising safety, and would shorten treatment duration and length of hospital stay. If widely adopted, treatment with these features would have the potential to decrease resource utilization and costs of treating NAS, as well as to improve psychosocial and developmental outcomes in infants exposed to opioids in utero. Lastly, treatment protocols should be standardized per institution, and re-evaluated as new outcomes data become available.

ACKNOWLEDGMENTS

John N van den Anker is in part supported by NIH grants (R01HD060543, K24DA027992, R01HD048689 and U54HD071601) and European Union FP7 grants TINN (223614), TINN2 (260908), NEUROSIS (223060), and GRIP (261060).

REFERENCES

1. Schneck H. Narcotic withdrawal symptoms in the newborn infant resulting from maternal addiction. J Pediatr 1958;52:584–7.
2. Dikshit SK. Narcotic withdrawal syndrome in newborns. Indian J Pediatr 1961; 28:11–5.
3. McCarthy JE, Siney C, Shaw NJ, et al. Outcome predictors in pregnant opiate and polydrug users. Eur J Pediatr 1999;158(9):748–9.
4. Swortfiguer D, Cissoko H, Giraudeau B, et al. Neonatal consequences of benzo-diazepines used during the last month of pregnancy. Arch Pediatr 2005;12(9): 1327–31.
5. ACOG Committee on Practice Bulletins–Obstetrics. ACOG Practice Bulletin: clinical management guidelines for obstetrician-gynecologists number 92, April 2008. Use of psychiatric medications during pregnancy and lactation. Obstet Gynecol 2008;111(4):1001–20.
6. Koren G, Matsui D, Einarson A, et al. Is maternal use of selective serotonin re-uptake inhibitors in the third trimester of pregnancy harmful to neonates? CMAJ 2005;172(11):1457–9.
7. Law KL, Stroud LR, LaGasse LL, et al. Smoking during pregnancy and newborn neurobehavior. Pediatrics 2003;111(6 Pt 1):1318–23.
8. Anand KJ, Willson DF, Berger J, et al. Tolerance and withdrawal from prolonged opioid use in critically ill children. Pediatrics 2010;125(5):e1208–25.
9. American Academy of Pediatrics Committee on Drugs. Neonatal drug with-drawal. Pediatrics 1998;101(6):1079–88.
10. SAMHSA (Substance Abuse, and Mental Health Services Administration). Results from the 2010 national survey on drug use and health: summary of national findings, NSDUH Series H-41. Rockville, (MD): HHS; 2011.
11. Finnegan LP, Kandall SR. In: Lowinson JH, Ruiz P, Millman RB, et al, editors. Maternal and neonatal effects of alcohol and drugs. Philadelphia: Lippincott Wil-liams & Wilkins; 2005. p. 805–39.
12. Kennare R, Heard A, Chan A. Substance use during pregnancy: risk factors and obstetric and perinatal outcomes in South Australia. Aust N Z J Obstet Gynaecol 2005;45(3):220–5.
13. Kandall SR, Albin S, Lowinson J, et al. Differential effects of maternal heroin and methadone use on birthweight. Pediatrics 1976;58(5):681–5.
14. Bell J, Harvey-Dodds L. Pregnancy and injecting drug use. BMJ 2008; 336(7656):1303–5.
15. Hulse GK, Milne E, English DR, et al. The relationship between maternal use of heroin and methadone and infant birth weight. Addiction 1997;92(11):1571–9.
16. Finnegan LP, Reeser DS, Connaughton JF Jr. The effects of maternal drug dependence on neonatal mortality. Drug Alcohol Depend 1977;2(2):131–40.
17. Manchikanti L, Fellows B, Ailinani H, et al. Therapeutic use, abuse, and nonmed-ical use of opioids: a ten-year perspective. Pain Physician 2010;13(5):401–35.
18. Pennsylvania Department of Health. Bureau of Health Statistics & Research Data From The Annual Hospital Questionnaire Reporting Period: July 1, 2008 Through June 30, 2009 Report 14. 2009;2010(10/11):1.
19. Burns L, Mattick RP. Using population data to examine the prevalence and corre-lates of neonatal abstinence syndrome. Drug Alcohol Rev 2007;26(5):487–92.
20. National Pregnancy and Health Survey. NIDA research monograph: Estimated percentage and numbers (in thousands) of infants exposed prenatally to se-lected substances: Table 4-2. 1996;No. 96-3819:37.

21. Patrick SW, Schumacher RE, Benneyworth BD, et al. Neonatal abstinence syndrome and associated health care expenditures: United States, 2000-2009. JAMA 2012;307(18):1934–40.

22. O'Donnell M, Nassar N, Leonard H, et al. Increasing prevalence of neonatal withdrawal syndrome: population study of maternal factors and child protection involvement. Pediatrics 2009;123(4):e614–21.

23. Cleary BJ, Donnelly J, Strawbridge J, et al. Methadone dose and neonatal abstinence syndrome-systematic review and meta-analysis. Addiction 2010;105(12): 2071–84.

24. Jones HE, Harrow C, O'Grady KE, et al. Neonatal abstinence scores in opioid-exposed and nonexposed neonates: a blinded comparison. J Opioid Manag 2010;6(6):409–13.

25. Stine SM, Heil SH, Kaltenbach K, et al. Characteristics of opioid-using pregnant women who accept or refuse participation in a clinical trial: screening results from the MOTHER study. Am J Drug Alcohol Abuse 2009;35(6):429–33.

26. Jansson LM, Dipietro JA, Elko A, et al. Maternal vagal tone change in response to methadone is associated with neonatal abstinence syndrome severity in exposed neonates. J Matern Fetal Neonatal Med 2007;20(9):677–85.

27. Holbrook A, Kaltenbach K. Gender and NAS: does sex matter? Drug Alcohol Depend 2010;112(1–2):156–9.

28. Unger A, Jagsch R, Bawert A, et al. Are male neonates more vulnerable to neonatal abstinence syndrome than female neonates? Gend Med 2011;8(6):355–64.

29. Leeman LM, Brown SA, Albright B, et al. Association between intrapartum fetal heart rate patterns and neonatal abstinence syndrome in methadone exposed neonates. J Matern Fetal Neonatal Med 2011;24(7):955–9.

30. Jansson LM, Dipietro JA, Elko A, et al. Infant autonomic functioning and neonatal abstinence syndrome. Drug Alcohol Depend 2010;109(1–3):198–204.

31. Almario CV, Seligman NS, Dysart KC, et al. Risk factors for preterm birth among opiate-addicted gravid women in a methadone treatment program. Am J Obstet Gynecol 2009;201(3):326.e1–6.

32. Cleary BJ, Donnelly JM, Strawbridge JD, et al. Methadone and perinatal outcomes: a retrospective cohort study. Am J Obstet Gynecol 2011;204(2):139.e1–9.

33. Liu AJ, Jones MP, Murray H, et al. Perinatal risk factors for the neonatal abstinence syndrome in infants born to women on methadone maintenance therapy. Aust N Z J Obstet Gynaecol 2010;50(3):253–8.

34. Seligman NS, Salva N, Hayes EJ, et al. Predicting length of treatment for neonatal abstinence syndrome in methadone-exposed neonates. Am J Obstet Gynecol 2008;199(4):396.e1–7.

35. Dysart K, Hsieh HC, Kaltenbach K, et al. Sequela of preterm versus term infants born to mothers on a methadone maintenance program: differential course of neonatal abstinence syndrome. J Perinat Med 2007;35(4):344–6.

36. Jansson LM, Di Pietro JA, Elko A, et al. Pregnancies exposed to methadone, methadone and other illicit substances, and poly-drugs without methadone: a comparison of fetal neurobehaviors and infant outcomes. Drug Alcohol Depend 2012;122(3):213–9.

37. Wesson DR, Smith DE, Ling W, et al. Sedative-hypnotics. In: Lowinson JH, Ruiz P, Millman RB, et al, editors. Substance abuse: a comprehensive textbook. 4th edition. Philadelphia: Lippincott Williams & Wilkins; 2005. p. 302–12.

38. Myllynen P, Vahakangas K. An examination of whether human placental perfusion allows accurate prediction of placental drug transport: studies with diazepam. J Pharmacol Toxicol Methods 2002;48(3):131–8.

39. McGrath C, Buist A, Norman TR. Treatment of anxiety during pregnancy: effects of psychotropic drug treatment on the developing fetus. Drug Saf 1999;20(2):171–86.
40. Wikner BN, Stiller CO, Kallen B, et al. Use of benzodiazepines and benzodiazepine receptor agonists during pregnancy: maternal characteristics. Pharmacoepidemiol Drug Saf 2007;16(9):988–94.
41. Czeizel AE, Eros E, Rockenbauer M, et al. Short-term oral diazepam treatment during pregnancy: a population-based teratological case-control study. Clin Drug Investig 2003;23(7):451–62.
42. Eros E, Czeizel AE, Rockenbauer M, et al. A population-based case-control teratologic study of nitrazepam, medazepam, tofisopam, alprazolum and clonazepam treatment during pregnancy. Eur J Obstet Gynecol Reprod Biol 2002; 101(2):147–54.
43. Dolovich LR, Addis A, Vaillancourt JM, et al. Benzodiazepine use in pregnancy and major malformations or oral cleft: meta-analysis of cohort and case-control studies. BMJ 1998;317(7162):839–43.
44. Mandelli M, Morselli PL, Nordio S, et al. Placental transfer to diazepam and its disposition in the newborn. Clin Pharmacol Ther 1975;17(5):564–72.
45. Iqbal MM, Sobhan T, Ryals T. Effects of commonly used benzodiazepines on the fetus, the neonate, and the nursing infant. Psychiatr Serv 2002;53(1):39–49.
46. Oei J, Lui K. Management of the newborn infant affected by maternal opiates and other drugs of dependency. J Paediatr Child Health 2007;43(1–2):9–18.
47. Choo RE, Huestis MA, Schroeder JR, et al. Neonatal abstinence syndrome in methadone-exposed infants is altered by level of prenatal tobacco exposure. Drug Alcohol Depend 2004;75(3):253–60.
48. Winklbaur B, Baewert A, Jagsch R, et al. Association between prenatal tobacco exposure and outcome of neonates born to opioid-maintained mothers. Implications for treatment. Eur Addict Res 2009;15(3):150–6.
49. Gray TR, Choo RE, Concheiro M, et al. Prenatal methadone exposure, meconium biomarker concentrations and neonatal abstinence syndrome. Addiction 2010;105(12):2151–9.
50. Arendt RE, Short EJ, Singer LT, et al. Children prenatally exposed to cocaine: developmental outcomes and environmental risks at seven years of age. J Dev Behav Pediatr 2004;25(2):83–90.
51. Frank DA, Augustyn M, Knight WG, et al. Growth, development, and behavior in early childhood following prenatal cocaine exposure: a systematic review. JAMA 2001;285(12):1613–25.
52. Schempf AH. Illicit drug use and neonatal outcomes: a critical review. Obstet Gynecol Surv 2007;62(11):749–57.
53. Hunt RW, Tzioumi D, Collins E, et al. Adverse neurodevelopmental outcome of infants exposed to opiate in-utero. Early Hum Dev 2008;84(1):29–35.
54. Jones HE, Kaltenbach K, O'Grady KE. The complexity of examining developmental outcomes of children prenatally exposed to opiates. A response to Hunt et al. Adverse neurodevelopmental outcome of infants exposed to opiates in-utero. Early Human Development (2008, 84, 29–35). Early Hum Dev 2009; 85(4):271–2.
55. Bandstra ES, Morrow CE, Mansoor E, et al. Prenatal drug exposure: infant and toddler outcomes. J Addict Dis 2010;29(2):245–58.
56. Lester BM, Lagasse LL. Children of addicted women. J Addict Dis 2010;29(2): 259–76.
57. Kaltenbach K, Finnegan LP. Neonatal abstinence syndrome, pharmacotherapy and developmental outcome. Neurobehav Toxicol Teratol 1986;8(4):353–5.

58. Messinger DS, Bauer CR, Das A, et al. The maternal lifestyle study: cognitive, motor, and behavioral outcomes of cocaine-exposed and opiate-exposed infants through three years of age. Pediatrics 2004;113(6):1677–85.

59. Farid WO, Dunlop SA, Tait RJ, et al. The effects of maternally administered methadone, buprenorphine and naltrexone on offspring: review of human and animal data. Curr Neuropharmacol 2008;6(2):125–50.

60. Nandakumar N, Sankar VS. What is the best evidence based management of neonatal abstinence syndrome? Arch Dis Child Fetal Neonatal Ed 2006;91(6): F463.

61. Sarkar S, Donn SM. Management of neonatal abstinence syndrome in neonatal intensive care units: a national survey. J Perinatol 2006;26(1):15–7.

62. O'Grady MJ, Hopewell J, White MJ. Management of neonatal abstinence syndrome: a national survey and review of practice. Arch Dis Child Fetal Neonatal Ed 2009;94(4):F249–52.

63. Crocetti MT, Amin DD, Jansson LM. Variability in the evaluation and management of opiate-exposed newborns in Maryland. Clin Pediatr (Phila) 2007; 46(7):632–5.

64. Lipsitz PJ. A proposed narcotic withdrawal score for use with newborn infants. A pragmatic evaluation of its efficacy. Clin Pediatr (Phila) 1975;14(6):592–4.

65. Green M, Suffet F. The Neonatal Narcotic Withdrawal Index: a device for the improvement of care in the abstinence syndrome. Am J Drug Alcohol Abuse 1981;8(2):203–13.

66. Zahorodny W, Rom C, Whitney W, et al. The neonatal withdrawal inventory: a simplified score of newborn withdrawal. J Dev Behav Pediatr 1998;19(2): 89–93.

67. Finnegan LP, Kaltenbach K. In: Hoekelman RA, Friedman SB, Nelson N, et al, editors. Neonatal abstinence syndrome. St Louis (MO): Mosby; 1992. p. 1367–78.

68. Jones HE, Johnson RE, Jasinski DR, et al. Buprenorphine versus methadone in the treatment of pregnant opioid-dependent patients: effects on the neonatal abstinence syndrome. Drug Alcohol Depend 2005;79(1):1–10.

69. Jones HE, Kaltenbach K, Heil SH, et al. Neonatal abstinence syndrome after methadone or buprenorphine exposure. N Engl J Med 2010;363(24):2320–31.

70. Kraft WK, Dysart K, Greenspan JS, et al. Revised dose schema of sublingual buprenorphine in the treatment of the neonatal opioid abstinence syndrome. Addiction 2011;106(3):574–80.

71. Agthe AG, Kim GR, Mathias KB, et al. Clonidine as an adjunct therapy to opioids for neonatal abstinence syndrome: a randomized, controlled trial. Pediatrics 2009;123(5):e849–56.

72. Zimmermann-Baer U, Notzli U, Rentsch K, et al. Finnegan neonatal abstinence scoring system: normal values for first 3 days and weeks 5-6 in non-addicted infants. Addiction 2010;105(3):524–8.

73. van Sleuwen BE, Engelberts AC, Boere-Boonekamp MM, et al. Swaddling: a systematic review. Pediatrics 2007;120(4):e1097–106.

74. Jansson LM. Neonatal abstinence syndrome. Acta Paediatr 2008;97(10):1321–3.

75. Oei J, Feller JM, Lui K. Coordinated outpatient care of the narcotic-dependent infant. J Paediatr Child Health 2001;37(3):266–70.

76. Coyle MG, Ferguson A, Lagasse L, et al. Diluted tincture of opium (DTO) and phenobarbital versus DTO alone for neonatal opiate withdrawal in term infants. J Pediatr 2002;140(5):561–4.

77. Osborn DA, Jeffery HE, Cole MJ. Opiate treatment for opiate withdrawal in newborn infants. Cochrane Database Syst Rev 2010;(10):CD002059.

78. Osborn DA, Jeffery HE, Cole MJ. Sedatives for opiate withdrawal in newborn infants. Cochrane Database Syst Rev 2010;(10):CD002053.
79. Hudak ML, Tan RC. Neonatal drug withdrawal. Pediatrics 2012;129(2):e540–60.
80. Jansson LM, Velez M. Neonatal abstinence syndrome. Curr Opin Pediatr 2012; 24(2):252–8.
81. Johnson K, Gerada C, Greenough A. Treatment of neonatal abstinence syndrome. Arch Dis Child Fetal Neonatal Ed 2003;88(1):F2–5.
82. Colombini N, Elias R, Busuttil M, et al. Hospital morphine preparation for abstinence syndrome in newborns exposed to buprenorphine or methadone. Pharm World Sci 2008;30(3):227–34.
83. Jones HC. Shorter dosing interval of opiate solution shortens hospital stay for methadone babies. Fam Med 1999;31(5):327–30.
84. Bouwmeester NJ, Hop WC, van Dijk M, et al. Postoperative pain in the neonate: age-related differences in morphine requirements and metabolism. Intensive Care Med 2003;29(11):2009–15.
85. Bouwmeester NJ, Anderson BJ, Tibboel D, et al. Developmental pharmacokinetics of morphine and its metabolites in neonates, infants and young children. Br J Anaesth 2004;92(2):208–17.
86. Barrett DA, Barker DP, Rutter N, et al. Morphine, morphine-6-glucuronide and morphine-3-glucuronide pharmacokinetics in newborn infants receiving diamorphine infusions. Br J Clin Pharmacol 1996;41(6):531–7.
87. Ferrari A, Coccia CP, Bertolini A, et al. Methadone—metabolism, pharmacokinetics and interactions. Pharmacol Res 2004;50(6):551–9.
88. Yang F, Tong X, McCarver DG, et al. Population-based analysis of methadone distribution and metabolism using an age-dependent physiologically based pharmacokinetic model. J Pharmacokinet Pharmacodyn 2006;33(4):485–518.
89. Madden JD, Chappel JN, Zuspan F, et al. Observation and treatment of neonatal narcotic withdrawal. Am J Obstet Gynecol 1977;127(2):199–201.
90. Lainwala S, Brown ER, Weinschenk NP, et al. A retrospective study of length of hospital stay in infants treated for neonatal abstinence syndrome with methadone versus oral morphine preparations. Adv Neonatal Care 2005;5(5):265–72.
91. Backes CH, Backes CR, Gardner D, et al. Neonatal abstinence syndrome: transitioning methadone-treated infants from an inpatient to an outpatient setting. J Perinatol 2011. [Epub ahead of print]. http://dx.doi.org/10.1038/jp.2011.114.
92. Gowing L, Ali R, White JM. Buprenorphine for the management of opioid withdrawal. Cochrane Database Syst Rev 2009;(3):CD002025.
93. Kraft WK, Gibson E, Dysart K, et al. Sublingual buprenorphine for treatment of neonatal abstinence syndrome: a randomized trial. Pediatrics 2008;122(3): e601–7.
94. Kuhlman JJ Jr, Levine B, Johnson RE, et al. Relationship of plasma buprenorphine and norbuprenorphine to withdrawal symptoms during dose induction, maintenance and withdrawal from sublingual buprenorphine. Addiction 1998; 93(4):549–59.
95. Anagnostis EA, Sadaka RE, Sailor LA, et al. Formulation of buprenorphine for sublingual use in neonates. Journal of Pediatric Pharmacology & Therapeutics 2011;16(4):281–4.
96. Jackson L, Ting A, McKay S, et al. A randomised controlled trial of morphine versus phenobarbitone for neonatal abstinence syndrome. Arch Dis Child Fetal Neonatal Ed 2004;89(4):F300–4.
97. Pitlick W, Painter M, Pippenger C. Phenobarbital pharmacokinetics in neonates. Clin Pharmacol Ther 1978;23(3):346–50.

98. Finnegan LP, Michael H, Leifer B. The use of phenobarbital in treating abstinence in newborns exposed in utero to psychoactive agents. NIDA Res Monogr 1984;49:329.
99. Wu D, Kraft WK, Ehrlich ME, et al. Sublingual bioavailability of buprenorphine in newborns with neonatal abstinence syndrome—a case study on physiological and developmental changes using SIMCYP. Presented at the American College of Clinical Pharmacology meeting. Philadelphia (PA), 2009. Available at: http://jdc.jefferson.edu/petfp/24/. Accessed August 10, 2012.
100. Xie HG, Cao YJ, Gauda EB, et al. Clonidine clearance matures rapidly during the early postnatal period: a population pharmacokinetic analysis in newborns with neonatal abstinence syndrome. J Clin Pharmacol 2011;51(4):502–11.
101. Wachman EM, Brown MS, Paul JA, et al. Single nucleotide polymorphisms and variability in severity of neonatal abstinence syndrome. Pediatric Academic Societies 2012.
102. Mass SB. Supporting breastfeeding in the United States: the Surgeon General's call to action. Curr Opin Obstet Gynecol 2011;23(6):460–4.
103. Jansson LM, Choo R, Velez ML, et al. Methadone maintenance and breastfeeding in the neonatal period. Pediatrics 2008;121(1):106–14.
104. Abdel-Latif ME, Pinner J, Clews S, et al. Effects of breast milk on the severity and outcome of neonatal abstinence syndrome among infants of drug-dependent mothers. Pediatrics 2006;117(6):e1163–9.
105. McQueen KA, Murphy-Oikonen J, Gerlach K, et al. The impact of infant feeding method on neonatal abstinence scores of methadone-exposed infants. Adv Neonatal Care 2011;11(4):282–90.
106. Liu AJ, Nanan R. Methadone maintenance and breastfeeding in the neonatal period. Pediatrics 2008;121(4):869.
107. Grimm D, Pauly E, Poschl J, et al. Buprenorphine and norbuprenorphine concentrations in human breast milk samples determined by liquid chromatography-tandem mass spectrometry. Ther Drug Monit 2005;27(4):526–30.
108. Marquet P, Chevrel J, Lavignasse P, et al. Buprenorphine withdrawal syndrome in a newborn. Clin Pharmacol Ther 1997;62(5):569–71.
109. Ilett KF, Hackett LP, Gower S, et al. Estimated dose exposure of the neonate to buprenorphine and its metabolite norbuprenorphine via breastmilk during maternal buprenorphine substitution treatment. Breastfeed Med 2011. [Epub ahead of print].
110. Lindemalm S, Nydert P, Svensson JO, et al. Transfer of buprenorphine into breast milk and calculation of infant drug dose. J Hum Lact 2009;25(2):199–205.
111. Johnson RE, Jones HE, Fischer G. Use of buprenorphine in pregnancy: patient management and effects on the neonate. Drug Alcohol Depend 2003;70(Suppl 2):S87–101.
112. Lejeune C, Aubisson S, Simmat-Durand L, et al. Withdrawal syndromes of newborns of pregnant drug abusers maintained under methadone or high-dose buprenorphine: 246 cases. Ann Med Interne (Paris) 2001;152(Suppl 7):21–7 [in French].
113. Loustauneau A, Auriacombe M, Daulouede JP, et al. Is buprenorphine a potential alternative to methadone for treating pregnant drug users? Inventory of clinical data in the literature. Ann Med Interne (Paris) 2002;153(Suppl 7):2S31–2S36 [in French].
114. SAMHSA (Substance Abuse, and Mental Health Services Administration). SAMHSA clinical guidelines for the use of buprenorphine in the treatment of opioid addiction: treatment improvement protocol series, No. 40. Rockville (MD): USDHHS; 2004.

115. Skorpen F, Laugsand EA, Klepstad P, et al. Variable response to opioid treatment: any genetic predictors within sight? Palliat Med 2008;22(4):310–27.
116. Troisi A, Frazzetto G, Carola V, et al. Social hedonic capacity is associated with the A118G polymorphism of the mu-opioid receptor gene (OPRM1) in adult healthy volunteers and psychiatric patients. Soc Neurosci 2011;6(1):88–97.
117. Campa D, Gioia A, Tomei A, et al. Association of ABCB1/MDR1 and OPRM1 gene polymorphisms with morphine pain relief. Clin Pharmacol Ther 2008; 83(4):559–66.
118. Rakvag TT, Ross JR, Sato H, et al. Genetic variation in the catechol-O-methyltransferase (COMT) gene and morphine requirements in cancer patients with pain. Mol Pain 2008;4:64.
119. Tammimaki AE, Mannisto PT. Are genetic variants of COMT associated with addiction? Pharmacogenet Genomics 2010;20(12):717–41.
120. Gertler R, Brown HC, Mitchell DH, et al. Dexmedetomidine: a novel sedative-analgesic agent. Proc (Bayl Univ Med Cent) 2001;14(1):13–21.
121. Oschman A, McCabe T, Kuhn RJ. Dexmedetomidine for opioid and benzodiazepine withdrawal in pediatric patients. Am J Health Syst Pharm 2011;68(13): 1233–8.
122. Gowing L, Farrell M, Ali R, et al. Alpha2-adrenergic agonists for the management of opioid withdrawal. Cochrane Database Syst Rev 2009;(2):CD002024.
123. De Cock RF, Piana C, Krekels EH, et al. The role of population PK-PD modelling in paediatric clinical research. Eur J Clin Pharmacol 2011;67(Suppl 1):5–16.
124. Hoder EL, Leckman JF, Poulsen J, et al. Clonidine treatment of neonatal narcotic abstinence syndrome. Psychiatry Res 1984;13(3):243–51.
125. Leikin JB, Mackendrick WP, Maloney GE, et al. Use of clonidine in the prevention and management of neonatal abstinence syndrome. Clin Toxicol (Phila) 2009; 47(6):551–5.
126. Esmaeili A, Keinhorst AK, Schuster T, et al. Treatment of neonatal abstinence syndrome with clonidine and chloral hydrate. Acta Paediatr 2010;99(2):209–14.

Update on Pain Assessment in Sick Neonates and Infants

Monique van Dijk, PhD[a,b,*], Dick Tibboel, MD, PhD[a]

KEYWORDS

- Pain measurement • Critically ill • Neonates • Infants • Review

KEY POINTS

- Newly introduced behavioral and multidimensional pain assessment tools have limited added value because they largely overlap with existing tools.
- Although most research focuses primarily on acute pain, clinical practice also presents the challenge of assessing prolonged and/or persisting pain.
- Many institutions have not yet adopted pain assessment as the fifth vital sign. The reasons for this noncompliance have not yet been elucidated.
- The effectiveness of behavioral pain assessment is still a matter of debate and its use as primary end point in analgesia-related trials has recently been challenged.
- Pain assessment should not be implemented as a stand-alone procedure but should come with pain treatment instructions.

PROLOGUE

To understand how complicated pain assessment in neonates and young infants is, this article presents 3 scenarios: a 25-week-old neonate with sepsis in the neonatal intensive care unit (NICU) in Rotterdam, the Netherlands; an infant with Down syndrome after major cardiac surgery in the cardiac intensive care unit (CICU) in Dublin, Ireland; and a 5-month-old malnourished baby with meningitis and pneumonia on the pediatric ward in Cape Town, South Africa. To start with, who can tell how much pain these children experience? They cannot tell us. These clinical situations are different from the research settings in which validation studies of pain assessment tools usually take place. The challenge is to bridge the gap between research and clinical practice and devise a method that is suitable in all circumstances and conditions, if such a method is possible.

[a] Intensive Care, Department of Pediatric Surgery, Erasmus MC-Sophia Children's Hospital, Room Sk 1276, Dr Molewaterplein 60, 3015 GJ, Rotterdam, The Netherlands; [b] Division of Neonatology, Department of Pediatrics, Erasmus MC-Sophia Children's Hospital, Room Sk 1276, Dr Molewaterplein 60, 3015 GJ, Rotterdam, The Netherlands
* Corresponding author.
E-mail address: m.vandijk.3@erasmusmc.nl

Pediatr Clin N Am 59 (2012) 1167–1181
http://dx.doi.org/10.1016/j.pcl.2012.07.012
0031-3955/12/$ – see front matter © 2012 Elsevier Inc. All rights reserved.

pediatric.theclinics.com

This article first identifies the framework of patient groups, severity of illness, and type of pain. It then describes psychometric studies of new and existing instruments published in the past 5 years, and describes how pain assessment in these vulnerable patients differs between the research setting and clinical practice.

PATIENT GROUPS

For the purpose of this article, the term neonates refers to all newborns requiring intensive care, be it for premature birth with its associated health challenges, congenital anomalies requiring surgery, or other perinatal problems. The term infants, derived from the Latin word infans, meaning unable to speak or speechless, usually refers to children up to 24 months of age, a definition that this article follows. It also includes studies on neonates and infants with neurologic impairments, a group of patients too often excluded from reports on pain assessment.

SEVERITY OF ILLNESS

Being sick has various gradations in terms of severity. It is known from earlier studies that severity of illness may affect the way neonates and infants express pain. Several risk of mortality scores, such as the Clinical Risk Index for Babies (CRIB)[1,2] and the Pediatric Index of Mortality (PIM and PIM-II)[3,4] and the Score for Neonatal Acute Physiology (SNAPPE II and III),[5] are considered proxy measures for severity of illness in neonates and infants. In a longitudinal study in 35 preterm newborns, Williams and colleagues,[6] found lower pain scores during heel lance in the more severely ill newborns. In extremely low gestational age infants this resulted in a dampened facial response to heel lancing.[7,8] In contrast with these studies, Valeri and colleagues[9] observed that pain responses to heel lance did not differ between newborns with high CRIB scores and those with lower CRIB scores.

However, because these risk of mortality scores take into account only physiologic parameters at the beginning of hospital admission or directly after birth, they may not fully encompass the severity of illness that affects pain expression in the course of the admission, such as in patients who develop necrotizing enterocolitis or sepsis, or those requiring major surgery. A multicenter study evaluating severity of illness in more than 3000 infants between 0 and 2 months old in health facilities in Bangladesh, Bolivia, Ghana, India, Pakistan, and South Africa[10] offered a new perspective that is worth investigating in the intensive care unit (ICU) setting. The investigators identified 7 clinical signs predictive of severe illness, 4 of which are behavioral: lethargy, movement only when stimulated, grunting, and stiff limbs. The other 3 signs included a history of difficult feeding, a history of convulsion, and temperature greater than 37.5°C or less than 35.5°C. There is no reason not to use some of these signs for patients in a NICU or pediatric intensive care unit (PICU). In short, verification is needed of whether the cutoff values used for pain assessment in neonates and children remain valid when the patient is severely ill. If so, practitioners need to be educated about such differences, recognize signs of severe illness, and be able to apply the pain assessment tools appropriately.

TYPES OF PAIN

1. Procedural pain, for instance as caused by heel lancing, usually serves as the gold standard paradigm to validate pain assessment instruments and to evaluate pain-reducing interventions such as the administration of sucrose and breastfeeding. In clinical practice, children undergo many (up to an average of 10–14 per day) potentially painful procedures, often performed without pain-reducing interventions.[11–14]

2. Postoperative pain is usually defined as pain experienced in the first 24 to 48 hours after surgery. The supposed advantage of this type of pain is the context; health care providers expect this type of pain and specifically monitor it. Although several randomized controlled trials have detailed optimal dosages of opioids for postoperative pain management for different age groups, the large interindividual variability in morphine requirements remains a challenge in achieving rapid pain control in each setting.[15,16] Proper guidelines should prevent underdosing and overdosing and it is the responsibility of the health care providers to follow guidelines or, if necessary, communicate admissible deviations from these guidelines in individual cases (**Fig. 1**).

3. Chronic pain, usually defined as pain lasting for more than 3 months, does not apply to newborns and infants because they have not lived long enough to fit these temporal criteria.[17] With regard to hospitalized neonates and infants, it is better to talk about prolonged or persisting pain. So far, health care providers have not reached consensus on a new definition.[17] Prolonged or persisting pain is primarily caused by disease, for example necrotizing enterocolitis or peritonitis. However, some therapies cause prolonged pain (eg, mechanical ventilation with occasionally multiple endotracheal intubations, nasogastric tube insertions, and occasional chest drains).

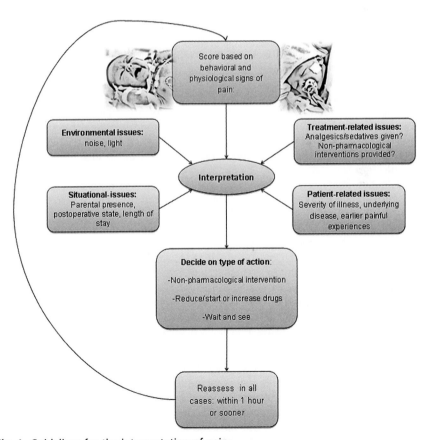

Fig. 1. Guidelines for the interpretation of pain.

PAIN ASSESSMENT

Two recent reviews describe the history of research on pain assessment in neonates and preterm neonates.[18,19] The first, by Ranger and colleagues[18] (2007), gives an overview of the existing controversies, such as the whether physiologic or behavioral responses should be assessed, and the possible influences of illness, postnatal age, gestational age, and behavioral state on pain expression. The other, by Holsti and colleagues[19] (2011), describes the evolution of pain assessment in preterm neonates from a more behaviorally oriented towards a brain-oriented approach using electroencephalography (EEG). However, both reviews underscore that many pain assessment techniques are not yet readily available at the bedside of most newborn patients. They require complex infrastructure and time-fixed data monitoring integrating all variables. However, these requirements cannot easily be met in day-to-day clinical practice.

Pain assessment in neonates at risk for neurologic impairment was addressed by Stevens and colleagues[20] in 2007. They evaluated the pain response to a heel stick in cohorts of infants with low, moderate, and high risk for neurologic impairment. All infants responded to heel lance, although the response magnitude with respect to facial expression and cry differed between the cohorts.

PAIN ASSESSMENT TOOLS

This article uses the term pain assessment tool rather than pain measurement instrument or pain assessment instrument; these terms are interchangeable.

Since the 1980s, there has been a proliferation of pain assessment tools for preverbal infants; they were reviewed in several publications between 1999 and 2004.[21–24] What has been developed since then? Most of these tools were validated for acute pain only. In recent years, there has been a shift toward the assessment of prolonged or persisting pain.[17,18,25] The Neurologic Outcomes and Preemptive Analgesia in Neonates (NEOPAIN) trial in preterm ventilated neonates found that facial expressions of pain, high activity levels, poor response to handling, and poor synchrony with ventilation were good indicators of pain because they occurred more often in those receiving placebo compared with those infants administered morphine.[26]

A qualitative study among health care providers elicited potential indicators for infant chronic pain such as no reaction when subjected to acute pain to hyperreactivity, lack of social interaction, inability to settle or to respond to comforting, and physiologic signs.[17]

Two validated pain assessment tools for prolonged or persisting pain are currently available: the EDIN (Échelle Douleur Inconfort Nouveau-Né [Neonatal Pain and Discomfort Scale])[27] for premature neonates, and the COMFORT behavior scale[28] for patients between 0 and 3 years old.

To our knowledge, 6 new pain assessment tools have been published since 2006; 2 contain behavioral items only, and 4 are multidimensional, incorporating both behavioral and physiologic items. **Table 1** gives an overview of these instruments.

1. Holsti and colleagues[29] found that finger splay and fisting were indicators of acute pain during heel lance. In addition, they developed and validated the Behavioral Indicators of Infant Pain (BIIP) scale, adding these hand actions to the indicators behavioral state and facial expression.[30,31] User instruction of this scale is provided at http://www.developmentalcare.net/. These indicators are also included in the behavioral assessment of stress as conducted in the Newborn Individualized Developmental Care and Assessment Program (NIDCAP).[29]

Table 1
Overview of new scales that have been validated since 2006

Tool, Year	Indicators	Type of Pain/Patients	Results
Behavioral Tools			
BIIP,[30,31] 2007 and 2008	(1) Behavioral state, (2) facial expression, (3) hand actions (finger splay and fisting)	Study 1: heel lance, n = 92; GA 24–31 wk Study 2: heel lance vs diaper change, n = 69; GA 24–32 wk	Internal consistency 0.82 Interrater reliability 0.80–0.92 Correlation with NIPS 0.64 Correlation with heart rate 0.45 Study 2 BIIP scores were statistically significantly higher during blood collection than during diaper change
COMFORTneo,[32] 2009	(1) Behavioral state, (2) calmness/agitation, (3) respiratory response or crying (spontaneously breathing children), (4) body movement, (5) facial tension, (6) muscle tone	Prolonged pain in n = 286 neonates GA 24.6–42.6 wk	Internal consistency 0.84–0.88 Interrater reliability 0.79 Correlation with NRS pain 0.52
Multidimensional Tools			
MAPS,[33,44] 2007	(1) Vital signs, (2) breathing pattern, (3) facial expression, (4) body movements, (5) state of arousal	Postoperative pain, n = 43; infants 0–31 mo old	Internal consistency 0.68 Interrater reliability 0.68–0.84
N-PASS,[34,35] 2008, 2010	(1) Crying irritability, (2) behavior state, (3) facial expression, (4) extremities tone, (5) vital signs, heart rate, RR, BP, Sao_2	Study 1: ventilated and/or postoperative n = 46; 23–40 wk Study 2: heel lance, n = 42; GA 23–40 wk	Internal consistency 0.85–0.95 Interrater reliability 0.88–0.93 Correlation with PIPP 0.61–0.83 Scores during heel lance statistically sign higher than for sham procedures
FANS,[36] 2010	(1) Heart rate, (2) bradycardia or desaturation, (3) limb movements, (4) vocal expression	Heel lance, n = 67; GA 30–35 wk	Internal consistency 0.72 Interrater reliability 0.92 Correlation FANS and DAN 0.88
PASPI,[37] 2011	(1) Behavioral state, (2) facial expression, (3) heart rate, (4) oxygen saturation, (5) hand behavior (splay and fisting)	Heel lance, n = 60; preterm 27.6–36.3 GA	Internal consistency 0.84 Interrater reliability 0.88–0.93 Correlation with VAS between 0.74 and 0.83 Correlation with PIPP 0.74 and 0.83

Abbreviations: BIIP, Behavioral Indicators of Infant Pain; BP, blood pressure; DAN, Douleur Aiguë du Nouveau-Né; FANS, Faceless Acute Neonatal Pain Scale; GA, gestational age; MAPS, Multidimensional Assessment of Pain Scale; NIPS, Neonatal Infant Pain Scale; NRS, Numeric Rating Scale; N-PASS, Neonatal Pain, Agitation, and Sedation Scale; PASPI, Pain Assessment Scale for Preterm Infants; PIPP, Premature Infant Pain Profile; RR, respiration rate; Sao_2, arterial oxygen saturation; VAS, visual analogue scale.

2. The COMFORTneo scale is an adaptation of the COMFORT behavior scale and is intended to better represent characteristics of preterm neonates.[32] It was generally validated in a large cohort of neonates and concurrent validity was established with the Numeric Rating Scale Pain and Distress. The COMFORTneo scale assesses pain and distress and is also able to identify oversedation.

3. The Multidimensional Assessment Pain Scale (MAPS) was validated for postoperative pain assessment in neonates and infants. The psychometric evaluation was performed in a small sample and the association with the existing FLACC (Faces, Legs, Arms, Cry, and Consolability) scale was visually presented with Bland and Altman plots.[33,34]

4. The Neonatal Pain, Agitation, and Sedation Scale (N-PASS) is intended to assess distress and acute and prolonged pain.[34,35] Information about this scale is available on http://www.n-pass.com/.

5. The Faceless Acute Neonatal Pain Scale (FANS) was developed because, in some cases, it is impossible to observe the facial expression of newborns because of protection against bright lights and noninvasive mask ventilation.[36]

6. The Pain Assessment Scale for Preterm Infants (PASPI) is similar to the BIIP: oxygen saturation and heart rate are added to the 4 items of the BIIP.[37]

In recent years, some existing scales have been studied as well. The Premature Infant Pain Profile (PIPP) seems to be the most studied of the tools for acute pain assessment.[38] A systematic review yielded 62 studies on the PIPP, 14 of which concerned its psychometric properties.[39] The COMFORT behavior scale was recently also validated for postoperative pain assessment in infants with Down syndrome[28] and in patients between 0 and 5 years old with burns.[40] The original COMFORT scale, which also assesses heart rate and mean arterial pressure, is still being used, although 2 studies found that these physiologic parameters could be left out without loss of information.[41,42] However, a study in full-term infants after cardiac surgery suggested that the physiologic items had added value.[43]

PHYSIOLOGIC ASSESSMENT UPDATE

Since the 1980s, a variety of physiologic parameters have served to estimate pain intensity of acute painful procedures. Heart rate and blood pressure are often included in multidimensional scales. In some scales, heart rate and blood pressure are compared against their baseline value. For instance, they use an increase of more than 20% from baseline (eg, N-PASS scale) or a decrease of heart rate of 10 beats per minute (MAPS) as a sign of pain. It would be worthwhile to obtain more information about the results of these physiologic items, although studies rarely go into more detail.[34,35,37,43,44]

A new and promising line of research focuses on physiologically oriented tools and tools that try to link pain expression to pain neurobiology. There are 2 major challenges. The first is the discrepancy between the response in the central nervous system elicited by the primary nociceptive stimulus and the behavioral response.[45,46] The second is the relation between EEG and functional magnetic resonance imaging changes and conscious experience of the painful stimulus.

HEART RATE VARIABILITY

Heart rate variability (HRV; the variation in the interval between heart beats) is mediated primarily by the changing levels of parasympathetic and sympathetic outflow from the central nervous system to the sinoatrial node of the heart. Term newborns showed decreased HRV and increased heart rate during heel lance.[47] More recently, Faye and colleagues[48] applied the High-Frequency Variability Index (HFVI) in 28 full-term newborns after surgery. The HFVI correlated (r = 0.7) significantly with the EDIN scale; thus the investigators concluded that postoperative pain was associated with a decreased high-frequency HRV. Most scientific work on HRV now uses power spectral density (PSD) analysis to relate the simple measurement of beat-to-beat variability to the state of the autonomic nervous system or vagal tone. Padhye and colleagues[49] found that HRV in 38 infants decreased during heel lance or venipuncture, but to a lesser extent in mechanically ventilated infants, which the investigators could not explain.

SKIN CONDUCTANCE

During the last 5 years, several studies have explored more objective approaches to pain assessment, such as skin conductance (SC) measurement. SC measurement is a method based on stress-induced sweating of the hand palms and/or foot soles.[50] Sweat glands are stimulated by sympathetic excitatory efferent neurons and sweat is released within 1 to 2 seconds of excitation, increasing SC because of a reduction of skin resistance. SC can be monitored continuously; the device calculates mean peaks per second over an interval of 10 to 60 seconds. The SC studies in newborns and infants published since 2006 are listed in **Table 2**. A study by Hullett and colleagues[51] suggests that SC measurement shows good sensitivity but moderate specificity for postoperative pain in children from 1 to 6 years old. Other studies showed that SC is correlated with body temperature in infants[53] and administration of glucose as an analgesic before heel lancing in neonates,[54] and that measurement is sensitive for movement artifacts.[55,56] The tool is not yet ready for clinical practice because of the wide range of reported sensitivity and specificity.

Table 2
Pediatric SC studies including newborns or infants

Study	Patient Group and Type of Pain	Results, Conclusions
Harrison et al,[52] 2006	N = 21; GA 25–40 wk, postnatal age 1–4 mo	SC highly variable, not statistically significantly different between painful and nonpainful procedures
Hullet et al,[51] 2009	N = 165; 1–6 y, postoperative pain	Compared with FLACC, sensitivity 90% and specificity 64%, discriminating between no to minor pain and moderate to severe pain
Valkenburg et al,[53] 2012	N = 11; infants postnatal age 13–76 d without evident pain	Skin temperature was statistically significantly correlated with SC values in all patients
Munsters et al,[54] 2012	N = 10; GA 22.4–34.3 wk, postnatal age 1–47 d, heel lancing compared with feeding, orogastric tube placement, and routine care	Routine care did not give any changes in SC. SC increased during heel lance in all infants. Oral glucose administration before heel lance unexpectedly increased SC in all infants

NIRS

NIRS is a noninvasive assessment of brain function through the intact skull. It detects changes in blood hemoglobin concentrations associated with neural activity. Bartocci and colleagues (2006)[57] studied 29 preterm neonates at 28 to 36 weeks of gestation and found that standardized tactile stimuli (skin disinfection) and venipuncture elicited specific hemodynamic responses in the somatosensory cortex, implying conscious sensory perception in preterm neonates.

Slater and colleagues[45] applied NIRS and the PIPP during heel lance and in some infants found cortical pain responses with NIRS registration without a change in facial expression. The investigators suggest that, in some cases, NIRS is more sensitive to assess pain than a behavioral pain assessment tool. Emotions were stirred by a study in the *Lancet* in which Slater and colleagues showed that sucrose during heel stick reduced behavioral pain scores (PIPP) but not activity in neonatal brain recorded with EEG or spinal cord nociceptive circuits assessed with spinal nociceptive reflex withdrawal activity.[46]

ANALGESIC STUDIES

Pain assessment tools need to be validated before they are implemented in daily clinical practice. Proper validation is just as important when tools are used in analgesic trials. Such efforts have greatly been supported by legislature promoting drug trials in children. In the United States (Food and Drug Administration Modernization Act in 1997, Best Pharmaceuticals for Children Act in 2002, and Pediatric Research Equity Act in 2003), legislation came into force to promote drug development and the authorization of medicines for use in pediatric patients. Similar legislation was introduced in the European Union in January 2007 (The Pediatric Regulation) (full texts on www.fda. gov and www.ema.europe.eu). Core outcome measures for children and adolescents have been established under the auspices of the Initiative on Methods, Measurement, and Pain Assessment in Clinical Trials (IMMPACT), but measures for neonates and infants are not yet available.[58]

Recently, a US Food and Drug Administration scientific workshop proposed rescue medication as a surrogate end point for analgesic trials in neonates and infants, although it was emphasized that behavioral measures remain the most useful for clinical research in this age group.[59] Placebo-controlled analgesic trials would be ethically problematic if more than minor pain were administered and effective analgesic therapy is available. The workshop members suggested a trial design in which nurse-controlled analgesia provides immediate rescue and reduced use of analgesia would be a surrogate primary efficacy end point. Basal infusions are not used in this setup; differences in cumulative rescue dosing between drug and placebo groups are primary end points, and pain scores are secondary end points. In this study design, long-acting opioids are preferably avoided because of their long duration of action and the influence of active metabolites. These suggestions ignore the concept of preemptive analgesia. Also, optimal dosing regimens of continuous intravenous (IV) morphine and IV paracetamol after major surgery, or during other therapies such as total body cooling, still need to be studied.[60]

FROM RESEARCH TO CLINICAL PRACTICE: HOW TO USE PAIN ASSESSMENT

In 1999, the Veterans Health Administration launched the Pain as the 5th Vital Sign initiative,[61] which was later also supported by the American Pain Society. The argument was that, if pain assessments were to be performed as frequently as heart rate, temperature, respiratory rate, and blood pressure measurements, patients would benefit. The Joint Commission on Accreditation of Health Care Organizations issued pain management standards in 2000 including pain assessment and regular reassessment next to educating patients and their families about pain management. But did all these initiatives result in improvements? Franck and Bruce[62] performed a systematic review in 2009 to find evidence for the usefulness of standard pain assessments in the pediatric setting. Fourteen studies were selected that either evaluated the effect of pain assessment on patient outcomes (n = 10) or the effect of pain assessment on process outcomes (n = 12). All studies had marked differences, including different interventions applied, different pain assessment instruments used, different implementation strategies, and different levels of compliance with the interventions. It was difficult to draw firm conclusions. The only conclusion made was that pain assessment is not yet evidence based. However, there is general consensus in the literature on the necessity of pain assessment in hospitalized neonates and infants.[25,63,64] Another issue is the level of compliance with pain assessment, which has been low in many settings.[65–67]

IMPLEMENTATION OF PAIN ASSESSMENT

In general, implementing guidelines is challenging.[68–70] Pain assessment guidelines normally describe the preferred pain assessment tool and criteria with respect to frequency of scoring. However, the availability of such guidelines does not necessarily translate into appropriate usage. Several studies have addressed ways to improve compliance. A survey among 272 pediatric nurses elicited potential barriers to optimal pain management.[71] The top 5 barriers mentioned included insufficient physician (MD) orders, insufficient MD orders before procedures, insufficient time to premedicate patients before procedures, low priority given to pain management by MDs, and parents' reluctance to have their children receive pain medication. These barriers did not include the role of the nurses themselves, but they were interviewed. This reminds us of one of our own surveys in MDs and nurses a few years ago. Almost everyone said that pain assessment in preverbal infants was important and should be done on a regular basis. However, the gap between this positive attitude and what is done in practice is large. **Fig. 1** shows how we think pain assessment tools should be applied in clinical practice, which is the first step in the process of evaluating whether pain treatment is needed. The second step is to interpret the situation using indicators from the environment, patient, and response to therapies. Combining this with the pain score then allows the determination of what action to undertake.

In clinical practice, it is not helpful to implement pain assessment as a stand-alone procedure. It should come with guidelines that define the actions to be taken if pain assessment indicates pain, which means that pain assessment should be linked to its treatment, and this makes pain guidelines a multidisciplinary responsibility. A multidisciplinary team should develop treatment algorithms or decision trees from the following criteria.

CRITERIA FOR A PAIN TREATMENT ALGORITHM

- Developed or accepted by the medical and nursing staff of the unit
- As simple and unambiguous as possible
- Pain assessment results in guided treatment decisions
- Cutoff values dictate increase or decrease in the amount of administered analgesics
- Reassessment after treatment changes

Several prerequisites must be met before pain assessment can be introduced successfully in a hospital setting.[69,72] First, on the managerial level, there must be outspoken commitment to dedicate time to introduce and maintain pain management strategies. Second, stakeholders, including neonatologists and nurses, need to be involved. Guidelines can be developed using the Appraisal of Guidelines for Research and Evaluation (AGREE) instrument.[73] For example, Spence and colleagues[72] described how they developed a guideline for newborn pain management using this instrument.

DISCUSSION

In spite of a plethora of pain assessment tools for acute pain, there is still a need for better pain assessment strategies for prolonged pain in the NICU and PICU environments. New pain assessment tools show considerable overlap with existing tools.[74] The assessment of pain in infants with neurologic impairment has proved difficult and requires more investigation.[20] One particular challenge is the question of how to interpret arm and hand movements and facial expressions. Are these movements and expressions manifestations of pain, of neurologic impairment, or a combination of both? This challenge of correct interpretation is even greater in asphyxiated neonates receiving hypothermia.

With respect to psychometric evaluations, we would like to see a shift away from correlating similar tools, which results in flattering high correlations.

The existing behavioral assessment tools should be further studied and compared with physiologically oriented tools. Validation should at least include sensitivity to change, and optimal cutoff scores should be calculated from real data. Validation studies should go beyond the heel prick/lance paradigm. Berde and McGrath[75] (2009) presented criteria for candidate physiologic measures of pain intensity. From our own experience, we know how important it is to follow such criteria. We introduced the Bispectral Index Monitor (BIS) as a promising device to establish the level of sedation in preverbal children. It took some time before we realized that the standard BIS algorithm was not applicable to children less than 6 months of age and therefore we discontinued the use of this device in this age group.

FUTURE DIRECTIONS

Worley and colleagues[76] recently introduced a multimodal approach to pain measurements in infants that consists of simultaneous monitoring of the brain (NIRS and EEG), reflex withdrawal (EMG), behavioral activity (video recordings), and autonomic activity (heart rate, oxygen saturation, and respiratory rate). This integrated approach objectively visualizes the central nervous system in combination with validated assessment tools and will result in novel ways to divide the different types of pain in neonates and young infants and its treatment.

Because there are currently no appropriately validated pain assessment tools for prolonged pain, many will probably be developed during the coming years that will all be comparable with each other.

We therefore urge the international pediatric pain community to perform multicenter studies investigating checklists in extremely premature neonates during their hospital stay, neonates with necrotizing enterocolitis (from the onset to surgery and recovery), neonates and infants requiring prolonged mechanical ventilation, and critically ill infants. At the same time, all painful procedures in these infants need to be documented to establish the effect of persisting and prolonged pain on their behavior. In addition, such a checklist should also include signs of well-being. **Table 3** presents

Table 3
Checklist of signs that indicate prolonged pain neonates and infants[a]

	Pain	*Well-Being*
Behavioral signs from observation		
Facial tension or constant grimacing, blank face		
Cry, moaning, verbal complaints		
Fussy, alert, inability to settle		
Lethargic, shutting down, social withdrawal		
Dysregulated sleep		
Relaxed asleep		
Smile, laughing		
Playing		
Behavioral signs after gentle touch		
Tense body		
Clenched fists (difficult to open with finger)		
Sensitive to touch, irritable, poor responses to handling		
Relaxed body posture		
Other signs		
Poor synchrony with ventilation		

[a] Based on literature and own work,[17,25,26] the italics denote behavioral signs associated with well-being.

such a checklist, although the item descriptions need to be further detailed. The items presented are based on different studies[17,25,26] and on our own experience in 3 different children's hospitals in Rotterdam, the Netherlands; Dublin, Ireland; and Cape Town, South Africa.

REFERENCES

1. The CRIB (clinical risk index for babies) score: a tool for assessing initial neonatal risk and comparing performance of neonatal intensive care units. The International Neonatal Network. Lancet 1993;342:193.
2. Parry G, Tucker J, Tarnow-Mordi W, et al. CRIB II: an update of the clinical risk index for babies score. Lancet 2003;361:1789.
3. Shann F, Pearson G, Slater A, et al. Paediatric index of mortality (PIM): a mortality prediction model for children in intensive care. Intensive Care Med 1997;23:201.
4. Slater A, Shann F, Pearson G, et al. PIM2: a revised version of the paediatric index of mortality. Intensive Care Med 2003;29:278.
5. Richardson DK, Corcoran JD, Escobar GJ, et al. SNAP-II and SNAPPE-II: simplified newborn illness severity and mortality risk scores. J Pediatr 2001;138:92.
6. Williams AL, Khattak AZ, Garza CN, et al. The behavioral pain response to heelstick in preterm neonates studied longitudinally: description, development, determinants, and components. Early Hum Dev 2009;85:369.
7. Grunau RE, Holsti L, Haley DW, et al. Neonatal procedural pain exposure predicts lower cortisol and behavioral reactivity in preterm infants in the NICU. Pain 2005;113:293.
8. Johnston CC, Stevens BJ. Experience in a neonatal intensive care unit affects pain response. Pediatrics 1996;98:925.

9. Valeri BO, Gaspardo CM, Martinez FE, et al. Does the neonatal clinical risk for illness severity influence pain reactivity and recovery in preterm infants? Eur J Pain 2012;16:727.

10. Young Infants Clinical Signs Study Group. Clinical signs that predict severe illness in children under age 2 months: a multicentre study. Lancet 2008; 371:135.

11. Carbajal R, Rousset A, Danan C, et al. Epidemiology and treatment of painful procedures in neonates in intensive care units. JAMA 2008;300:60.

12. Harrison D, Loughnan P, Manias E, et al. Analgesics administered during minor painful procedures in a cohort of hospitalized infants: a prospective clinical audit. J Pain 2009;10:715.

13. Simons SH, van Dijk M, Anand KS, et al. Do we still hurt newborn babies? A prospective study of procedural pain and analgesia in neonates. Arch Pediatr Adolesc Med 2003;157:1058.

14. Stevens BJ, Abbott LK, Yamada J, et al. Epidemiology and management of painful procedures in children in Canadian hospitals. CMAJ 2011;183:E403.

15. Knibbe CA, Krekels EH, van den Anker JN, et al. Morphine glucuronidation in preterm neonates, infants and children younger than 3 years. Clin Pharmacokinet 2009;48:371.

16. Tibboel D, Anand KJ, van den Anker JN. The pharmacological treatment of neonatal pain. Semin Fetal Neonatal Med 2005;10:195.

17. Pillai Riddell RR, Stevens BJ, McKeever P, et al. Chronic pain in hospitalized infants: health professionals' perspectives. J Pain 2009;10:1217–25.

18. Ranger M, Johnston CC, Anand KJ. Current controversies regarding pain assessment in neonates. Semin Perinatol 2007;31:283.

19. Holsti L, Grunau RE, Shany E. Assessing pain in preterm infants in the neonatal intensive care unit: moving to a 'brain-oriented' approach. Pain Manag 2011;1:171.

20. Stevens B, McGrath P, Gibbins S, et al. Determining behavioural and physiological responses to pain in infants at risk for neurological impairment. Pain 2007; 127:94.

21. Duhn LJ, Medves JM. A systematic integrative review of infant pain assessment tools. Adv Neonatal Care 2004;4:126.

22. Franck LS, Greenberg CS, Stevens B. Pain assessment in infants and children. Pediatr Clin North Am 2000;47:487.

23. Stevens BJ, Pillai Riddell RR, Oberlander TF, et al. Assessment of pain in neonates and infants. In: Anand KJ, Stevens BJ, McGrath PJ, editors. Pain in neonates and infants, vol. 5, 3rd edition. Amsterdam: Elsevier; 2007. p. 67.

24. van Dijk M, Peters J, Bouwmeester J, et al. Are postoperative pain instruments useful for specific groups of vulnerable infants? Clin Perinatol 2002;29:469.

25. Anand KJ. Pain assessment in preterm neonates. Pediatrics 2007;119:605.

26. Boyle EM, Freer Y, Wong CM, et al. Assessment of persistent pain or distress and adequacy of analgesia in preterm ventilated infants. Pain 2006;124:87.

27. Debillon T, Zupan V, Ravault N, et al. Development and initial validation of the EDIN scale, a new tool for assessing prolonged pain in preterm infants. Arch Dis Child Fetal Neonatal Ed 2001;85:F36.

28. Valkenburg AJ, Boerlage AA, Ista E, et al. The COMFORT-Behavior scale is useful to assess pain and distress in 0- to 3-year-old children with Down syndrome. Pain 2011;152:2059.

29. Holsti L, Grunau RE, Oberlander TF, et al. Specific Newborn Individualized Developmental Care and Assessment Program movements are associated with

acute pain in preterm infants in the neonatal intensive care unit. Pediatrics 2004; 114:65.

30. Holsti L, Grunau RE. Initial validation of the behavioral indicators of infant pain (BIIP). Pain 2007;132(3):264–72.
31. Holsti L, Grunau RE, Oberlander TF, et al. Is it painful or not? Discriminant validity of the Behavioral Indicators of Infant Pain (BIIP) scale. Clin J Pain 2008;24:83.
32. van Dijk M, Roofthooft DW, Anand KJ, et al. Taking up the challenge of measuring prolonged pain in (premature) neonates: the COMFORTneo scale seems promising. Clin J Pain 2009;25:607.
33. Ramelet AS, Rees NW, McDonald S, et al. Clinical validation of the multidimensional assessment of pain scale. Paediatr Anaesth 2007;17:1156.
34. Hummel P, Lawlor-Klean P, Weiss MG. Validity and reliability of the N-PASS assessment tool with acute pain. J Perinatol 2010;30:474.
35. Hummel P, Puchalski M, Creech SD, et al. Clinical reliability and validity of the N-PASS: Neonatal Pain, Agitation and Sedation Scale with prolonged pain. J Perinatol 2008;28:55.
36. Milesi C, Cambonie G, Jacquot A, et al. Validation of a neonatal pain scale adapted to the new practices in caring for preterm newborns. Arch Dis Child Fetal Neonatal Ed 2010;95(4):F263–6.
37. Liaw JJ, Yang L, Chou HL, et al. Psychometric analysis of a Taiwan-version pain assessment scale for preterm infants. J Clin Nurs 2012;21:89.
38. Stevens BJ, Johnston CC, Petryshen P, et al. Premature infant pain profile: development and initial validation. Clin J Pain 1996;12:13.
39. Stevens B, Johnston C, Taddio A, et al. The Premature Infant Pain Profile: evaluation 13 years after development. Clin J Pain 2010;26:813.
40. de Jong A, Baartmans M, Bremer M, et al. Reliability, validity and clinical utility of three types of pain behavioural observation scales for young children with burns aged 0-5 years. Pain 2010;150(3):561–7.
41. Carnevale FA, Razack S. An item analysis of the COMFORT scale in a pediatric intensive care unit. Pediatr Crit Care Med 2002;3:177.
42. van Dijk M, de Boer JB, Koot HM, et al. The reliability and validity of the COMFORT scale as a postoperative pain instrument in 0 to 3-year-old infants. Pain 2000;84:367.
43. Franck LS, Ridout D, Howard R, et al. A comparison of pain measures in newborn infants after cardiac surgery. Pain 2011;152:1758.
44. Ramelet AS, Rees N, McDonald S, et al. Development and preliminary psychometric testing of the Multidimensional Assessment of Pain Scale: MAPS. Paediatr Anaesth 2007;17:333.
45. Slater R, Cantarella A, Franck L, et al. How well do clinical pain assessment tools reflect pain in infants? PLoS Med 2008;5:e129.
46. Slater R, Cornelissen L, Fabrizi L, et al. Oral sucrose as an analgesic drug for procedural pain in newborn infants: a randomised controlled trial. Lancet 2010; 376(9748):1225–32.
47. Lindh V, Wiklund U, Håkannson S. Heel lancing in term new-born infants: an evaluation of pain by frequency domain analysis of heart rate variability. Pain 1999;80:143.
48. Faye PM, De Jonckheere J, Logier R, et al. Newborn infant pain assessment using heart rate variability analysis. Clin J Pain 2010;26:777.
49. Padhye NS, Williams AL, Khattak AZ, et al. Heart rate variability in response to pain stimulus in VLBW infants followed longitudinally during NICU stay. Dev Psychobiol 2009;51:638.

50. Storm H. The development of a software program for analyzing skin conductance changes in preterm infants. Clin Neurophysiol 2001;112:1562.

51. Hullett B, Chambers N, Preuss J, et al. Monitoring electrical skin conductance: a tool for the assessment of postoperative pain in children? Anesthesiology 2009;111:513.

52. Harrison D, Boyce S, Loughnan P, et al. Skin conductance as a measure of pain and stress in hospitalised infants. Early human development 2006;82(9): 603–8.

53. Valkenburg AJ, Niehof SP, van Dijk M, et al. Skin conductance peaks could result from changes in vital parameters unrelated to pain. Pediatr Res 2012; 71:375.

54. Munsters J, Wallstrom L, Agren J, et al. Skin conductance measurements as pain assessment in newborn infants born at 22–27 weeks gestational age at different postnatal age. Early Hum Dev 2012;88:21.

55. Choo EK, Magruder W, Montgomery CJ, et al. Skin conductance fluctuations correlate poorly with postoperative self-report pain measures in school-aged children. Anesthesiology 2010;113:175.

56. Storm H. Why do similar studies conclude differently when they are performed with nearly the same protocol and the same skin conductance technology and on the same population of patients? Anesthesiology 2011;114:464.

57. Bartocci M, Bergqvist LL, Lagercrantz H, et al. Pain activates cortical areas in the preterm newborn brain. Pain 2006;122:109.

58. McGrath PJ, Walco GA, Turk DC, et al. Core outcome domains and measures for pediatric acute and chronic/recurrent pain clinical trials: PedIMMPACT recommendations. J Pain 2008;9:771.

59. Berde CB, Walco GA, Krane EJ, et al. Pediatric analgesic clinical trial designs, measures, and extrapolation: report of an FDA scientific workshop. Pediatrics 2012;129:354.

60. van den Anker JN, Tibboel D. Pain relief in neonates: when to use intravenous paracetamol. Arch Dis Child 2011;96:573.

61. Veterans Health Administration. Pain as the fifth vital sign toolkit. Revised edition. Geriatric and Extended Care Committee; 2000. Available at: http://www.va.gov/PAINMANAGEMENT/docs/TOOLKIT.pdf. Accessed August 8, 2012.

62. Franck LS, Bruce E. Putting pain assessment into practice: why is it so painful? Pain Res Manag 2009;14:13.

63. Batton DG, Barrington KJ, Wallman C. Prevention and management of pain in the neonate: an update. Pediatrics 2006;118:2231.

64. Finley A, Franck LS, Grunau RE, et al. Why children's pain matters. Seattle: International Association for the study of pain; 2005.

65. Drendel AL, Brousseau DC, Gorelick MH. Pain assessment for pediatric patients in the emergency department. Pediatrics 2006;117:1511.

66. Ceelie I, de Wildt SN, de Jong M, et al. Protocolized post-operative pain management in infants; do we stick to it? Eur J Pain 2012;16:760.

67. Losacco V, Cuttini M, Greisen G, et al. Heel blood sampling in European neonatal intensive care units: compliance with pain management guidelines. Arch Dis Child Fetal Neonatal Ed 2011;96:F65.

68. Grol R. Has guideline development gone astray? Yes. BMJ 2010;340:c306.

69. Grol R, Grimshaw J. From best evidence to best practice: effective implementation of change in patients' care. Lancet 2003;362:1225.

70. MacLaren J, Kain ZN. Research to practice in pediatric pain: what are we missing? Pediatrics 2008;122:443.

71. Czarnecki ML, Simon K, Thompson JJ, et al. Barriers to pediatric pain management: a nursing perspective. Pain Manag Nurs 2011;12:154.
72. Spence K, Henderson-Smart D, New K, et al. Evidenced-based clinical practice guideline for management of newborn pain. J Paediatr Child Health 2010;46:184.
73. Agree Collaboration. Development and validation of an international appraisal instrument for assessing the quality of clinical practice guidelines: the AGREE project. Qual Saf Health Care 2003;12:18.
74. Thewissen L, Allegaert K. Analgosedation in neonates: do we still need additional tools after 30 years of clinical research? Arch Dis Child Educ Pract Ed 2011; 96:112.
75. Berde C, McGrath P. Pain measurement and Beecher's challenge: 50 years later. Anesthesiology 2009;111:473.
76. Worley A, Fabrizi L, Boyd S, et al. Multi-modal pain measurements in infants. J Neurosci Methods 2012;205:252.

The Impact of Extracorporeal Life Support and Hypothermia on Drug Disposition in Critically Ill Infants and Children

Enno D. Wildschut, MD, PhD[a],*, Annewil van Saet, MD, PhD[a,b],
Pavla Pokorna, MD[a,c], Maurice J. Ahsman, PharmD, PhD[d],
John N. Van den Anker, MD, PhD[a,e,f,g], Dick Tibboel, MD, PhD[a]

KEYWORDS

- Infant • Extracorporeal membrane oxygenation • Sedation • Analgesia
- Pharmacology • Pharmacokinetics • Pharmacodynamics • Hypothermia

KEY POINTS

- Extracorporeal membrane oxygenation (ECMO) increases volume of distribution and reduces clearance of most drugs.
- Lipophilic drugs in particular are sequestered by the ECMO circuits.
- Sequestration of drugs is to a large extent circuit dependent.
- Hypothermia influences volume of distribution and decreases clearance.
- Hypothermia superimposed on ECMO most likely decreases clearance further, especially for drugs with a high hepatic clearance.
- Therapeutic drug monitoring is recommended for drugs with a small therapeutic window.

Disclosures: The authors have no financial disclosures concerning the contents of this paper.
Conflict of interests: The authors declare that they have no competing or conflicting interests.
[a] Department of Pediatric Surgery, Intensive Care, Erasmus MC-Sophia Children's Hospital, Dr. Molewaterplein 60, 3015 GJ Rotterdam, The Netherlands; [b] Department of Cardio-Thoracic Anesthesiology, Erasmus MC, Dr. Molewaterplein 60, 3015 GJ Rotterdam, The Netherlands; [c] Faculty of Medicine, Department of Pediatrics, PICU/NICU, Charles University, ke Karlovu 2, Praha 2, 121 00 Prague, Czech Republic; [d] LAP&P Consultants BV, Archimedesweg 31, 2333 CM, Leiden, The Netherlands; [e] Division of Pediatric Clinical Pharmacology, Children's National Medical Center, Sheikh Zayed Campus for Advanced Children's Medicine, 111 Michigan Avenue, NW, Washington, DC 20010, USA; [f] Department of Pediatrics, School of Medicine and Health Sciences, The George Washington University, Washington, DC, USA; [g] Department of Pharmacology & Physiology, School of Medicine and Health Sciences, The George Washington University, Washington, DC, USA
* Corresponding author. Department of Pediatric Surgery, Intensive Care, Erasmus MC-Sophia Children's Hospital, Dr Molewaterplein 60, 3015 GJ Rotterdam, The Netherlands.
E-mail address: e.wildschut@erasmusmc.nl

INTRODUCTION

Extracorporeal life support (ECLS) or extracorporeal membrane oxygenation (ECMO) is a technique providing life support in severe but potentially reversible cardiorespiratory failure in patients with an expected mortality greater than 80%.[1] ECLS has been used as prolonged cardiopulmonary support in neonates since 1976[2] with a proven survival benefit in neonates and adults.[3,4]

ECMO provides extracorporeal gas exchange and circulatory support by pumping blood from the patient through an artificial circuit comprising tubing, a pump, an oxygenator, and a heater. The oxygenator is used to oxygenate the blood and extract carbon dioxide. Blood is drawn from a venous access site, preferably a central catheter positioned in the right atrium, and returned either into the right atrium via a double-lumen catheter (venovenous ECMO) for respiratory support or via the carotid artery (venoarterial ECMO) for cardiopulmonary support.

Up to July, 2011, 46,509 patients worldwide have received ECMO support, including 29,839 neonates, 11,779 pediatric patients, and 4891 adult patients (Extracorporeal Life Support Organization registry report, July, 2011). ECMO support is used in a variety of diagnoses in the pediatric population. Cardiac failure is the primary reason for ECMO in 45% of all cases. Diagnoses include cardiopulmonary resuscitation (CPR), cardiomyopathy, cardiomyositis, postcardiothoracic surgery, and sepsis. Pulmonary failure caused by viral or bacterial pneumonia and acute respiratory distress syndrome constitutes the major cause for pulmonary ECMO support. In 10% of all cases, ECMO was initiated during the course of CPR. There are increasing reports of ECMO in severe accidental hypothermia and prolonged refractory CPR.[5-10]

Although it may be lifesaving in critically ill patients, ECMO treatment is associated with several complications and mortality. Overall survival after ECMO support is 62%, and mortality is primarily associated with the underlying disease and complications of/during ECMO such as bleeding, renal failure, and infections.[11-15] Prolonged ECMO support (>10 days) is associated with increased complications (such as nosocomial infections[16-25]) and poor outcome.[15,26]

Neurologic complications are frequent in ECMO patients, with intracranial hemorrhage, infarction, or seizures occurring in 7.4%, 5.7%, and 8.4% of all ECMO patients.[27]

Therapeutic hypothermia is an established therapy to prevent secondary neurologic damage in adults after cardiac arrest as well as in neonates after severe asphyxia.[28-34] The use of therapeutic hypothermia in the pediatric setting remains controversial.[35-37] However, several small studies have explored feasibility and safety of therapeutic hypothermia in the pediatric population.[38-40] At least 1 study included ECMO patients.[38] There are several publications of sustained therapeutic hypothermia in both neonates and infants during ECMO, showing that it is at least feasible.[38,41-44] Although randomized controlled trials (RCTs) in the pediatric setting are lacking, the resuscitation guidelines of the American Heart Association state that mild hypothermia may be considered in children who remain comatose after resuscitation.[45] An RCT evaluating standard hypothermia in neonates on ECMO is being conducted in the United Kingdom to evaluate the effect of hypothermia on neurologic outcome.[41] Hypothermia is used in pediatric postresuscitation patients awaiting RCTs, including ECMO patients.

Pharmacokinetic Changes in ECMO

The use of ECMO is associated with major pharmacokinetic (PK) and pharmacodynamic (PD) changes.[46-49] Patients on ECMO generally receive more than 10 different drugs per day.[50] These patients are heparinized to prevent clotting of the ECMO circuit, receive sedatives and analgesics to alleviate pain and discomfort, diuretics to manage fluid overload, and antibiotics or antiviral medication to treat infections.[50]

ECMO increases the circulating volume of the patient because of the added blood volume necessary to fill the circuit. Total circulating volume may be increased by 5% to more than 100% depending on patient and circuit size. The added volume influences blood composition, coagulation, circulation, and PK. Decreased protein levels, especially albumin, increase the unbound fraction of protein-bound drugs, thereby influencing volume of distribution (Vd) and total body clearance (Cl). Depending on the ECMO mode, organ perfusion and organ function are altered, which alters drug absorption, distribution, metabolism, and elimination.[46]

Profound changes in amount and composition of drug-metabolizing enzymes, organ function, and body composition take place in early infancy. Both total body water and extracellular water content change rapidly within the first months of life. Changes in body water and body fat are most dramatic in the first year of life but continue up to puberty. This situation results in age-specific and drug-specific PK changes.[51,52] Both hepatic and renal Cl are subject to changes in the first month of life. Hepatic metabolism via cytochrome P450 (CYP) and uridine diphosphate glucuronosyltransferase (UGT) are markedly different in the newborn period compared with the pediatric and adult population. Most CYP enzymes reach mature levels at 1 year of age, with higher than adult levels in children younger than 10 years. Renal Cl increases from the newborn period to mature values in the first year of life.[52]

Patients on ECMO are critically ill, which in itself changes PK and PD.[53-55] CYP enzymes are downregulated during inflammation, resulting in reduced Cl of drugs cleared by the liver.[56-58] ECMO increases the inflammatory response by activating inflammatory cytokines, which could further decrease CYP metabolism.[59] Whether ECMO patients differ in this regard compared with patients who are critically ill but not on ECMO remains to be determined.

These changes should be taken into account when evaluating PK changes during ECMO treatment in the pediatric population.

A recent review[46] has evaluated the changes in PK and PD during ECMO. With the use of nonlinear mixed modeling (NONMEM) and liquid chromatography mass spectrometry (LC-MS), sparse sampling strategies are used to access PK in infants on ECMO. Most available studies show altered PK with changes in Vd as well as Cl.[60-74] Typically, Vd is increased between 5% and 400% for most drugs, whereas Cl is decreased between 0% and 50% compared with patients who are not on ECMO, resulting in prolonged elimination half-life.[46]

A major factor in the changed Vd is adsorption of drugs within the ECMO system components. Several studies have reported drug loss up to 99% for some drugs in in vitro setups. Lipophilic drugs in particular are sequestered to a high degree by the ECMO circuit,[75-83] with a strong correlation between lipophilicity expressed as logP and adsorption rates.[77] There is a large difference in adsorption rates between silicone-based membranes and microporous membranes.[77,83] The use of newer circuits with microporous membranes may result in markedly different PK profiles in patients. New systems such as the iLA Activve ECMO circuit (Novalung, Hechingen, Germany) are being used in the pediatric population (Wildschut, personal communication, 2012). It is unclear how these newer systems and oxygenators affect drug disposition.

Incorporating continuous renal replacement therapy into the ECMO circuits influences drug disposition by increasing hemodilution and drug sequestration. Depending on water solubility, molecule size and protein-binding drugs can be cleared via hemofiltration or dialysis.[84] The unbound fraction can be used as a crude estimation for the sieving coefficient and the subsequent expected effect of hemofiltration.[84] Therefore, Cl may be increased for these drugs during dialysis, whereas for other drugs it may be decreased.

Although there are increasing data on PK changes, we are still limited by sparse data and small data sets, which make it difficult to effectively predict PK for our patients. Most PK data are from neonatal studies with large ECMO circuits consisting of PVC tubing and silicone-based membranes.

PK Changes in Hypothermia

Hypothermia is associated with significant changes in physiology as well as absorption, distribution, and elimination of drugs. As a consequence, changes in PK and PD may occur.[47–49] A recent review by van den Broek and colleagues[47] summarized the studies on changes in PK and PD during hypothermia in animals, adults, and children.

Hypothermia decreases cardiac output[85] and changes organ perfusion by redistribution of blood flow from the extremities, kidneys, and liver to the brain and heart. Furthermore, intravascular volume is decreased by hemoconcentration, thereby influencing PK.[86–88] Renal blood flow is also decreased during hypothermia in animal studies. Elimination of drugs by glomerular filtration subsequently decreases. It is unclear if tubular excretion and reabsorption are affected as well.[47]

Hypothermia changes the solubility of carbon dioxide in blood. When blood samples are not corrected for patient temperature (alpha-stat method) the patient Pco_2 (partial pressure of carbon dioxide) is lower by 0.82% compared with the measured value, with a subsequent higher pH than the obtained value. Potentially, there is a risk of higher pH values during hypothermia if clinicians use normal Pco_2 and pH targets and blood gas analysis without temperature correction (pH-stat method).[89] Ionization of drugs may be altered by changes in pH. The Vd of drugs with pK_a between 7 and 8 may be altered. Weak bases show in an increased Vd and weak acids show decreased Vd when pH is not corrected. Lipid solubility is affected by temperature as well. Lower temperature decreases lipid solubility, thereby influencing Vd for lipophilic drugs. The effects on overall PK is probably small in mild hypothermia (32–34°C).[47]

Overall, ECMO seems to increase Vd, whereas the effects of hypothermia result in decreased Vd for most drugs.

Both ECMO and hypothermia seem to decrease renal and hepatic drug Cl. Combining ECMO and hypothermia may result in increased plasma levels and subsequent adverse effects. During rewarming, changes may reverse and may be even more profound in the ECMO population compared with the non-ECMO population.

PK Changes in Cardiopulmonary Bypass

There are no PK or PD data in ECMO patients during hypothermia, in the adult, pediatric, or neonatal population. However, by combining the available data, including PK data, during hypothermic cardiopulmonary bypass (CPB), we have tried to predict the possible effects on the PK of several drugs in the pediatric ECMO population. A recent review summarized the available PK data in pediatric and adult patients during CPB. (van Saet, 2012, submitted for publication).

CPB is significantly different from ECMO not only in duration (hours vs days) and system size but also in the use of mild to deep hypothermia (normally 34°C down to 18°C) and circulatory arrest or selective brain perfusion. Cardiac output or flow rates during ECMO may be significantly different from those targeted during hypothermic CPB, thus changing organ perfusion and subsequent organ function. PK in CPB may therefore be markedly different compared with PK during ECMO and should be translated to the ECMO population with caution.

However, the comparison of PK between normothermic and hypothermic CPB may give vital clues in PK changes caused by hypothermia during ECMO. **Table 1** gives an overview of the general effects of ECMO, CPB, and hypothermia on PK parameters. The next section discusses possible changes in PK or PD of different drugs in infants on ECMO. The changes for individual drugs are summarized in **Table 2**.

Sedative and Analgesic Drugs

Data on sedation and analgesia in ECMO patients are available only from newborn studies. Higher needs of sedative drugs have been reported for these patients.[110,112,127,145] Midazolam, fentanyl, and morphine are the drugs most commonly used and studied in the ECMO population.

Midazolam
Midazolam is a lipophilic drug (logP 3.9) with high protein binding (97%). Midazolam is metabolized in the liver by CYP3A4 and CYP3A5 to a hydroxylated metabolite (1-OH-midazolam) with subsequent metabolism to 1-OH-midazolam-glucuronide by UGTs. Both metabolites are pharmacologically active when 1-OH-midazolam is nearly equipotent to the parent drug.

There are no PK studies of midazolam in older children on ECMO. PK studies in neonates and young infants on ECMO show a 3-fold to 4-fold increase in Vd after initiation of ECMO for midazolam. This increase can be attributed mainly to hemodilution and sequestration of midazolam by the ECMO circuit. Mulla and colleagues[60] described a reduced Cl for midazolam, resulting in accumulation of midazolam 48 hours after initiation of ECMO in term neonates. In the study by Ahsman and colleagues,[117] midazolam Cl in term neonates increased over time, possibly reflecting maturation of the CYP drug-metabolizing enzymes and therefore hepatic Cl. In contrast, renal Cl of the glucoronidated active metabolite of hydroxymidazolam was decreased.[117]

In animal studies of postcardiac arrest, hypothermia midazolam Vd and Cl are decreased.[146,147] In healthy adult volunteers, midazolam Cl but not Vd was affected by induced mild hypothermia.[113] In an adult population with traumatic brain injury with mild hypothermia (32–34°C), midazolam concentrations increased 5-fold during

Table 1
Overall effect on PK by different treatment modalities

		ECMO	CPB	Hypothermia
Absorption	Gastrointestinal tract	?	?	↓
Vd		↑	↑	—/↓
	Extracellular water	↑	↑	↑↓
	Drug adsorption	↑	↑	?
	Blood volume	↓	↓	↓
	Protein binding	?	?	↓
	Ionization	?	?	↑
Cl		↓	↓	↓
	Organ perfusion	?	↓	↓
	Kidney	?	↓	↓
	Liver	?	↓	↓
	Enzymatic Cl	↓	↓	↓
Receptor		?	?	↓

Abbreviations: ↓, decreased; ↑, increased; ?, unknown.

Table 2
Changes of PK for different drugs in different treatment modalities

Drugs	ECMO	Hypothermia	CPB
Cardiovascular Drugs			
Amiodarone	Increased dose[90]		
Bumetanide	Vd ↑[74]		
Esmolol	Increased dose[91]		
Furosemide	No change[92]		
Nesiritide	Increased dose[93]		
Nicardipine	Vd–, Cl–[94,95]		
Prostaglandin E_1	Increased dose[96]		
Sildenafil	Vd ↑, Cl ↑[97]		
Antimicrobial Drugs			
Caspofungin	No change[98]		
Caspofungin	Low plasma levels[99]		
Cefazolin			Vd ↑, Cl ↓[100]
Cefotaxime	Vd ↑, Cl–[101]		
Cefuroxime			No change[102]
Gentamicin	Vd ↑, Cl ↓[63–67]	Cl ↓[103–105]	Vd ↑[100]
Oseltamivir	Vd–, CL–[106]		
Ribavirin	Vd ↑[107]		
Ticarcillin-clavulanic acid	No change[108]		
Vancomycin	Vd ↑, Cl ↓[69,70]		No change[109]
Vancomycin	No change[68]		
Voriconazole	Vd ↑, Cl ↓[98,99,111]		
Neurological Drugs			
Midazolam	Vd ↑, Cl ↓[60,112]	Cl ↓, Vd ↑[113,114]	Vd ↑, Cl ↓[115,116]
Midazolam	Vd ↑, Cl ↑[117,118]		
Fentanyl	High doses[110]	Cl ↓, Vd ↓[119,120]	Vd ↓, Cl ↓[121–123]
Morphine	No change[62]	Cl ↓,[124] Vd ↓[126]	
Morphine	Vd ↑, Cl ↓[61,127,128]		
Phenobarbital	Vd ↑[129]	Cl ↓[130]	
Phenytoin		Cl ↓, Vd–[131,132]	
Pentobarbital		Vd ↓,[133] Cl ↓[134]	
Propofol		Cl ↓[135]	V ↑, Cl–[116,136] Cl ↑[137]
Topiramate		Cl ↓[138]	
Neuromuscular Blocking Drugs			
Cisatracurium			Cl–, Cl ↓[139]
Pancuronium		Vd ↓, Cl ↓[140]	Vd ↑, Cl ↓[141,142]
Vecuronium		Cl ↓[143]	Cl ↓[144]
Miscellaneous			
Ranitidine	Vd ↑, Cl ↓[72]		
Theophylline	Vd ↑, Cl ↓[73]	Vd ↓[103]	

hypothermia, with a subsequent decrease in plasma levels during rewarming. PK evaluation showed a 2-fold increase in Vd with a more than 100-fold decrease in Cl during the hypothermic phase.[114] During the hypothermic phase of CPB, midazolam plasma levels increase in pediatric patients.[115]

Initiation of ECMO greatly increases Vd by hemodilution and drug adsorption to the circuit. Although the effects of hypothermia on Vd remain contradictory, it seems that these changes are small compared with the effect of adsorption to the ECMO system. An initial reduction of plasma concentrations should be expected. Reduced Cl during ECMO and hypothermia greatly increases risk of adverse effects, and efforts should be made to reduce midazolam infusions when possible based on clear treatment protocols. During slow rewarming, increased Cl lowers plasma levels, necessitating increased midazolam infusions when discomfort is noted.

Fentanyl

Fentanyl is a lipophilic drug (logP 4) with a high hepatic extraction ratio. Fentanyl is sequestered to a high degree by the ECMO circuit.[77] Koren and colleagues[81] reported drug sequestration of fentanyl in ECMO circuits, with a subsequent need for high fentanyl infusion rates. High fentanyl infusion rates have been reported by others as well, indicating altered PK or PD in these patients, but clear PK data in neonates and children on ECMO are lacking.[110,148]

Animal studies have shown increased fentanyl plasma levels in hypothermia models mostly caused by reduced hepatic blood flow and a reduction of CYP3A enzyme function.[119,120] During deep hypothermia (18–25°C), Cl seems to be greatly reduced.[119] Several studies show an initial decrease of fentanyl plasma concentrations during CPB caused by increased Vd by hemodilution and drug sequestration to the CPB circuit components. Plasma concentrations remain stable during hypothermic CPB, indicating reduced Cl.[121–123]

The high adsorption rate of fentanyl in ECMO circuits may necessitate high doses. Changes in ECMO circuits with reduced capacity to adsorb drugs probably reduce fentanyl needs. Reduced Cl during hypothermia with subsequent increased Cl during rewarming requires careful monitoring of patients. Rapid reduction of plasma levels may lead to agitation or opioid withdrawal symptoms.

Morphine

Morphine has a low protein binding and is metabolized by the liver to active metabolites morphine-6-glucuronide by the enzyme UGT2B7 and morphine-3-glucuronide by UGT2B7 and the enzyme-family UGT1A.

Morphine is widely used in neonatal intensive care as an analgesic and sedative during mechanical ventilation and ECMO. In 1994, Dagan and colleagues[127] reported decreased morphine Cl in neonates on ECMO, with a concomitant 2-fold increase after decannulation. Geiduschek and colleagues[62] found a similar change in Cl of morphine in 11 newborns on ECMO. Almost half of the patients showed increased Cl over time, possibly reflecting age-related maturation of drug-metabolizing enzyme activity. However, Geiduschek and colleagues found no significant decrease of morphine levels directly after cannulation. These investigators concluded therefore that PK of morphine was not significantly altered during ECMO.

In 2006, Peters and colleagues reported a 2-fold increase of Vd for morphine in neonates on ECMO compared with postoperative patients not treated with ECMO. Furthermore, Cl was decreased at the start of ECMO but increased over time, with normal Cl for age at day 14. The Cl of morphine-3-glucuronide and morphine-6-glucuronide is related to creatinine Cl.[61,128]

Bansinath and colleagues[126] and Alcaraz and colleagues[149] found decreased Vd and total body Cl in a dog model of moderate hypothermia (30°C). In a neonatal trial assessing whole-body therapeutic hypothermia in postasphyxiated neonates, significantly higher morphine plasma levels were found in the hypothermic treatment group.[124] Apart from these changes in PK, there is evidence that morphine affinity for the μ opioid receptor is reduced by hypothermia.[125,150]

The increased Vd found in ECMO patients is partly caused by dilution. Morphine sequestration is substantially less compared with more lipophilic drugs such as fentanyl and midazolam, explaining in part the reduced effect on Vd. Altered Cl may reflect severity of disease more than specific ECMO-related changes. The use of hypothermia in ECMO patients probably leads to higher than expected plasma levels, with a subsequent decrease in plasma levels during the rewarming phase.

Propofol

Propofol is a highly protein-bound (95%–99%) and highly lipophilic drug (logP 3.8). It is mainly metabolized in the liver by glucuronidation at the C_1-hydroxyl end. Hydroxylation of the benzene ring to 4-hydroxypropofol may also occur via CYP2B6 and 2C9. In children, propofol is not used for long-term sedation because of the possible occurrence of propofol infusion syndrome.[151,152]

There are no in vivo data on propofol during ECMO in either the pediatric or adult population. In vitro studies show high adsorption rates by ECMO systems.[78,80] This situation most likely results in increased Vd when used in ECMO patients. Propofol concentrations were lower than expected in a pediatric CPB population.[136] In adults, propofol concentrations decrease by 30% to 67% during CPB.[116,153,154] There are indications that propofol PK or PD is affected by hypothermia. When using bispectral index to titrate propofol dosing on CPB, mild hypothermia reduces propofol requirements almost 2-fold in adults.[154,155]

In pediatric ECMO patients, higher doses of propofol bolus injections are probably caused by the increased Vd caused by hemodilution and drug adsorption to the ECMO circuit components. When used as a continuous infusion during hypothermia, increased plasma levels may occur.

Neuromuscular Blocking Agents

Neuromuscular blocking agents are used during hypothermia to prevent shivering. There are no PK data on neuromuscular blocking agents in children on ECMO. Several agents have been studied during CPB. Miller and colleagues[156] found a decreased Vd by 40% with stable Cl for pancuronium during mild hypothermia in cats.[140] Vecuronium Cl during hypothermia is unaltered in rats but seems to be decreased in human adults.[143] Lower plasma levels with decreased Cl during mild and deep hypothermia are found in children on CPB. Overall, vecuronium requirements were greatly reduced during hypothermia as a result of altered PD.[144] Cisatracurium PK does not seem to be greatly altered in infants on mild hypothermic CPB, although dose requirements decrease during hypothermia.[139,157]

Overall, there is evidence that PK, and especially PD, of neuromuscular blocking agents is altered during hypothermia. How PK is altered during ECMO is unknown and drugs should be titrated to effect.

Antimicrobial Drugs

Antibiotic use in ECMO patients is high, with a reported 71% use of antibiotic prophylaxis and 40% prolonged antibiotic use during ECMO. Infection rates in the pediatric

ECMO population vary between 9% and 14%.[16,158] Nosocomial or ongoing infections remain a significant problem and are associated with increased mortality.[158]

PK data on antibiotics on ECMO are limited; only vancomycin, gentamicin, and cefotaxime have been studied in detail.

Sequestration of antimicrobial drugs by the ECMO circuit is less pronounced compared with more lipophilic drugs.

Most antibiotics are excreted via the kidney. Addition of hemofiltration potentially increases Cl for drugs with a high unbound fraction.

Efficacy of antibiotics the effectiveness of which depends on peak concentrations (such as aminoglycosides) may be reduced by increased Vd. The risk of adverse events related to high trough levels may be increased because of reduced Cl. Antibiotics the effectiveness of which depends on time greater than minimal inhibitory concentration (MIC) (such as cefalosporins and vancomycin) may be affected by differences in drug Cl as well as Vd. Both undertreatment and toxicity need to be considered when dosing antibiotics on ECMO.

To guide antibiotic dosing regimens in ECMO patients, PK models that take into account ECMO-related PK changes need to be developed.

Gentamicin

Gentamicin is an aminoglycoside antibiotic with high water solubility (logP −3) and low protein binding (0%–30%). It is mainly eliminated unchanged via the kidneys.

Five studies examined gentamicin in infants on ECMO. All found an increased Vd, ranging from 0.51 L/kg[67] to 0.748 L/kg[63–66] compared with 0.45 L/kg in post-ECMO patients and critically non-ECMO patients.[65,66] Cl on ECMO was decreased compared with the Cl in the post-ECMO period.[65,66] It is unclear whether this decrease is because of ECMO itself or because of improvement in the clinical condition. When compared with term septic neonates, gentamicin Cl on ECMO seems to be unaffected or slightly decreased.[63–67,159] All studies showed an increased elimination half-life of 10 hours compared with 5 to 6 hours in non-ECMO patients.[160]

Different dosing regimens were used in the studies. None reflect the current dose recommendations.

Induced hypothermia to 29°C was associated with decreased Vd and Cl in pigs.[103] However, mild hypothermia of 35°C did not affect PK in juvenile pigs.[104] Liu and colleagues[105] confirmed these latter findings in 55 neonates cooled to 34°C after asphyxia.

During CPB and deep hypothermia (18–25°C), gentamicin Vd increased 2-fold, whereas Cl decreased. It is unclear if these effects reflect the influence of hypothermia or CPB. The increased Vd reflects the findings in infants on ECMO and can mostly be contributed to dilution. The possible decrease in peak concentrations with prolonged elimination necessitates the use of therapeutic drug monitoring (TDM) for these patients, especially during hypothermia or renal replacement therapy, in which serum creatinine does not accurately reflect renal function. The kinetically guided maintenance dosing of gentamicin based on plasma concentration after the first dose should be optimized despite high interindividual PK parameter variability, especially in neonates treated for perinatal asphyxia with therapeutic hypothermia and multiorgan dysfunction syndrome.[161]

Vancomycin

Vancomycin is a glycopeptide with a high water solubility (logP −3.1) and moderate protein binding (55%). This drug exerts a high renal Cl by glomerular filtration.

Vd is either increased or unaffected by ECMO. Cl was decreased, but primarily correlated to renal function.[68–71] There are no trials assessing the effect of hypothermia on vancomycin Cl. A decrease in renal perfusion likely results in a decreased vancomycin Cl. Especially in patients who have had a cardiac arrest with a high risk of acute renal injury, this decrease could lead to toxic plasma levels. In children on CPB, vancomycin plasma levels decrease by 45% on initiation of CPB. Overall Vd and Cl do not seem to be greatly affected.[109]

Based on the available literature, vancomycin dosing intervals should be based on age and renal function. Drug monitoring should be used to adjust dosing.

Cephalosporins
Cefotaxime, cefuroxime, cefazolin Cephalosporins are widely used in pediatric patients, including those on ECMO. PK of cefotaxime during ECMO and of cefuroxime during CPB is altered but plasma levels are more than the MIC using normal dosing regimens.[101,102] Cefotaxime Cl was found to be increased during ECMO compared with the pre-ECMO and post-ECMO period, possibly reflecting improved hepatic or renal perfusion during ECMO or Cl via hemofiltration.[101] A possible decrease in Cl caused by hypothermia increases plasma levels, negating the effects of ECMO. Cefazolin plasma levels remained greater than MIC in infants during CPB after bolus infusions before the start of bypass.[100] Because of the large therapeutic window of cefotaxime, the chance of reaching toxic effects is small. For cefotaxime and cefazolin, dose adjustments do not seem to be necessary during ECMO and hypothermia.

Oseltamivir
In the recent H1N1 influenza pandemic, ECMO support was successfully initiated in children and adults, with survival rates of 70%.[162–164] Oseltamivir is the drug of choice in H1N1 influenza, whereas alternatives such as inhaled zanamivir or intravenous zanamivir have not been evaluated in critically ill children. A case report describing 3 patients with H1N1 influenza supported with ECMO showed that adequate oseltamivir plasma levels were achieved in 2 of 3 patients. More specifically, a 2-fold dose increase of 4 mg/kg/d (vs 2 mg/kg/d) resulted in a 2-fold increase in plasma levels. The influence of the ECMO circuit seems to be limited in this small case series. One patient with profuse gastric retentions and hematemesis failed to achieve adequate plasma concentrations of oseltamivir and oseltamivir carboxylate, probably reflecting insufficient intestinal absorption of the parent drug.[106]

Oseltamivir is metabolized in the liver by esterases. Bioavailability is about 75% after oral administration. There are indications that oral absorption of some drugs may be reduced during hypothermia in animal studies.[165] The active metabolite oseltamivir carboxylate is eliminated by the kidney. Hypothermia could influence bioavailability and elimination of oseltamivir and oseltamivir carboxylate. There is no evidence to alter the standard dosing regimen in hypothermic ECMO patients.

Miscellaneous

Heparin
Coagulation is affected by hypothermia. Enzymatic reactions in the coagulation cascade are decreased, resulting in prolonged activated partial thromboplastin time (aPTT) and prothrombin time.[166,167] Platelet activation and aggregation are influenced by hypothermia. Some experimental studies show decreased platelet function and aggregation,[168–170] whereas others show increased platelet aggregation during mild and moderate hypothermia in adults.[171,172] Ramaker and colleagues[173] found increased clotting times with normal or enhanced thrombus strength using thromboelastography.

ECMO activates the coagulation cascade, resulting in consumption and activation of clotting factors. This situation leads to clotting factor deficiencies, impaired platelet function, thrombocytopenia, and fibrinolysis.[174]

All ECMO patients receive heparin to reduce the risk of thromboembolic complications. Heparin infusions are titrated to either activated clotting time, aPTT, or antifactor Xa. Heparin Cl is increased during ECMO by adsorption of heparin by the ECMO circuit. Higher heparin doses on ECMO are necessary to maintain anticoagulation.[175,176]

Anticoagulation targets may be different during therapeutic hypothermia on ECMO. Careful monitoring using multiple tests helps to titrate heparin infusions in these patients.

Phenobarbital

Phenobarbital is a long-acting barbiturate mainly eliminated via the liver by CYP 2C19. It is partly bound to protein (20%–45%) with a logP of 1.47. Phenobarbital PK data during ECMO are limited to a single case report. A slightly Vd (1.2 L/kg) with a normal serum elimination half-life (92 hours) resulted in low but still therapeutic serum concentrations. Dose recommendations cannot be made based on this single case report, but clinicians should be aware that higher loading doses may be required.[129] In hypothermic children, Cl and Vd of pentobarbital and phenobarbital seem to be reduced.[130,133]

Filippi and colleagues[177] described increased plasma levels of phenobarbital with decreased Cl in neonates treated for perinatal asphyxia with therapeutic hypothermia. Barbiturates are primarily metabolized in the liver by the hepatic microsomal enzyme system. The metabolites are excreted in the urine and, less commonly, in the feces. Reduction of enzymatic processes and redistribution of blood flow influence PK, possibly negating the decreased plasma levels reported during ECMO. TDM is advised in these patients to monitor plasma levels during cooling and rewarming to prevent toxicity and withdrawal.

SUMMARY

Almost 10% of all pediatric ECMO runs occur during or shortly after CPR. With the increased use of therapeutic hypothermia, most of these patients are cooled during their ECMO run. Evidence-based dose regimens are still lacking for many regularly used drugs in children on ECMO, either with or without hypothermia. Our understanding of PK changes is insufficient to prepare a predictive model. The combination of routine sparse sampling, drug assay via LC-MS, and a PK analysis using NONMEM in combination with validated PD end points such as the COMFORT behavioral scale[178] or face, legs, arms, cry, consolability (FLACC)[179] and a numeric rating scale to assess discomfort and pain allow the study of drug behavior in these vulnerable patients without harm to the individual.

Overall, Vd changes occur rapidly at start of ECMO as a result of hemodilution and adsorption of drugs by the ECMO system. Initial changes in Vd may necessitate higher doses to achieve adequate plasma concentrations. If Vd is increased and stays unchanged, steady state levels are affected only by the dose rate and Cl rate.

Changes in PK are drug and circuit dependent, with more dramatic changes found with lipophilic drugs and silicone oxygenators. Differences in ECMO circuits used, patient populations, and diseases may influence PK and PD further. Changes in Vd as a result of hypothermia are difficult to predict during ECMO, but seem to be small compared with the changes caused by adsorption of drugs to the ECMO circuit. Cl may be more dramatically changed by combining ECMO with therapeutic hypothermia. Both organ perfusion and enzymatic reactions are reduced by hypothermia. Most data on PK of drugs during hypothermia show decreased Cl with higher plasma levels. Particularly during rewarming, clinicians need to be vigilant and expect rapid decreases in plasma levels of most sedatives.

The greatest changes are:

- Increased Vd, especially for lipophilic drugs on initiation of ECMO
- Decreased Cl as a result of ECMO and hypothermia, especially of drugs dependent on enzymatic reactions
- Reduced renal Cl as a result of reduced renal perfusion during ECMO and hypothermia for drugs cleared by glomerular filtration

ACKNOWLEDGMENTS

John N van den Anker is in part supported by NIH grants (R01HD060543, K24DA027992, R01HD048689 and U54HD071601) and European Union FP7 grants TINN (223614), TINN2 (260908), NEUROSIS (223060), and GRIP (261060).

REFERENCES

1. Organization EELS. General Guidelines for all ECLS Cases. Version 1:1. April 2009. Available at: http://www.elso.med.umich.edu/WordForms/ELSO%20Guidelines%20General%20All%20ECLS%20Version1.1.pdf. Accessed January 1, 2010.
2. Bartlett RH, Gazzaniga AB, Jefferies MR, et al. Extracorporeal membrane oxygenation (ECMO) cardiopulmonary support in infancy. Trans Am Soc Artif Intern Organs 1976;22:80–93.
3. UK collaborative randomised trial of neonatal extracorporeal membrane oxygenation. UK Collaborative ECMO Trail Group. Lancet 1996;348(9020):75–82.
4. Peek GJ, Mugford M, Tiruvoipati R, et al. Efficacy and economic assessment of conventional ventilatory support versus extracorporeal membrane oxygenation for severe adult respiratory failure (CESAR): a multicentre randomised controlled trial. Lancet 2009;374(9698):1351–63.
5. Coskun KO, Popov AF, Schmitto JD, et al. Extracorporeal circulation for rewarming in drowning and near-drowning pediatric patients. Artif Organs 2010;34(11):1026–30.
6. Ruttmann E, Weissenbacher A, Ulmer H, et al. Prolonged extracorporeal membrane oxygenation-assisted support provides improved survival in hypothermic patients with cardiocirculatory arrest. J Thorac Cardiovasc Surg 2007;134(3):594–600.
7. Guenther U, Varelmann D, Putensen C, et al. Extended therapeutic hypothermia for several days during extracorporeal membrane-oxygenation after drowning and cardiac arrest Two cases of survival with no neurological sequelae. Resuscitation 2009;80(3):379–81.
8. Kane DA, Thiagarajan RR, Wypij D, et al. Rapid-response extracorporeal membrane oxygenation to support cardiopulmonary resuscitation in children with cardiac disease. Circulation 2010;122(Suppl 11):S241–8.
9. Fiser RT, Morris MC. Extracorporeal cardiopulmonary resuscitation in refractory pediatric cardiac arrest. Pediatr Clin North Am 2008;55(4):929–41, x.
10. Prodhan P, Fiser RT, Dyamenahalli U, et al. Outcomes after extracorporeal cardiopulmonary resuscitation (ECPR) following refractory pediatric cardiac arrest in the intensive care unit. Resuscitation 2009;80(10):1124–9.
11. Swaniker F, Kolla S, Moler F, et al. Extracorporeal life support outcome for 128 pediatric patients with respiratory failure. J Pediatr Surg 2000;35(2):197–202.
12. Pathan N, Ridout DA, Smith E, et al. Predictors of outcome for children requiring respiratory extra-corporeal life support: implications for inclusion and exclusion criteria. Intensive Care Med 2008;34(12):2256–63.

13. Shah SA, Shankar V, Churchwell KB, et al. Clinical outcomes of 84 children with congenital heart disease managed with extracorporeal membrane oxygenation after cardiac surgery. ASAIO J 2005;51(5):504–7.
14. Zwischenberger JB, Nguyen TT, Upp JR Jr, et al. Complications of neonatal extracorporeal membrane oxygenation. Collective experience from the Extracorporeal Life Support Organization. J Thorac Cardiovasc Surg 1994;107(3):838–48 [discussion: 48–9].
15. Karimova A, Brown K, Ridout D, et al. Neonatal extracorporeal membrane oxygenation: practice patterns and predictors of outcome in the UK. Arch Dis Child Fetal Neonatal Ed 2009;94(2):F129–32.
16. Brown KL, Ridout DA, Shaw M, et al. Healthcare-associated infection in pediatric patients on extracorporeal life support: the role of multidisciplinary surveillance. Pediatr Crit Care Med 2006;7(6):546–50.
17. Coffin SE, Bell LM, Manning M, et al. Nosocomial infections in neonates receiving extracorporeal membrane oxygenation. Infect Control Hosp Epidemiol 1997;18(2):93–6.
18. Costello JM, Morrow DF, Graham DA, et al. Systematic intervention to reduce central line-associated bloodstream infection rates in a pediatric cardiac intensive care unit. Pediatrics 2008;121(5):915–23.
19. Douglass BH, Keenan AL, Purohit DM. Bacterial and fungal infection in neonates undergoing venoarterial extracorporeal membrane oxygenation: an analysis of the registry data of the extracorporeal life support organization. Artif Organs 1996;20(3):202–8.
20. Elerian LF, Sparks JW, Meyer TA, et al. Usefulness of surveillance cultures in neonatal extracorporeal membrane oxygenation. ASAIO J 2001;47(3):220–3.
21. O'Neill JM, Schutze GE, Heulitt MJ, et al. Nosocomial infections during extracorporeal membrane oxygenation. Intensive Care Med 2001;27(8): 1247–53.
22. Schutze GE, Heulitt MJ. Infections during extracorporeal life support. J Pediatr Surg 1995;30(6):809–12.
23. Steiner CK, Stewart DL, Bond SJ, et al. Predictors of acquiring a nosocomial bloodstream infection on extracorporeal membrane oxygenation. J Pediatr Surg 2001;36(3):487–92.
24. Alsoufi B, Al-Radi OO, Gruenwald C, et al. Extra-corporeal life support following cardiac surgery in children: analysis of risk factors and survival in a single institution. Eur J Cardiothorac Surg 2009;35(6):1004–11 [discussion: 11].
25. Alsoufi B, Al-Radi OO, Nazer RI, et al. Survival outcomes after rescue extracorporeal cardiopulmonary resuscitation in pediatric patients with refractory cardiac arrest. J Thorac Cardiovasc Surg 2007;134(4):952–959.e2.
26. Kumar TK, Zurakowski D, Dalton H, et al. Extracorporeal membrane oxygenation in postcardiotomy patients: factors influencing outcome. J Thorac Cardiovasc Surg 2010;140(2):330–336.e2.
27. Hervey-Jumper SL, Annich GM, Yancon AR, et al. Neurological complications of extracorporeal membrane oxygenation in children. J Neurosurg Pediatr 2011; 7(4):338–44.
28. Hypothermia after Cardiac Arrest Study Group. Mild therapeutic hypothermia to improve the neurologic outcome after cardiac arrest. N Engl J Med 2002;346(8): 549–56.
29. Bernard SA, Gray TW, Buist MD, et al. Treatment of comatose survivors of out-of-hospital cardiac arrest with induced hypothermia. N Engl J Med 2002;346(8): 557–63.

30. Nolan JP, Morley PT, Hoek TL, et al. Therapeutic hypothermia after cardiac arrest. An advisory statement by the Advancement Life Support Task Force of the International Liaison Committee on Resuscitation. Resuscitation 2003; 57(3):231–5.

31. Gluckman PD, Wyatt JS, Azzopardi D, et al. Selective head cooling with mild systemic hypothermia after neonatal encephalopathy: multicentre randomised trial. Lancet 2005;365(9460):663–70.

32. Eicher DJ, Wagner CL, Katikaneni LP, et al. Moderate hypothermia in neonatal encephalopathy: efficacy outcomes. Pediatr Neurol 2005;32(1):11–7.

33. Shankaran S, Pappas A, Laptook AR, et al. Outcomes of safety and effectiveness in a multicenter randomized, controlled trial of whole-body hypothermia for neonatal hypoxic-ischemic encephalopathy. Pediatrics 2008;122(4): e791–8.

34. Azzopardi D, Brocklehurst P, Edwards D, et al, The TOBY Study. Whole body hypothermia for the treatment of perinatal asphyxial encephalopathy: a randomised controlled trial. BMC Pediatr 2008;8:17.

35. Sanchez de Toledo J, Bell MJ. Complications of hypothermia: interpreting 'serious,' 'adverse,' and 'events' in clinical trials. Pediatr Crit Care Med 2010; 11(3):439–41.

36. Baltagi S, Fink EL, Bell MJ. Therapeutic hypothermia: ready...fire...aim? How small feasibility studies can inform large efficacy trials. Pediatr Crit Care Med 2011;12(3):370–1.

37. Statler KD, Bratton SL. Therapeutic hypothermia and pediatric cardiac arrests: vexing questions. Pediatr Crit Care Med 2010;11(1):151–3.

38. Fink EL, Clark RS, Kochanek PM, et al. A tertiary care center's experience with therapeutic hypothermia after pediatric cardiac arrest. Pediatr Crit Care Med 2010;11(1):66–74.

39. Topjian A, Hutchins L, DiLiberto MA, et al. Induction and maintenance of therapeutic hypothermia after pediatric cardiac arrest: efficacy of a surface cooling protocol. Pediatr Crit Care Med 2011;12(3):e127–35.

40. Bourdages M, Bigras JL, Farrell CA, et al. Cardiac arrhythmias associated with severe traumatic brain injury and hypothermia therapy. Pediatr Crit Care Med 2010;11(3):408–14.

41. Field DJ, Firmin R, Azzopardi DV, et al. Neonatal ECMO Study of Temperature (NEST)–a randomised controlled trial. BMC Pediatr 2010;10:24.

42. Horan M, Ichiba S, Firmin RK, et al. A pilot investigation of mild hypothermia in neonates receiving extracorporeal membrane oxygenation (ECMO). J Pediatr 2004;144(3):301–8.

43. Ichiba S, Killer HM, Firmin RK, et al. Pilot investigation of hypothermia in neonates receiving extracorporeal membrane oxygenation. Arch Dis Child Fetal Neonatal Ed 2003;88(2):F128–33.

44. Massaro A, Rais-Bahrami K, Chang T, et al. Therapeutic hypothermia for neonatal encephalopathy and extracorporeal membrane oxygenation. J Pediatr 2010;157(3):499–501.e1.

45. American Heart Association. 2005 American Heart Association (AHA) guidelines for cardiopulmonary resuscitation (CPR) and emergency cardiovascular care (ECC) of pediatric and neonatal patients: pediatric advanced life support. Pediatrics 2006;117(5):e1005–28.

46. Wildschut ED, Ahsman MJ, Houmes RJ, et al. Pharmacotherapy in neonatal and pediatric extracorporeal membrane oxygenation (ECMO). Curr Drug Metab 2012;13(6):767–77.

47. van den Broek MP, Groenendaal F, Egberts AC, et al. Effects of hypothermia on pharmacokinetics and pharmacodynamics: a systematic review of preclinical and clinical studies. Clin Pharmacokinet 2010;49(5):277–94.
48. Zanelli S, Buck M, Fairchild K. Physiologic and pharmacologic considerations for hypothermia therapy in neonates. J Perinatol 2011;31(6):377–86.
49. Arpino PA, Greer DM. Practical pharmacologic aspects of therapeutic hypothermia after cardiac arrest. Pharmacotherapy 2008;28(1):102–11.
50. Buck ML. Pharmacokinetic changes during extracorporeal membrane oxygenation: implications for drug therapy of neonates. Clin Pharmacokinet 2003;42(5): 403–17.
51. de Wildt SN. Profound changes in drug metabolism enzymes and possible effects on drug therapy in neonates and children. Expert Opin Drug Metab Toxicol 2011;7(8):935–48.
52. Kearns GL, Abdel-Rahman SM, Alander SW, et al. Developmental pharmacology–drug disposition, action, and therapy in infants and children. N Engl J Med 2003;349(12):1157–67.
53. Vet NJ, de Hoog M, Tibboel D, et al. The effect of critical illness and inflammation on midazolam therapy in children. Pediatr Crit Care Med 2012;13(1): e48–50.
54. Peeters MY, Bras LJ, DeJongh J, et al. Disease severity is a major determinant for the pharmacodynamics of propofol in critically ill patients. Clin Pharmacol Ther 2008;83(3):443–51.
55. Lopez SA, Mulla H, Durward A, et al. Extended-interval gentamicin: population pharmacokinetics in pediatric critical illness. Pediatr Crit Care Med 2010;11(2): 267–74.
56. Morgan ET. Regulation of cytochromes P450 during inflammation and infection. Drug Metab Rev 1997;29(4):1129–88.
57. Carcillo JA, Doughty L, Kofos D, et al. Cytochrome P450 mediated-drug metabolism is reduced in children with sepsis-induced multiple organ failure. Intensive Care Med 2003;29(6):980–4.
58. Vet NJ, de Hoog M, Tibboel D, et al. The effect of inflammation on drug metabolism: a focus on pediatrics. Drug Discov Today 2011;16(9–10):435–42.
59. Peek GJ, Firmin RK. The inflammatory and coagulative response to prolonged extracorporeal membrane oxygenation. ASAIO J 1999;45(4):250–63.
60. Mulla H, McCormack P, Lawson G, et al. Pharmacokinetics of midazolam in neonates undergoing extracorporeal membrane oxygenation. Anesthesiology 2003;99(2):275–82.
61. Peters JW, Anderson BJ, Simons SH, et al. Morphine pharmacokinetics during venoarterial extracorporeal membrane oxygenation in neonates. Intensive Care Med 2005;31(2):257–63.
62. Geiduschek JM, Lynn AM, Bratton SL, et al. Morphine pharmacokinetics during continuous infusion of morphine sulfate for infants receiving extracorporeal membrane oxygenation. Crit Care Med 1997;25(2):360–4.
63. Bhatt-Mehta V, Johnson CE, Schumacher RE. Gentamicin pharmacokinetics in term neonates receiving extracorporeal membrane oxygenation. Pharmacotherapy 1992;12(1):28–32.
64. Cohen P, Collart L, Prober CG, et al. Gentamicin pharmacokinetics in neonates undergoing extracorporal membrane oxygenation. Pediatr Infect Dis J 1990; 9(8):562–6.
65. Dodge WF, Jelliffe RW, Zwischenberger JB, et al. Population pharmacokinetic models: effect of explicit versus assumed constant serum concentration assay

error patterns upon parameter values of gentamicin in infants on and off extracorporeal membrane oxygenation. Ther Drug Monit 1994;16(6):552–9.

66. Munzenberger PJ, Massoud N. Pharmacokinetics of gentamicin in neonatal patients supported with extracorporeal membrane oxygenation. ASAIO Trans 1991;37(1):16–8.

67. Southgate WM, DiPiro JT, Robertson AF. Pharmacokinetics of gentamicin in neonates on extracorporeal membrane oxygenation. Antimicrob Agents Chemother 1989;33(6):817–9.

68. Buck ML. Vancomycin pharmacokinetics in neonates receiving extracorporeal membrane oxygenation. Pharmacotherapy 1998;18(5):1082–6.

69. Mulla H, Pooboni S. Population pharmacokinetics of vancomycin in patients receiving extracorporeal membrane oxygenation. Br J Clin Pharmacol 2005; 60(3):265–75.

70. Amaker RD, DiPiro JT, Bhatia J. Pharmacokinetics of vancomycin in critically ill infants undergoing extracorporeal membrane oxygenation. Antimicrob Agents Chemother 1996;40(5):1139–42.

71. Hoie EB, Swigart SA, Leuschen MP, et al. Vancomycin pharmacokinetics in infants undergoing extracorporeal membrane oxygenation. Clin Pharm 1990; 9(9):711–5.

72. Wells TG, Heulitt MJ, Taylor BJ, et al. Pharmacokinetics and pharmacodynamics of ranitidine in neonates treated with extracorporeal membrane oxygenation. J Clin Pharmacol 1998;38(5):402–7.

73. Mulla H, Nabi F, Nichani S, et al. Population pharmacokinetics of theophylline during paediatric extracorporeal membrane oxygenation. Br J Clin Pharmacol 2003;55(1):23–31.

74. Wells TG, Fasules JW, Taylor BJ, et al. Pharmacokinetics and pharmacodynamics of bumetanide in neonates treated with extracorporeal membrane oxygenation. J Pediatr 1992;121(6):974–80.

75. Hynynen M. Binding of fentanyl and alfentanil to the extracorporeal circuit. Acta Anaesthesiol Scand 1987;31(8):706–10.

76. Mehta NM, Halwick DR, Dodson BL, et al. Potential drug sequestration during extracorporeal membrane oxygenation: results from an ex vivo experiment. Intensive Care Med 2007;33(6):1018–24.

77. Wildschut ED, Ahsman MJ, Allegaert K, et al. Determinants of drug absorption in different ECMO circuits. Intensive Care Med 2010;36(12):2109–16.

78. Mulla H, Lawson G, von Anrep C, et al. In vitro evaluation of sedative drug losses during extracorporeal membrane oxygenation. Perfusion 2000;15(1):21–6.

79. Dagan O, Klein J, Gruenwald C, et al. Preliminary studies of the effects of extracorporeal membrane oxygenator on the disposition of common pediatric drugs. Ther Drug Monit 1993;15(4):263–6.

80. Hynynen M, Hammaren E, Rosenberg PH. Propofol sequestration within the extracorporeal circuit. Can J Anaesth 1994;41(7):583–8.

81. Koren G, Crean P, Klein J, et al. Sequestration of fentanyl by the cardiopulmonary bypass (CPBP). Eur J Clin Pharmacol 1984;27(1):51–6.

82. Rosen D, Rosen K, Davidson B, et al. Fentanyl uptake by the Scimed membrane oxygenator. J Cardiothorac Anesth 1988;2(5):619–26.

83. Rosen DA, Rosen KR, Silvasi DL. In vitro variability in fentanyl absorption by different membrane oxygenators. J Cardiothorac Anesth 1990;4(3):332–5.

84. Bouman CS. Antimicrobial dosing strategies in critically ill patients with acute kidney injury and high-dose continuous veno-venous hemofiltration. Curr Opin Crit Care 2008;14(6):654–9.

85. Gebauer CM, Knuepfer M, Robel-Tillig E, et al. Hemodynamics among neonates with hypoxic-ischemic encephalopathy during whole-body hypothermia and passive rewarming. Pediatrics 2006;117(3):843–50.
86. Delin NA, Kjartansson KB, Pollock L, et al. Redistribution of regional blood flow in hypothermia. J Thorac Cardiovasc Surg 1965;49:511–6.
87. Metz C, Holzschuh M, Bein T, et al. Moderate hypothermia in patients with severe head injury: cerebral and extracerebral effects. J Neurosurg 1996;85(4):533–41.
88. Lazenby WD, Ko W, Zelano JA, et al. Effects of temperature and flow rate on regional blood flow and metabolism during cardiopulmonary bypass. Ann Thorac Surg 1992;53(6):957–64.
89. Tarr TJ, Snowdon SL. Blood/gas solubility coefficient and blood concentration of enflurane during normothermic and hypothermic cardiopulmonary bypass. J Cardiothorac Vasc Anesth 1991;5(2):111–5.
90. Kendrick JG, Macready JJ, Kissoon N. Amiodarone treatment of junctional ectopic tachycardia in a neonate receiving extracorporeal membrane oxygenation. Ann Pharmacother 2006;40(10):1872–5.
91. Robinson B, Eshaghpour E, Ewing S, et al. Hypertrophic obstructive cardiomyopathy in an infant of a diabetic mother: support by extracorporeal membrane oxygenation and treatment with beta-adrenergic blockade and increased intravenous fluid administration. ASAIO J 1998;44(6):845–7.
92. van der Vorst MM, den Hartigh J, Wildschut E, et al. An exploratory study with an adaptive continuous intravenous furosemide regimen in neonates treated with extracorporeal membrane oxygenation. Crit Care 2007;11(5):R111.
93. Smith T, Rosen DA, Russo P, et al. Nesiritide during extracorporeal membrane oxygenation. Paediatr Anaesth 2005;15(2):152–7.
94. Sell LL, Cullen ML, Lerner GR, et al. Hypertension during extracorporeal membrane oxygenation: cause, effect, and management. Surgery 1987;102(4):724–30.
95. McBride BF, White CM, Campbell M, et al. Nicardipine to control neonatal hypertension during extracorporeal membrane oxygen support. Ann Pharmacother 2003;37(5):667–70.
96. Stone DM, Frattarelli DA, Karthikeyan S, et al. Altered prostaglandin E1 dosage during extracorporeal membrane oxygenation in a newborn with ductal-dependent congenital heart disease. Pediatr Cardiol 2006;27(3):360–3.
97. Ahsman MJ. Determinants of pharmacokinetic variability during extracorporeal membrane oxygenation: a roadmap to rational pharmacotherapy in children. Rotterdam (The Netherlands): Erasmus MC; 2010.
98. Spriet I, Annaert P, Meersseman P, et al. Pharmacokinetics of caspofungin and voriconazole in critically ill patients during extracorporeal membrane oxygenation. J Antimicrob Chemother 2009;63(4):767–70.
99. Ruiz S, Papy E, Da Silva D, et al. Potential voriconazole and caspofungin sequestration during extracorporeal membrane oxygenation. Intensive Care Med 2009;35(1):183–4.
100. Haessler D, Reverdy ME, Neidecker J, et al. Antibiotic prophylaxis with cefazolin and gentamicin in cardiac surgery for children less than ten kilograms. J Cardiothorac Vasc Anesth 2003;17(2):221–5.
101. Ahsman MJ, Wildschut ED, Tibboel D, et al. Pharmacokinetics of cefotaxime and desacetylcefotaxime in infants during extracorporeal membrane oxygenation. Antimicrob Agents Chemother 2010;54(5):1734–41.
102. Knoderer CA, Saft SA, Walker SG, et al. Cefuroxime pharmacokinetics in pediatric cardiovascular surgery patients undergoing cardiopulmonary bypass. J Cardiothorac Vasc Anesth 2011;25(3):425–30.

103. Koren G, Barker C, Bohn D, et al. Influence of hypothermia on the pharmacokinetics of gentamicin and theophylline in piglets. Crit Care Med 1985;13(10): 844–7.

104. Satas S, Hoem NO, Melby K, et al. Influence of mild hypothermia after hypoxia-ischemia on the pharmacokinetics of gentamicin in newborn pigs. Biol Neonate 2000;77(1):50–7.

105. Liu X, Borooah M, Stone J, et al. Serum gentamicin concentrations in encephalopathic infants are not affected by therapeutic hypothermia. Pediatrics 2009; 124(1):310–5.

106. Wildschut ED, de Hoog M, Ahsman MJ, et al. Plasma concentrations of oseltamivir and oseltamivir carboxylate in critically ill children on extracorporeal membrane oxygenation support. PLoS One 2010;5(6):e10938.

107. Aebi C, Headrick CL, McCracken GH, et al. Intravenous ribavirin therapy in a neonate with disseminated adenovirus infection undergoing extracorporeal membrane oxygenation: pharmacokinetics and clearance by hemofiltration. J Pediatr 1997;130(4):612–5.

108. Lindsay CA, Bawdon R, Quigley R. Clearance of ticarcillin-clavulanic acid by continuous venovenous hemofiltration in three critically ill children, two with and one without concomitant extracorporeal membrane oxygenation. Pharmacotherapy 1996;16(3):458–62.

109. Hatzopoulos FK, Stile-Calligaro IL, Rodvold KA, et al. Pharmacokinetics of intravenous vancomycin in pediatric cardiopulmonary bypass surgery. Pediatr Infect Dis J 1993;12(4):300–4.

110. Leuschen MP, Willett LD, Hoie EB, et al. Plasma fentanyl levels in infants undergoing extracorporeal membrane oxygenation. J Thorac Cardiovasc Surg 1993; 105(5):885–91.

111. Bruggemann RJ, Antonius T, Heijst A, et al. Therapeutic drug monitoring of voriconazole in a child with invasive aspergillosis requiring extracorporeal membrane oxygenation. Ther Drug Monit 2008;30(6):643–6.

112. Mulla H, Lawson G, Peek GJ, et al. Plasma concentrations of midazolam in neonates receiving extracorporeal membrane oxygenation. ASAIO J 2003; 49(1):41–7.

113. Hostler D, Zhou J, Tortorici MA, et al. Mild hypothermia alters midazolam pharmacokinetics in normal healthy volunteers. Drug Metab Dispos 2010;38(5):781–8.

114. Fukuoka N, Aibiki M, Tsukamoto T, et al. Biphasic concentration change during continuous midazolam administration in brain-injured patients undergoing therapeutic moderate hypothermia. Resuscitation 2004;60(2):225–30.

115. Kern FH, Ungerleider RM, Jacobs JR, et al. Computerized continuous infusion of intravenous anesthetic drugs during pediatric cardiac surgery. Anesth Analg 1991;72(4):487–92.

116. Dawson PJ, Bjorksten AR, Blake DW, et al. The effects of cardiopulmonary bypass on total and unbound plasma concentrations of propofol and midazolam. J Cardiothorac Vasc Anesth 1997;11(5):556–61.

117. Ahsman MJ, Hanekamp M, Wildschut ED, et al. Population pharmacokinetics of midazolam and its metabolites during venoarterial extracorporeal membrane oxygenation in neonates. Clin Pharmacokinet 2010;49(6):407–19.

118. Wildschut ED, Hanekamp MN, Vet NJ, et al. Feasibility of sedation and analgesia interruption following cannulation in neonates on extracorporeal membrane oxygenation. Intensive Care Med 2010;36(9):1587–91.

119. Koren G, Barker C, Goresky G, et al. The influence of hypothermia on the disposition of fentanyl–human and animal studies. Eur J Clin Pharmacol 1987;32(4):373–6.

120. Fritz HG, Holzmayr M, Walter B, et al. The effect of mild hypothermia on plasma fentanyl concentration and biotransformation in juvenile pigs. Anesth Analg 2005;100(4):996–1002.

121. Newland MC, Leuschen P, Sarafian LB, et al. Fentanyl intermittent bolus technique for anesthesia in infants and children undergoing cardiac surgery. J Cardiothorac Anesth 1989;3(4):407–10.

122. Koska AJ 3rd, Romagnoli A, Kramer WG. Effect of cardiopulmonary bypass on fentanyl distribution and elimination. Clin Pharmacol Ther 1981;29(1): 100–5.

123. Kussman BD, Zurakowski D, Sullivan L, et al. Evaluation of plasma fentanyl concentrations in infants during cardiopulmonary bypass with low-volume circuits. J Cardiothorac Vasc Anesth 2005;19(3):316–21.

124. Roka A, Melinda KT, Vasarhelyi B, et al. Elevated morphine concentrations in neonates treated with morphine and prolonged hypothermia for hypoxic ischemic encephalopathy. Pediatrics 2008;121(4):e844–9.

125. Puig MM, Warner W, Tang CK, et al. Effects of temperature on the interaction of morphine with opioid receptors. Br J Anaesth 1987;59(11):1459–64.

126. Bansinath M, Turndorf H, Puig MM. Influence of hypo and hyperthermia on disposition of morphine. J Clin Pharmacol 1988;28(9):860–4.

127. Dagan O, Klein J, Bohn D, et al. Effects of extracorporeal membrane oxygenation on morphine pharmacokinetics in infants. Crit Care Med 1994;22(7): 1099–101.

128. Peters JW, Anderson BJ, Simons SH, et al. Morphine metabolite pharmacokinetics during venoarterial extra corporeal membrane oxygenation in neonates. Clin Pharmacokinet 2006;45(7):705–14.

129. Elliott ES, Buck ML. Phenobarbital dosing and pharmacokinetics in a neonate receiving extracorporeal membrane oxygenation. Ann Pharmacother 1999; 33(4):419–22.

130. Kadar D, Tang BK, Conn AW. The fate of phenobarbitone in children in hypothermia and at normal body temperature. Can Anaesth Soc J 1982;29(1):16–23.

131. Iida Y, Nishi S, Asada A. Effect of mild therapeutic hypothermia on phenytoin pharmacokinetics. Ther Drug Monit 2001;23(3):192–7.

132. Bhagat H, Bithal PK, Chouhan RS, et al. Is phenytoin administration safe in a hypothermic child? J Clin Neurosci 2006;13(9):953–5.

133. Schaible DH, Cupit GC, Swedlow DB, et al. High-dose pentobarbital pharmacokinetics in hypothermic brain-injured children. J Pediatr 1982;100(4):655–60.

134. Kalser SC, Kelly MP, Forbes EB, et al. Drug metabolism in hypothermia. Uptake, metabolism and biliary excretion of pentobarbital-2-C14 by the isolated, perfused rat liver in hypothermia and euthermia. J Pharmacol Exp Ther 1969; 170(1):145–52.

135. Leslie K, Sessler DI, Bjorksten AR, et al. Mild hypothermia alters propofol pharmacokinetics and increases the duration of action of atracurium. Anesth Analg 1995;80(5):1007–14.

136. Absalom A, Amutike D, Lal A, et al. Accuracy of the 'Paedfusor' in children undergoing cardiac surgery or catheterization. Br J Anaesth 2003;91(4):507–13.

137. Bailey JM, Mora CT, Shafer SL. Pharmacokinetics of propofol in adult patients undergoing coronary revascularization. The Multicenter Study of Perioperative Ischemia Research Group. Anesthesiology 1996;84(6):1288–97.

138. Filippi L, la Marca G, Fiorini P, et al. Topiramate concentrations in neonates treated with prolonged whole body hypothermia for hypoxic ischemic encephalopathy. Epilepsia 2009;50(11):2355–61.

139. Withington D, Menard G, Varin F. Cisatracurium pharmacokinetics and pharmacodynamics during hypothermic cardiopulmonary bypass in infants and children. Paediatr Anaesth 2011;21(3):341–6.

140. Miller RD, Agoston S, van der Pol F, et al. Hypothermia and the pharmacokinetics and pharmacodynamics of pancuronium in the cat. J Pharmacol Exp Ther 1978;207(2):532–8.

141. d'Hollander AA, Duvaldestin P, Henzel D, et al. Variations in pancuronium requirement, plasma concentration, and urinary excretion induced by cardiopulmonary bypass with hypothermia. Anesthesiology 1983;58(6):505–9.

142. Wierda JM, van der Starre PJ, Scaf AH, et al. Pharmacokinetics of pancuronium in patients undergoing coronary artery surgery with and without low dose dopamine. Clin Pharmacokinet 1990;19(6):491–8.

143. Caldwell JE, Heier T, Wright PM, et al. Temperature-dependent pharmacokinetics and pharmacodynamics of vecuronium. Anesthesiology 2000;92(1):84–93.

144. Withington D, Menard G, Harris J, et al. Vecuronium pharmacokinetics and pharmacodynamics during hypothermic cardiopulmonary bypass in infants and children. Can J Anaesth 2000;47(12):1188–95.

145. Arnold JH, Truog RD, Scavone JM, et al. Changes in the pharmacodynamic response to fentanyl in neonates during continuous infusion. J Pediatr 1991;119(4):639–43.

146. Empey PE, Miller TM, Philbrick AH, et al. Mild hypothermia decreases fentanyl and midazolam steady-state clearance in a rat model of cardiac arrest. Crit Care Med 2012;40(4):1221–8.

147. Zhou J, Empey PE, Bies RR, et al. Cardiac arrest and therapeutic hypothermia decrease isoform-specific cytochrome P450 drug metabolism. Drug Metab Dispos 2011;39(12):2209–18.

148. Arnold JH, Truog RD, Orav EJ, et al. Tolerance and dependence in neonates sedated with fentanyl during extracorporeal membrane oxygenation. Anesthesiology 1990;73(6):1136–40.

149. Alcaraz C, Bansinath M, Turndorf H, et al. Cardiovascular effects of morphine during hypothermia. Arch Int Pharmacodyn Ther 1989;297:133–47.

150. Simantov R, Snowman AM, Snyder SH. Temperature and ionic influences on opiate receptor binding. Mol Pharmacol 1976;12(6):977–86.

151. Cremer OL. The propofol infusion syndrome: more puzzling evidence on a complex and poorly characterized disorder. Crit Care 2009;13(6):1012.

152. Okamoto MP, Kawaguchi DL, Amin AN. Evaluation of propofol infusion syndrome in pediatric intensive care. Am J Health Syst Pharm 2003;60(19):2007–14.

153. Hiraoka H, Yamamoto K, Okano N, et al. Changes in drug plasma concentrations of an extensively bound and highly extracted drug, propofol, in response to altered plasma binding. Clin Pharmacol Ther 2004;75(4):324–30.

154. Yoshitani K, Kawaguchi M, Takahashi M, et al. Plasma propofol concentration and EEG burst suppression ratio during normothermic cardiopulmonary bypass. Br J Anaesth 2003;90(2):122–6.

155. Mathew PJ, Puri GD, Dhaliwal RS. Propofol requirement titrated to bispectral index: a comparison between hypothermic and normothermic cardiopulmonary bypass. Perfusion 2009;24(1):27–32.

156. Beaufort AM, Wierda JM, Belopavlovic M, et al. The influence of hypothermia (surface cooling) on the time-course of action and on the pharmacokinetics of rocuronium in humans. Eur J Anaesthesiol Suppl 1995;11:95–106.

157. Withington DE, Menard G, Varin F. Cisatracurium pharmacokinetics and pharmacodynamics during hypothermic CPB in infants. Paediatr Anaesth 2000; 10(6):695.

158. Kaczala GW, Paulus SC, Al-Dajani N, et al. Bloodstream infections in pediatric ECLS: usefulness of daily blood culture monitoring and predictive value of biological markers. The British Columbia experience. Pediatr Surg Int 2009;25(2):169–73.

159. DiCenzo R, Forrest A, Slish JC, et al. A gentamicin pharmacokinetic population model and once-daily dosing algorithm for neonates. Pharmacotherapy 2003; 23(5):585–91.

160. Kinderen NKFb. Kinderformularium. Available at: http://www.kinderformularium.nl. Accessed January 1, 2011.

161. Martinkova J, Pokorna P, Zahora J, et al. Tolerability and outcomes of kinetically guided therapy with gentamicin in critically ill neonates during the first week of life: an open-label, prospective study. Clin Ther 2010;32(14):2400–14.

162. Davies A, Jones D, Bailey M, et al. Extracorporeal membrane oxygenation for 2009 influenza A(H1N1) acute respiratory distress syndrome. JAMA 2009; 302(17):1888–95.

163. Buckley E, Sidebotham D, McGeorge A, et al. Extracorporeal membrane oxygenation for cardiorespiratory failure in four patients with pandemic H1N1 2009 influenza virus and secondary bacterial infection. Br J Anaesth 2010; 104(3):326–9.

164. Bessereau J, Chenaitia H, Michelet P, et al. Acute respiratory distress syndrome following 2009 H1N1 virus pandemic: when ECMO come to the patient bedside. Ann Fr Anesth Reanim 2010;29(2):165–6.

165. Stavchansky S, Tung IL. Effects of hypothermia on drug absorption. Pharm Res 1987;4(3):248–50.

166. Rohrer MJ, Natale AM. Effect of hypothermia on the coagulation cascade. Crit Care Med 1992;20(10):1402–5.

167. Watts DD, Trask A, Soeken K, et al. Hypothermic coagulopathy in trauma: effect of varying levels of hypothermia on enzyme speed, platelet function, and fibrinolytic activity. J Trauma 1998;44(5):846–54.

168. Valeri CR, Feingold H, Cassidy G, et al. Hypothermia-induced reversible platelet dysfunction. Ann Surg 1987;205(2):175–81.

169. Valeri CR, MacGregor H, Cassidy G, et al. Effects of temperature on bleeding time and clotting time in normal male and female volunteers. Crit Care Med 1995;23(4):698–704.

170. Boldt J, Knothe C, Welters I, et al. Normothermic versus hypothermic cardiopulmonary bypass: do changes in coagulation differ? Ann Thorac Surg 1996;62(1): 130–5.

171. Hall MW, Goodman PD, Alston SM, et al. Hypothermia-induced platelet aggregation in heparinized flowing human blood: identification of a high responder subpopulation. Am J Hematol 2002;69(1):45–55.

172. Xavier RG, White AE, Fox SC, et al. Enhanced platelet aggregation and activation under conditions of hypothermia. Thromb Haemost 2007;98(6):1266–75.

173. Ramaker AJ, Meyer P, van der Meer J, et al. Effects of acidosis, alkalosis, hyperthermia and hypothermia on haemostasis: results of point-of-care testing with the thromboelastography analyser. Blood Coagul Fibrinolysis 2009;20(6):436–9.

174. Olivier P, D'Attellis N, Sirieix D, et al. Continuous infusion versus bolus administration of sufentanil and midazolam for mitral valve surgery. J Cardiothorac Vasc Anesth 1999;13(1):3–8.

175. Green TP, Isham-Schopf B, Irmiter RJ, et al. Inactivation of heparin during extracorporeal circulation in infants. Clin Pharmacol Ther 1990;48(2):148–54.

176. Oliver WC. Anticoagulation and coagulation management for ECMO. Semin Cardiothorac Vasc Anesth 2009;13(3):154–75.

177. Filippi L, la Marca G, Cavallaro G, et al. Phenobarbital for neonatal seizures in hypoxic ischemic encephalopathy: a pharmacokinetic study during whole body hypothermia. Epilepsia 2011;52(4):794–801.

178. van Dijk M, de Boer JB, Koot HM, et al. The reliability and validity of the COMFORT scale as a postoperative pain instrument in 0 to 3-year-old infants. Pain 2000;84(2–3):367–77.

179. Merkel SI, Voepel-Lewis T, Shayevitz JR, et al. The FLACC: a behavioral scale for scoring postoperative pain in young children. Pediatr Nurs 1997;23(3):293–7.

Ethical Issues in Neonatal and Pediatric Clinical Trials

Naomi Laventhal, MD, MA[a],*, Beth A. Tarini, MD, MS[b],
John Lantos, MD[c]

KEYWORDS

- Ethics • Informed consent • Risk-benefit assessment • Clinical trials
- Stem cell transplantation • Genetic testing • Hypoxic-ischemic encephalopathy

KEY POINTS

- Because neonates and children cannot consent to research, they are considered to be vulnerable research subjects for whom research is subject to unique and specific regulations.
- Adults may consent to risky studies that are not beneficial. For children, the risk must be minimal or the benefits must outweigh the risks.
- The concept of "minimal risk" is somewhat arbitrary. It is applied differently by different IRBs. The U.S. federal government is considering revisions of current research regulation guidelines for children.
- The three basic principles of research ethics-respect forpersons, minimization of risk, and justice in selection of research subjects-can be applied to pediatric research. Appropriately, they lead to more restrictive oversight of research for children than for adults.

THE ORIGINS OF PEDIATRIC RESEARCH ETHICS

The unique vulnerability of children as research subjects came to light when Henry Beecher[1] published a landmark article in the *New England Journal of Medicine* entitled, "Ethics and Clinical Research." Beecher's[1] article cataloged several research studies that he argued were ethically unacceptable. One of them was a study by Saul Krugman and colleagues, conducted at the Willowbrook State School, a residential facility for children with neurocognitive problems. In Krugman's studies, some children were deliberately infected with hepatitis to study the natural history of hepatitis

The authors do have no commercial or financial relationships to disclose.
[a] Division of Neonatal-Perinatal Medicine, Department of Pediatrics and Communicable Diseases, University of Michigan School of Medicine, 8-621 C&W Mott Hospital, 1540 East Hospital Drive, SPC 4254, Ann Arbor, MI 48109-4254, USA; [b] Child Health Evaluation and Research Unit, Department of Pediatrics and Communicable Diseases, University of Michigan School of Medicine, 300 North Ingalls, 6C11, Ann Arbor, MI 48109-5456, USA; [c] Department of pediatrics, Children's Mercy Bioethics Center, Children's Mercy Hospital, 2401 Gilham Road, Kansas City, MO 64108, USA
* Corresponding author.
E-mail address: naomilav@med.umich.edu

Pediatr Clin N Am 59 (2012) 1205–1220
http://dx.doi.org/10.1016/j.pcl.2012.07.007
0031-3955/12/$ – see front matter © 2012 Elsevier Inc. All rights reserved.

and better characterize different types of hepatitis, with the ultimate goal of developing a vaccine against hepatitis. Although these studies were done with parental permission, Beecher[1] argued that they were unacceptable because the risks to the children were too high and the informed consent process lacking: "Artificial induction of hepatitis was performed in an institution for mentally defective children in which a mild form of hepatitis was endemic. The parents gave consent for the intramuscular injection or oral administration of the virus, but nothing is said regarding what was told them concerning the appreciable hazards involved" (p. 1359).

Other critiques of Krugman's studies soon followed. In 1970, theologian Paul Ramsey[2] wrote of the Willowbrook studies: "Such use of captive populations of children for purely experimental purposes ought to be made legally impossible … stopped by legal acknowledgement of the moral invalidity of parental or legal proxy consent for the child to procedures having no relation to a child's own diagnosis or treatment."[2] Five years later, the *Lancet* published an exchange of letters about the Willowbrook studies. Steven Goldby[3] wrote that "it was indefensible to give potentially dangerous infected material to children, particularly those who were mentally retarded, with or without parental consent, when no benefit to the child could conceivably result." Krugman[4] (1971) himself wrote back, defending the studies on the grounds that the children involved did benefit, because:

> *(1) they were bound to be exposed to the same strains under the natural conditions existing in the institution; and (2) they would be admitted to a special, well-equipped, and well-staffed unit where they would be isolated from exposure to other infectious diseases which were prevalent in the institution—namely shigellosis, parasitic infections, and respiratory infections—thus, their exposure in the hepatitis unit would be associated with less risk than the type of institutional exposure where multiple infections could occur.[4]*

This debate polarized the research community. The editors of the *Lancet* criticized the Willowbrook studies[3] and suggested that they would no longer publish Krugman's papers. In contrast, the editors of the *Journal of the American Medical Association* published Krugman's follow-up studies, along with a laudatory editorial criticizing what they called the pious tone of the *Lancet* editorial and suggesting that Krugman's studies were ethically justifiable.[5] A decade later, medical historian David Rothman[6] (1982) wrote of Willowbrook that the parental consent was meaningless because "[t] he consent form that parents signed to allow their children to be infected with the virus read as though their children were to receive a vaccine against the virus." Furthermore, he argued, parents often consented to the studies to get their children out of the overcrowded wards at Willowbrook and into the superior accommodations of the research wing. Thus, he argued, the supposed benefit of better care in the research wing of Willowbrook was a coercive inducement to participate in the studies. Such a justification for research, he suggested, would specifically put poor children at risk of participating in the most risky research.

The debate about Krugman's Willowbrook studies exemplifies a central feature of the ongoing debates about pediatric research, specifically which studies are justifiable, for which populations of patients, and with what safeguards and oversights. Many children cannot participate in decisions about their participation in research. Even those who can participate in such decisions may not be able to fully understand the risks and benefits. Parents, physicians, and scientists all have an obligation to protect children from the harms of research, but they may also hope to discover new treatments or cures for childhood illnesses. The tension between the 2 goals of protection and progress is inevitable.

Reasonable people can disagree about the proper balance in any particular intervention. Those disagreements occasionally attract public scrutiny. Specific controversial studies become paradigm cases that serve as the basic building blocks of the unique body of moral philosophy that is the foundation of pediatric research ethics. This article reviews the current federal guidelines for research in children as well as some of the controversies that test the application of those guidelines.

ETHICS AND REGULATORY OVERSIGHT OF PEDIATRIC RESEARCH

Research that involves children has always been ethically problematic. The fundamental reason is straightforward. Research, by its nature, uses subjects as a means to the end of creating knowledge that can be generalized. In adults, the solution to this fundamental ethical problem is to get the voluntary, informed consent of the research subject. Children cannot consent on their own behalf. Instead, researchers, parents, and regulators must determine whether the risk/benefit ratio is acceptable to permit the research to go forward.

The regulations governing research conduct in the United States have always included special requirements and considerations for pediatric research subjects and other vulnerable populations. These special requirements call for a higher level of scrutiny and more stringent thresholds of protection than for less vulnerable populations.

Although the reasons for extra scrutiny of pediatric research are straightforward, the arguments for the necessity of doing research in children are also compelling. Children, and particularly infants, respond differently to drugs and other medical treatments than do adults. There are many stories of drugs that, although safe in adults, have serious and even fatal side effects in children.[7] Studies in children often require longer follow-up than studies in adults to determine whether innovative treatments have any long-term developmental effects.

The current regulatory guidelines for pediatric research define 4 levels of risk in research studies, each of which is subject to a different level of regulation and oversight (**Table 1**). The lowest level of risk is minimal risk. Minimal risk is defined as "the probability and magnitude of physical or psychological harm that is normally encountered in the daily lives, or in the routine medical or psychological examination, or health children" (National Commission, *Research Involving Children*[8,9]). Studies that involve only minimal risk can be performed, even if they do not offer any prospect of direct benefit to the research subjects. For such studies, researchers only need the permission of 1 parent and the assent of the child, if the child is old enough and cognitively capable of giving assent.

However, this categorization is problematic because it is vague. First, the definition does not specify whether these risks should be interpreted relative to normal, healthy children, or relative to the sick children who are like those to be enrolled in the study. The normal daily lives of sick children might include invasive procedures, treatments, and discomforts. Second, the daily life of a child can be risky. Children are at risk of injury when they ride a bike, play competitive sports, take ballet lessons, or climb trees, but these risks are different from those to which a child is exposed in a research study.

This vagueness creates variable interpretations by investigators and institutional review boards (IRBs).[10] In a survey study of IRB chairmen, Shah and colleagues[11] identified marked variation in assessment of the level of risk associated with different procedures; for example, allergy skin testing was found by 23% of those surveyed to be minimal risk, by 43% to convey a minor increase compared with minimal risk, and by 27% to impose more than a minor increase compared with minimal risk; similar variation was observed in assessment of potential for direct benefit.

Table 1
Pediatric research risk stratification

Classification	Definition	Stipulations	Informed Consent
No greater than minimal risk[a]	No requirement for benefit to subject	None	Adequate provisions made for soliciting assent of children and permission of 1 parent
Greater than minimal risk[a]; presents the prospect of direct benefit to the individual subjects	Intervention or procedure presents more than minimal risk and prospect of direct benefit for the individual subject Or: Monitoring procedure is likely to contribute to the subject's well-being	Risk justified by the anticipated benefit to subjects Relation of the anticipated benefit to the risk at least as favorable to the subjects as that presented by available alternative approaches	Adequate provisions made for soliciting assent of children and permission of 1 parent Child's assent can be overridden
Greater than minimal risk[a] with no prospect of direct benefit to individual subjects Likely to yield knowledge that can be generalized about the subject's disorder or condition (of vital importance for the understanding or amelioration of the disorder or condition)	Intervention or procedure has no prospect of direct benefit for the individual subject Or: Monitoring procedure not likely to contribute to the well-being of the subject	Risk represents a minor increase to minimal risk Presents experiences commensurate with those inherent in actual or expected medical, dental, psychological, social, or educational situations	
Greater than minor increase above minimal risk[a] with no prospect of direct benefit to subjects	Presents a reasonable opportunity to further the understanding, prevention, or alleviation of a serious problem affecting the health or welfare of children	Health and Human Services may approve after consultation with a panel of experts in pertinent disciplines and following opportunity for public review and comment	Adequate provisions made for soliciting assent of children and permission of both parents

[a] Minimal risk: the probability and magnitude of harm or discomfort anticipated in the research are not greater than those ordinarily encountered in daily life or during the performance of routine physical or psychological examinations or tests.

Data from Title Code of Federal Regulations, Title 45, Public Welfare, Department of Health and Human Services; Part 46, Protection of Human Subjects. Revised June 23, 2005, accessed May 8, 2012; and Ross LF. Children in medical research: access versus protection. Oxford (United Kingdom): Oxford University Press; 2006.

The second level of risk is a minor increase compared with minimal risk. Research with this level of risk, and with no prospect of direct benefit to the research subjects, may still be approved by an IRB, but only if the research is likely to yield knowledge that is of vital importance to understanding or ameliorating the child's disorder or condition. The research risks are acceptable if they are commensurate with those in the child's actual or expected medical, dental, psychological, social, or educational situations. For research in this category, the permission of both parents is required, as is the child's assent (again, if the child is developmentally capable of providing it).

The third risk category is for studies that involve risks that are greater than a minimal or even minor increase compared with minimal risk but that also include the prospect of direct benefit to the child. These studies were previously referred to as therapeutic research, but that term has gone out of favor. In such studies, the task of the IRB is to conduct a risk-benefit assessment and to determine whether the potential anticipated benefit justifies the risk. Although tangible, quantifiable information about the likelihood of these risks and benefits may be available, this assessment may be subjective.[12] Conduct of these studies requires the consent of 1 parent and the assent of the child.

Implicit in the ethical conduct of studies that are in this third risk category is the assumption of clinical equipoise. First described by Benjamin Freedman,[13] clinical equipoise is defined as "a state of genuine uncertainty on the part of the clinical investigator regarding the comparative therapeutic merits of each arm in a trial." However, as Freedman[13] also pointed out, these studies cannot be absent of merit: "Equipoise is an important concept in the conduct of ethically sound pediatric research, which must be conducted in pursuit of findings that are of scientific merit." According to Freedman,[13] clinical equipoise exists when there is "an honest, professional disagreement among expert clinicians about the preferred treatment." An ethically sound clinical trial should offer reasonable hope of resolving this disagreement. In contrast, if existing evidence clearly favors one treatment or another, or if the proposed trial is unlikely to disturb the state of equipoise, the trial should not proceed as designed. Research must be done in authentic pursuit of answers to valid clinical questions, and patients should not be subjected to research risks in the absence of genuine belief that the answer to the research question is unknown, which also applies to research that involves children. In the initial interpretation of the National Commission's recommendations for research involving children, Albert Jonsen[12] described the need for this research to be "valuable and necessary for the health and wellbeing of children."

The fourth risk category is the most complex and the most unusual. It is for studies that involve more than a minor increase above minimal risk, no prospect of direct benefit for the child, but that are judged to be so important in terms of the knowledge that they might yield, that they ought, perhaps, to be conducted anyway. Studies that meet these criteria must be likely to yield knowledge that will prevent or alleviate a serious health condition in childhood. IRBs cannot approve these studies. If an IRB determines that a proposed study meets these criteria, it must refer the study to the Federal Government, which will convene an expert panel to review the proposed study and to decide whether it may go forward. Such studies, if approved, require the permission of both parents and the assent of the child.

THE COMPLICATED CONCEPT OF ASSENT

All research in children requires the assent of the child. But what is assent? At what age is a child capable of assent? When should it be sought? As with minimal risk, answers to all of these questions are vague and variable. At the most basic level, assent is an affirmative agreement by the child to participate in research.

William Bartholome,[14] one of the strongest advocates for the necessity of assent, broke it down into 4 elements. (1) a developmentally appropriate understanding of the nature of the condition, (2) disclosure of the nature of the proposed intervention and what it will involve, (3) an assessment of the child's understanding of the information provided and the influences that affect the child's evaluation of the situation, and (4) a solicitation of the child's expression of willingness to accept the intervention. These elements notwithstanding, there is active debate about the definition of assent, its process, and the age at which a child can provide it. Roth-Cline and colleagues[15] point out the controversies about assent: "how to resolve disputes between children and their parents; the relationship between assent and consent; the quantity and quality of information to disclose to children and their families; how much and what information children desire and need, the necessity and methods for assessing both children's understanding of disclosed information and of the assent process itself; and what constitutes an effective, practical, and realistically applicable decision-making model." Unguru and colleagues[16] interviewed children aged 7 to 19 years about their experience in oncology trials and discovered that many children did not understand basic aspects of the research (for example, that there might be added risk compared with standard treatments), and did not think that they were able to play a significant role in decision making.

In the absence of validated processes for engaging children in meaningful, developmentally appropriate exchange of information about research participation, the process of obtaining assent before enrolling children in research studies is at risk for the same pitfalls that plague the informed consent process for adult research subjects, including cumbersome and legalistic documents and minimal critical evaluation of comprehension. Furthermore, for studies in which the anticipated benefit is thought to outweigh the risk, such as clinical trials of cancer chemotherapy, the parents may claim the right to override the child's dissent. In such studies, it is not clear whether the guiding moral framework should be the research paradigm or the ethical paradigms that govern non-research clinical care in which parents have the right to make decisions for their children.

IRB chairs are as variable in their interpretations of assent as they are in their interpretations of minimal risk. Whittle and colleagues[17] found that half of IRB chairs rely on the investigators' judgment about when assent must be sought; the other half had a required method for investigators to determine whether obtaining assent was appropriate, most commonly based on age, but the age cutoff for requiring investigators to obtain assent from the child ranged from less than or equal to 5 years to older than or equal to 10 years.

PROBLEMS WITH THE CURRENT REGULATORY FRAMEWORK

Despite the recognition of the importance of research oversight in protecting children in research studies, the existence of the federal regulations for child research participants have not brought harmony or efficiency to the process of bringing pediatric research protocols to fruition. The process of research oversight by IRBs remains cumbersome for reasons that are both logistic and ideological. The following problems are commonly identified as most obstructive to ongoing research in pediatric populations:

1. There is disconnect between the level of required scrutiny and the level of risk, such that minimal risk studies are still subjected to long and onerous review processes.
2. There is inter-institutional variation in interpretation of research protocols and regulations, which requires multicenter trials to submit the different protocols at the

participating centers, resulting in not only delayed but sometimes also weakened investigations.
3. There is vagueness in the regulations about the likelihood of benefit, burden of interventions, and acceptability, which leads to disagreements within an IRB and results in a prolonged review process.
4. There is a volunteer system of IRB reviewers, who may have limited background knowledge of the research subject area, incomplete understanding of the regulations, and limited time and resources to devote to methodological and thoughtful consideration of a proposed protocol.
5. The informed consent documents are cumbersome and lengthy, weighed down by boilerplate language included to protect institutions rather than inform and protect children and their parents. The emphasis is on an institutionally uniform and comprehensive informed consent document, which may detract from a more relevant and meaningful interactive process of discussing a study's potential risks and benefits with children and their parents.

These problems no doubt lead to investigator cynicism and development of protocols that "teach to the test", such that there is disconnect between the process of research oversight and a more meaningful protection of child research subjects. Protocol approval is not a guarantee that a study is ethical, and an ethically designed study is not guaranteed to be approved.

PROPOSED CHANGES TO REGULATIONS

In July 2011, the Office of the Secretary of the Department of Health and Human Services issued advance notice of proposed rulemaking (ANPRM), seeking comments on suggested changes to existing human subject protection regulations to make these rules more modern and effective (**Table 2**). These proposed changes were designed to include contemporary problems in research ethics, such as the use of biospecimens and electronic medical records, the need for systematic approaches across institutions regarding informed consent and scientific review, and categorization of exempt and minimal risk research. An exhaustive review of the proposed changes is beyond the scope of this article, but some of the proposed changes with the potential to directly affect pediatric research are briefly described:

1. There is currently no system for standardized data security protections; addressing this has the potential to ameliorate what many view to be excessively burdensome oversight of minimal risk studies, many of which are limited to chart review or evaluation of previously collected data or samples.
2. There is no consent required for use of deidentified existing biospecimens, which may ultimately be relinked to individual identifiers.
3. The common rule is only enforceable if research is funded by certain sources, introducing inconsistency in the way research is conducted in the United States with regard to ethical principles that ought to be universal.
4. There is no systematized way to report adverse events, minimizing the likelihood that important safety information will be consistently reported to regulatory bodies and investigators.
5. There are burdensome but inadequate requirements for informed consent, with inordinate amounts of attention and effort dedicated to the informed consent document, rather than focusing on requiring IRBs and investigators to present information to potential research subjects in an informative way.[18]

Table 2
Overview of proposed changes to federal regulatory framework for human subjects protection

Ensuring risk-based protections	Refinement of existing risk-based regulatory framework
	Calibration of the levels of review to the level of risk
	New mechanism for protecting subjects from informational risks
Streamlining IRB review of multisite studies	Use of single IRB review for domestic sites of multicenter studies
Improved informed consent	Improved consent forms
	Waiver of informed consent or documentation of informed consent in primary data collection
	Strengthened consent protections related to reuse or additional analysis of existing data and biospecimens
Strengthening data protections to minimize information risks	Consistent characterization of information with respect to potential for identification
	Standards for data security and information problems
Data collection to enhance system oversight	Establishment of an improved, more systematic approach for the collection and analysis of data on unanticipated problems and adverse events
Extension of federal regulations	Regulatory protections to all research, regardless of funding source, conducted at US institutions that receive federal funding from a common rule agency for human subjects research
Consistency across federal regulations	Improvement in the harmonization of regulations and related agency guidance

Adapted from The Office of the Secretary of the Department of Health and Human Services. Human subjects research protections: enhancing protections for research subjects and reducing burden, delay, and ambiguity for investigators; advance notice of proposed rulemaking. Fed Regist 2011;7(143):44512–31.

6. Multiple IRBs review the same protocol for multicenter studies, which can be cumbersome for local IRBs that may not have reviewers with the highly specialized expertise needed to evaluate some complex clinical trials,[19] and may delay or even thwart efforts to carry out timely multicenter clinical studies.[18] A streamlined process of centralized regulation and oversight has the potential to both improve the quality of research oversight and to support investigators conducting important multicenter trials.

CONTROVERSIAL RESEARCH IN CHILDREN

There are many examples of the difficulties in following the current regulations for pediatric research. This article briefly discusses 3: studies of genetic screening, the enrollment of healthy children in studies of sibling bone marrow donation, and the use of therapeutic hypothermia for neonates with asphyxia.

Genetic Testing Research in Children

Genetic testing research in children presents ethical challenges in pediatric research. Although genetic testing research encompasses different types of research that require distinction before any discussion about risks and benefits,[20] this article focuses on research that identifies active or future disease risk to the individual being tested. The ethical issues that surround testing for carrier status (when individuals carry a genetic change that does not cause concern for themselves but can be passed on to offspring) are important, but they are beyond the scope of this paper.

The first distinction of genetic testing research in children is whether the research involves genetic testing of symptomatic or asymptomatic (ie, healthy) children. For example, genetic testing studies may involve children with clinical findings (eg, congenital anomalies, developmental delay) that lack an underlying genetic diagnosis. Some of these studies recruit and study families with multiple members who have a similar constellation of symptoms and/or physical findings for which an underlying genetic cause is sought.[21] Others involve large cohorts of unrelated patients with diverse and complex phenotypes whose genomes are examined to identify genetic alterations that might explain the observed phenotype.[22]

For affected children and families who participate in these types of genetic testing research, the benefits of this kind of research (causal diagnosis that may inform future treatments and reproductive decisions) are deemed to outweigh the risks. There are greater concerns about the psychological harms of receiving the research results than on undergoing the research process (eg, consent for use of samples, privacy of results). For example, there are potential threats to individual and familial identity caused by the identification of a genetic condition (eg, parental/familial guilt,[23,24] or revealing information about other family members who might carry the same predisposition). Uncertainty about the causality of the research findings may be important. Parents might expect (and hope) for definitive answers about their child's illness. They may use the research findings in making future decisions about their child's health and their own future family planning. As a result, there has been a call for careful attention to the process of returning research results to these children and their families.[24]

Most genetic testing research among asymptomatic children has focused on mendelian disorders (ie, those caused by mutations in single genes and that are minimally influenced by environment) such as Huntington disease or Li-Fraumeni syndrome. In the coming decade, pediatric genetic testing research will face ethical challenges that result from the ability to sequence an individual's genome. This technology will allow research on genetic susceptibility testing (also referred to as predictive genomic testing) and lead to challenges related to incidental findings as vast quantities of information, some unanticipated, are generated. The term genomic reflects that this testing assesses disease risk for common complex diseases, such as type 2 diabetes. The term complex refers to the influence of both genetic (usually across multiple genes) and environmental factors on disease development. Unlike in mendelian diseases, in which the risk of disease is almost always 100%, genetic susceptibility testing provides disease risks that are modestly increased compared with that of the population, on the order of 10%.

In either type of genetic testing research of children (mendelian or common diseases) risk/benefit considerations are influenced by (1) the timing of disease onset (ie, childhood or adult), and (2) treatability of disease. Predicting an early-onset disease (ie, one that manifests during childhood) carries with it more potential urgency and relevance to the child's life than one that occurs during adulthood. This urgency is only increased when the disease can be cured or its complications can be mitigated. For example, although there is no cure for Li-Fraumeni syndrome, the child may benefit from regular cancer screening because the disease can carry a nearly 20% risk of childhood malignancy.[25] As the treatability of the disease decreases, the benefits of testing shift more to the psychosocial realm, such as helping to prepare for future health and life decisions (eg, long-term care insurance, childbearing). Any potential benefits from genetic testing research in childhood are significantly tempered when the child will not develop disease until adulthood. A commonly cited case is identification of children with Huntington disease. There is debate whether children's or adolescents' knowledge of their own predispositions to develop adult-onset disease status merits testing during childhood, rather than waiting until the child becomes a competent adult who can provide autonomous consent to participate in this kind of research.[26] Many professional societies recommend deferring such testing,[27] based on arguments that imposing this knowledge interferes with the child's right to an open future,[28,29] a term that captures children's right to preserve their future life options by limiting the decisions and information imposed on them by others.

Genetic susceptibility testing in children is an emerging field likely to generate significant debate and controversy in the pediatric ethics community. There has been strong opposition to this type of genetic testing research because of concerns that it causes significant psychological harm, specifically a fatalistic approach to health. The implications are that genetic risk is exceptional and that it differs in some fundamental ways from other clinical risk factors for disease such as blood pressure or obesity. Proponents of conducting research on, not providing clinical services for, genetic susceptibility testing point out that studies thus far have failed to support this concern[30] and that this testing involves diseases that frequently are adult onset, but for which early preventive behaviors may improve long-term health outcomes.[31] Here there is tension between protection and progress: on the individual level, research in this area should not subject children to unnecessary risk. However, not conducting the research may lead to inadvertent harm on a societal level, because the technology is likely to find its way into the clinical realm, whether or not it has been subjected to rigorous scientific evaluation.

Research on Healthy Children Who Donate Stem Cells to Siblings

As allogeneic hematopoietic stem cell transplantation has become standard treatment of several oncologic and hematologic illnesses that affect children, HLA-matched biologic siblings, who are also children, may be identified as potential stem cell donors for these pediatric patients.[32] The American Academy of Pediatrics has supported this process, which is now performed without much controversy in clinical practice. However, evaluating risks and benefits to a child of donating bone marrow to a sibling is difficult. How can the potential benefit of saving the life of a child by donating bone marrow to a sibling with cancer be quantified? Can this be considered to be direct benefit to the child? What kinds of risks to the donor are reasonable? In addition, scientific questions continue to emerge and evolve, bringing forth questions about the ethics of enrolling child stem cell donors in clinical research. When siblings are to donate stem cells in a research context, the IRB must apply the guidelines discussed earlier to categorize the risks and benefits. In this scenario, careful interpretation and application of existing regulations for research involving children becomes critical. If there is perceived direct benefit, then research that imposes more than a minor increase compared with minimal risk may be justified. Otherwise, the research should impart no more than minimal risk.

What should be the point of comparison for these donor children? Does it make sense to compare the potential burdens to a sibling donating bone marrow with those accrued by healthy children in day-to-day life? Ordinary life takes on a different meaning for a child who has a sibling with a serious cancer.

A recent protocol made the questions even more complex. Investigators proposed giving the donors granulocyte macrophage colony-stimulating factor (GM-CSF), a treatment generally thought to be safe but with potential long-term risks, to improve the likelihood of success for the recipient.[33] This proposed research was deemed to entail more than a minor increase above minimal risk with no prospect of direct benefit to the donor, and, in 2008, the US Food and Drug Administration Pediatric Advisory Committee's Pediatric Ethics Subcommittee reviewed this protocol and considered whether a third party should advocate for the donor, whether parental discretion can credibly be based on assessment of risk and benefit to the donor, and what implications the committee findings would have on future research on healthy sibling stem cell donation. The results of these deliberations are available online.[34] In brief, they concluded that:

1. The potential research represented more than a minor increase above minimal risk, excluding it from approval as minimal risk research that would not require direct benefit.
2. There were potential benefits, but these were indirect, excluding the research from approval as research with more than minimal risk but with potential direct benefit to the child.
3. Potential donors did not have a condition with respect to the protocol, excluding the possibility of approval as research that posed more than minimal risk but with the potential to ameliorate the participant's condition.
4. The protocol offered an opportunity to address a serious problem affecting the health of children, such that, in an invocation of the rare fourth category described earlier, potential donors would be allowed to participate provided that they had no identifiable risk factors for complications from GM-CSF administration, that an independent third party was available as an advocate for the potential donor, that the life-threatening nature of some of the potential risks (acute respiratory distress syndrome and leukemia) was disclosed in the informed consent document, and that all things being equal, preference should go to an older sibling donor.

Therapeutic Hypothermia for Perinatal Hypoxic-Ischemic Encephalopathy

Research on therapeutic hypothermia shows many of the ethical issues in pediatric research. The earliest clinical trials of hypothermia for babies with neonatal hypoxic-ischemic encephalopathy (HIE) were conducted in the late 1990s. The first study, by Gunn and colleagues[35] in New Zealand, was designed only to address safety and practicality. There was no anticipation of direct benefit for the babies. The study was approved by a regional ethics committee and parental consent was obtained.

A few years later, Shankaran and colleagues[36] proposed that it would be ethically acceptable to enroll babies in a prospective randomized trial. Although the criteria for approval are not included in published reports, we assume that the studies were assessed as having more than a minor increase compared with minimal risk, but with a prospect of direct benefit.

Over the next few years, many such randomized trials were conducted. A meta-analysis by the Cochrane Library in 2007 reported that, in 8 randomized controlled trials involving 638 term infants, therapeutic hypothermia resulted in a statistically significant and clinically important reduction in the combined outcome of mortality or major neurodevelopmental disability to 18 months of age (typical relative risk [RR] 0.76; 95% confidence interval [CI] 0.65, 0.89; typical risk difference [RD] −0.15; 95% CI −0.24, −0.07; number needed to treat [NNT] 7; 95% CI 4, 14). Cooling also resulted in statistically significant reductions in mortality (typical RR 0.74; 95% CI

0.58, 0.94; typical RD −0.09; 95% CI −0.16, −0.02; NNT 11; 95% CI 6, 50) and neuro-developmental disability in survivors (typical RR 0.68; 95% CI 0.51, 0.92; typical RD −0.13; 95% CI −0.23, −0.03; NNT 8; 95% CI 4, 33). Some adverse effects of hypothermia included an increase in the need for inotrope support of borderline significance and a significant increase in thrombocytopenia.[37]

At that point, the debate shifted. It was no longer a question of whether enough was known about the innovative therapy (hypothermia) to allow patients to be randomized. Instead, the debate shifted to being about whether the data were so compelling that it would no longer be acceptable to not treat babies with hypothermia.

The debate polarized the research community in neonatology. In 2005, the American Academy of Pediatrics Committee on the Fetus and Newborn noted that, "Therapeutic hypothermia is a promising therapy that should be considered investigational until the short-term safety and efficacy have been confirmed in the additional human trials underway. Long-term safety and efficacy remain to be defined."[38] That same year, Papile[39] wrote of hypothermia, "This treatment is best considered an experimental technique for which informed parental consent should be obtained. Widespread application of brain cooling in the care of neonates with hypoxic-ischemic encephalopathy would be premature." A few years later, Schulzke and colleagues[40] echoed these cautious sentiments: "Further research is necessary to minimize the uncertainty regarding efficacy and safety of any specific technique of cooling for any specific population." Kirpalani and colleagues[41] demanded, "...strong evidence of robust, consistent effects in highly valid studies that have enrolled adequate numbers of patients before mandating a new therapy for management of all relevant patients."

However, others took a different view. Wilkinson and associates,[42] writing in 2007, noted that, "We believe that the strength of the existing evidence warrants careful consideration of whether the risks to participants involved in continuing trials are justified." The next year, Gunn and colleagues[43] noted that, "robust evidence for benefit from current meta-analyses, the remarkable safety profile, the strong foundation in basic science, and supporting evidence from related disease states such as encephalopathy after cardiac arrest..." These investigators dictate that practicing physicians, in consultation with patients and families, should use hypothermia as a treatment of neonatal encephalopathy.

The debate about hypothermia shows the difficulty in deciding about 2 thresholds in the evaluation of an innovative therapy. The first is the threshold of deciding when enough is known about a new therapy to consider clinical trials in neonatal populations. That is, when is there enough evidence of both safety and efficacy to justify randomizing babies to standard or innovative therapy? The second threshold occurs as evidence from such trials accumulates. When enough known to be confident that the innovative therapy is better, worse, or equivalent to the standard therapy? For both thresholds, reasonable people (and reasonable IRBs) can disagree.

Establishing the second threshold has been easy to do for the patients who most resemble those studied in the therapeutic hypothermia trials. Initiating standard cooling therapy (3 days of cooling to a core temperature 33.5°C for 72 hours) for term (at least 36 weeks) infants with moderate or severe perinatal HIE within 6 hours of birth has become standard of care in neonatal intensive care units (NICUs) in developed countries[44–46]; this therapy, which was once only available in academic referral centers, has been adopted by growing numbers of community NICUs around the country. At least in theory, this practice is guided by highly specific published protocols and step-by-step instructions on how to offer safe and effective therapy.[47,48]

The dissemination of this knowledge has made cooling widely available to affected infants and obviates transfer to referral centers or enrollment in complicated research protocols, but only for those patients who meet the strict inclusion criteria. However, questions still remain about whether there is opportunity to further optimize the protocols to yield even greater reductions in the incidence of adverse outcomes (which remains high, even among infants who receive standard cooling therapy). What if, for example, cooling infants for longer than 3 days, or targeting an even lower core body temperature, could impart even more benefit without imposing more adverse effects? Questions also remain about whether this treatment could help a more diverse group of babies, such as those who are not recognized to have HIE until after the 6-hour window has passed, or those infants who are born prematurely. Another set of questions remains about whether therapeutic hypothermia is beneficial to infants who have the most severe HIE, and whether, for some infants, offering this treatment could redistribute poor outcomes from death to survival with significant neurologic impairment, an outcome that is viewed by some physicians and parents as a fate worse than death.[49] Although subgroup analyses of the larger clinical trials has not shown this to be the case, this method of analysis may not yield results that are as robust as a clinical trial designed a priori to evaluate the outcome in question[50]; however, at this point it is difficult to imagine that it would be ethically permissible to randomize infants with severe HIE to cooling or placebo.

Some of the residual questions about therapeutic hypothermia are being addressed by ongoing clinical trials; specifically, clinical trials are underway assessing the effect of cooling initiated up to 24 hours after birth, comparing the safety and efficacy of standard cooling with longer and/or deeper cooling, and evaluating cooling protocols for late preterm infants. Work is also underway to address strategies to initiate therapeutic hypothermia at smaller community hospitals and to continue it during transport to referral centers, as well as to evaluate the value of various adjuvant clinical therapies, all with the hope of reducing the incidence of death and disability for babies with HIE.

All of this research is resource intense, requires careful assessment of risk and benefit, and involves a laborious and often nuanced process of informed consent. At our center, we encounter the difficulties of trying to maintain an informed consent process that upholds the spirit of the principles of research ethics under significant time pressure (eg, studies of longer, deeper cooling require randomization before 6 hours of life) with major logistic obstacles, such as having these discussions on the telephone with women at referring hospitals who are immediately postpartum, discussing the sudden and unexpected illness of a newborn baby. Fully informing families with whom the investigator has no previous relationship of the potential risks and benefits associated with subtly different cooling protocols can be difficult in these circumstances. In placebo trials, such as the late cooling protocols, the concepts of equipoise and randomization must also be described in lay terms, because parents may not understand why it is not better to offer *any* therapy with the potential to help their baby.

Equipoise regarding the ongoing research questions about therapeutic hypothermia may also prove to be a major issue that affects the success of future trials as neonatologists consider the validity of generalizations from the initial cooling studies. Does it make sense for a physician to refer a 7-hour-old neonate to a different hospital for a cooling trial, when standard clinical cooling could be initiated at the birth hospital, obviating a potentially risky transport and separation of mother and baby? If cooling is safe and effective for infants born at or after 36 completed gestational weeks, is it unreasonable to offer it to a well-grown 35-week infant with HIE? What is the neonatologist's responsibility to refrain from offering off-label cooling, and, if these therapies are increasingly available off-label, why would a parent of an infant with HIE not choose that rather than a randomized trial?

SUMMARY

This article reviews 3 areas of controversy in pediatric research: research on genetic screening tests, research involving healthy children who donate stem cells to siblings, and research on therapeutic hypothermia for HIE. In each area, the challenge for researchers and policy makers is to use the framework of minimal risk, acceptable risk/benefit ratio, parental permission, and child assent to determine which study designs are morally acceptable. In each case, the application of basic principles to the practicalities of the research projects requires careful attention to the details of the study, flexibility in the application of the principles, and opens deliberation about the best way to conduct important research safely in a vulnerable patient population.

ACKNOWLEDGMENTS

Dr Tarini is supported by a K23 Mentored Patient-Oriented Research Career Development Award from the National Institute for Child Health and Human Development (K23HD057994). John Lantos is supported in part by a CTSA grant from the National Institute of Health (UL1 RR033179).

REFERENCES

1. Beecher HK. Ethics and clinical research. N Engl J Med 1966;274(24):1354–60.
2. Ramsey P. The patient as person; explorations in medical ethics. New Haven (CT): Yale University Press; 1970.
3. Goldby S. Experiments at the Willowbrook State School. Lancet 1971;297(7702): 749.
4. Krugman S. Experiments at the Willowbrook State School. Lancet 1971;1(7706): 966–7.
5. Prevention of viral hepatitis: mission impossible? JAMA 1971;217(1):70–1.
6. Rothman DJ. Were Tuskegee & Willowbrook 'studies in nature'? Hastings Cent Rep 1982;12(2):5–7.
7. Steinbrook R. Testing medications in children. N Engl J Med 2002;347(18): 1462–70.
8. National Commission for the Protection of Human Subjects of Biomedical and Behavioral Research. Report and recommendations on research involving children. Washington, DC: US Government Printing Office; 1977.
9. United State National Commission for the Protection of Human Subjects of Biomedical and Behavioral Research. Research involving children: report and recommendations. Bethesda (MD): The Commission; 1977.
10. Westra AE, Wit JM, Sukhai RN, et al. How best to define the concept of minimal risk. J Pediatr 2011;159(3):496–500.
11. Shah S, Whittle A, Wilfond B, et al. How do institutional review boards apply the federal risk and benefit standards for pediatric research? JAMA 2004;291(4):476–82.
12. Jonsen AR. Research involving children: recommendations of the National Commission for the Protection of Human Subjects of Biomedical and Behavioral Research. Pediatrics 1978;62(2):131–6.
13. Freedman B. Equipoise and the ethics of clinical research. N Engl J Med 1987; 317(3):141–5.
14. Bartholome W. Ethical issues in pediatric research. In: Vanderpool HY, editor. The ethics of research involving human subjects. Frederick (MD): University Publishing Group; 1996. p. 360–1.

15. Roth-Cline M, Gerson J, Bright P, et al. Ethical considerations in conducting pediatric research 1st Edition. Handb Exp Pharmacol 2011;205:219–44.

16. Unguru Y, Sill AM, Kamani N. The experiences of children enrolled in pediatric oncology research: implications for assent. Pediatrics 2010;125(4): e876–83.

17. Whittle A, Shah S, Wilfond B, et al. Institutional review board practices regarding assent in pediatric research. Pediatrics 2004;113(6):1747–52.

18. Human subjects research protections: enhancing protections for research subjects and reducing burden, delay, and ambiguity for investigators; advance notice of proposed rulemaking. Fed Regist 2011;76(143):44512–31.

19. Stark AR, Tyson JE, Hibberd PL. Variation among institutional review boards in evaluating the design of a multicenter randomized trial. J Perinatol 2010;30(3):163–9.

20. Ross LF, Moon MR. Ethical issues in genetic testing of children. Arch Pediatr Adolesc Med 2000;154(9):873–9.

21. Martin DM, Probst FJ, Camper SA, et al. Characterisation and genetic mapping of a new X linked deafness syndrome. J Med Genet 2000;37(11):836–41.

22. Mefford HC. Genotype to phenotype-discovery and characterization of novel genomic disorders in a "genotype-first" era. Genet Med 2009;11(12):836–42.

23. Lehmann A, Speight BS, Kerzin-Storrar L. Extended family impact of genetic testing: the experiences of X-linked carrier grandmothers. J Genet Couns 2011; 20(4):365–73.

24. Tabor HK, Cho MK. Ethical implications of array comparative genomic hybridization in complex phenotypes: points to consider in research. Genet Med 2007; 9(9):626–31.

25. Teplick A, Kowalski M, Biegel JA, et al. Educational paper: screening in cancer predisposition syndromes: guidelines for the general pediatrician. Eur J Pediatr 2011;170(3):285–94.

26. Wilfond B, Ross LF. From genetics to genomics: ethics, policy, and parental decision-making. J Pediatr Psychol 2009;34(6):639–47.

27. Nelson RM, Botkjin JR, Kodish ED, et al. Ethical issues with genetic testing in pediatrics. Pediatrics 2001;107(6):1451–5.

28. Davis DS. Genetic dilemmas and the child's right to an open future. Rutgers Law J 1997;28:549–92.

29. Wertz DC, Fanos JH, Reilly PR. Genetic testing for children and adolescents. Who decides? JAMA 1994;272(11):875–81.

30. Wade CH, Wilfond BS, McBride CM. Effects of genetic risk information on children's psychosocial wellbeing: a systematic review of the literature. Genet Med 2010;12(6):317–26.

31. Tarini BA, Tercyak KP, Wilfond BS. Commentary: children and predictive genomic testing: disease prevention, research protection, and our future. J Pediatr Psychol 2011;36(10):1113–21.

32. Committee on Bioethics. Children as hematopoietic stem cell donors. Pediatrics 2010;125(2):392–404.

33. Pulsipher MA, Nagler A, Iannone R, et al. Weighing the risks of G-CSF administration, leukopheresis, and standard marrow harvest: ethical and safety considerations for normal pediatric hematopoietic cell donors. Pediatr Blood Cancer 2006;46(4):422–33.

34. Summary PESM. 2008. Available at: http://www.fda.gov/ohrms/dockets/ac/08/slides/2008-4406s1-01.pdf. Accessed April 24, 2012.

35. Gunn AJ, Gluckman PD, Gunn TR. Selective head cooling in newborn infants after perinatal asphyxia: a safety study. Pediatrics 1998;102(4):885–92.

36. Shankaran S, Laptook A, Wright L, et al. Whole-body hypothermia for neonatal encephalopathy: animal observations as a basis for a randomized, controlled pilot study in term infants. Pediatrics 2002;110(2):377–85.

37. Jacobs S, Hunt R, Tarnow-Mordi W, et al. Cooling for newborns with hypoxic ischaemic encephalopathy. Cochrane Database Syst Rev 2007;(4):CD003311.

38. Blackmon LR, Stark AR, American Academy of Pediatrics Committee on Fetus and Newborn. Hypothermia: a neuroprotective therapy for neonatal hypoxic-ischemic encephalopathy. Pediatrics 2006;117(3):942–8.

39. Papile LA. Systemic hypothermia — A "cool" therapy for neonatal hypoxic-ischemic encephalopathy. N Engl J Med 2005;353(15):1619–20.

40. Schulzke S, Rao S, Patole S. A systematic review of cooling for neuroprotection in neonates with hypoxic ischemic encephalopathy - are we there yet? BMC Pediatr 2007;7(1):30.

41. Kirpalani H, Barks J, Thorlund K, et al. Cooling for neonatal hypoxic ischemic encephalopathy: do we have the answer? Pediatrics 2007;120(5):1126–30.

42. Wilkinson D, Casalaz D, Watkins A, et al. Hypothermia: a neuroprotective therapy for neonatal hypoxic-ischemic encephalopathy. Pediatrics 2007;119(2):422–3.

43. Gunn A, Hoehn T, Hansmann G, et al. Hypothermia: an evolving treatment for neonatal hypoxic ischemic encephalopathy. Pediatrics 2008;121(3):648–9.

44. Raghuveer TS, Cox AJ. Neonatal resuscitation: an update. Am Fam Physician 2011;83(8):911–8.

45. Hoehn T, Hansmann G, Bhrer C, et al. Therapeutic hypothermia in neonates. Review of current clinical data, ILCOR recommendations and suggestions for implementation in neonatal intensive care units. Resuscitation 2008;78(1):7–12.

46. Roehr CC, Hansmann G, Hoehn T, et al. The 2010 guidelines on neonatal resuscitation (AHA, ERC, ILCOR): similarities and differences - what progress has been made since 2005? Klin Padiatr 2011;223(5):299–307.

47. Barks JD. Technical aspects of starting a neonatal cooling program. Clin Perinatol 2008;35(4):765–75.

48. Jacobs SE, Morley CJ, Inder TE, et al. Whole-body hypothermia for term and near-term newborns with hypoxic-ischemic encephalopathy: a randomized controlled trial. Arch Pediatr Adolesc Med 2011;165(8):692–700.

49. Wyatt JS. Ethics and hypothermia treatment. Semin Fetal Neonatal Med 2010; 15(5):299–304.

50. Assmann SF, Pocock SJ, Enos LE, et al. Subgroup analysis and other (mis)uses of baseline data in clinical trials. Lancet 2000;355(9209):1064–9.

Index

Note: Page numbers of article titles are in **boldface** type.

Pediatr Clin N Am 59 (2012) 1221–1231
http://dx.doi.org/10.1016/S0031-3955(12)00148-4
0031-3955/12/$ – see front matter © 2012 Elsevier Inc. All rights reserved.

pediatric.theclinics.com

United States Postal Service

Statement of Ownership, Management, and Circulation
(All Periodicals Publications Except Requester Publications)

1. Publication Title Pediatric Clinics of North America	**2. Publication Number** 4 2 4 - 6 6 0 0	**3. Filing Date** 9/14/12

4. Issue Frequency Feb, Apr, Jun, Aug, Oct, Dec	**5. Number of Issues Published Annually** 6	**6. Annual Subscription Price** $191.00

7. Complete Mailing Address of Known Office of Publication *(Not printer) (Street, city, county, state, and ZIP+4®)*

Elsevier Inc.
360 Park Avenue South
New York, NY 10010-1710

Contact Person
Stephen R. Bushing

Telephone *(Include area code)*
215-239-3688

8. Complete Mailing Address of Headquarters or General Business Office of Publisher *(Not printer)*

Elsevier Inc., 360 Park Avenue South, New York, NY 10010-1710

9. Full Names and Complete Mailing Addresses of Publisher, Editor, and Managing Editor *(Do not leave blank)*

Publisher *(Name and complete mailing address)*

Kim Murphy, Elsevier, Inc., 1600 John F. Kennedy Blvd. Suite 1800, Philadelphia, PA 19103-2899

Editor *(Name and complete mailing address)*

Kerry Holland, Elsevier, Inc., 1600 John F. Kennedy Blvd. Suite 1800, Philadelphia, PA 19103-2899

Managing Editor *(Name and complete mailing address)*

Sarah Barth, Elsevier, Inc., 1600 John F. Kennedy Blvd. Suite 1800, Philadelphia, PA 19103-2899

10. Owner *(Do not leave blank. If the publication is owned by a corporation, give the name and address of the corporation immediately followed by the names and addresses of all stockholders owning or holding 1 percent or more of the total amount of stock. If not owned by a corporation, give the names and addresses of the individual owners. If owned by a partnership or other unincorporated firm, give its name and address as well as those of each individual owner. If the publication is published by a nonprofit organization, give its name and address.)*

Full Name	**Complete Mailing Address**
Wholly owned subsidiary of	1600 John F. Kennedy Blvd., Ste. 1800
Reed/Elsevier, US holdings	Philadelphia, PA 19103-2899

11. Known Bondholders, Mortgagees, and Other Security Holders Owning or Holding 1 Percent or More of Total Amount of Bonds, Mortgages, or Other Securities. If none, check box ☐ None

Full Name	**Complete Mailing Address**
N/A	

12. Tax Status *(For completion by nonprofit organizations authorized to mail at nonprofit rates) (Check one)*
The purpose, function, and nonprofit status of this organization and the exempt status for federal income tax purposes:
☐ Has Not Changed During Preceding 12 Months
☐ Has Changed During Preceding 12 Months *(Publisher must submit explanation of change with this statement)*

PS Form 3526, September 2007 (Page 1 of 3 (Instructions Page 3)) PSN 7530-01-000-9931 PRIVACY NOTICE: See our Privacy policy in www.usps.com

---

13. Publication Title Pediatric Clinics of North America		**14. Issue Date for Circulation Data Below** August 2012

15. Extent and Nature of Circulation		**Average No. Copies Each Issue During Preceding 12 Months**	**No. Copies of Single Issue Published Nearest to Filing Date**
a. Total Number of Copies *(Net press run)*		2742	2360
b. Paid Circulation (By Mail and Outside the Mail)	(1) Mailed Outside-County Paid Subscriptions Stated on PS Form 3541. *(Include paid distribution above nominal rate, advertiser's proof copies, and exchange copies)*	1318	1201
	(2) Mailed In-County Paid Subscriptions Stated on PS Form 3541 *(Include paid distribution above nominal rate, advertiser's proof copies, and exchange copies)*		
	(3) Paid Distribution Outside the Mails Including Sales Through Dealers and Carriers, Street Vendors, Counter Sales, and Other Paid Distribution Outside USPS®	844	860
	(4) Paid Distribution by Other Classes Mailed Through the USPS *(e.g. First-Class Mail®)*		
c. Total Paid Distribution *(Sum of 15b (1), (2), (3), and (4))*		2162	2061
d. Free or Nominal Rate Distribution (By Mail and Outside the Mail)	(1) Free or Nominal Rate Outside-County Copies Included on PS Form 3541	88	62
	(2) Free or Nominal Rate In-County Copies Included on PS Form 3541		
	(3) Free or Nominal Rate Copies Mailed at Other Classes Through the USPS (e.g. First-Class Mail)		
	(4) Free or Nominal Rate Distribution Outside the Mail (Carriers or other means)		
e. Total Free or Nominal Rate Distribution *(Sum of 15d (1), (2), (3) and (4))*		88	62
f. Total Distribution *(Sum of 15c and 15e)*		2250	2123
g. Copies not Distributed *(See instructions to publishers #4 (page #3))*		492	237
h. Total *(Sum of 15f and g)*		2742	2360
i. Percent Paid *(15c divided by 15f times 100)*		96.09%	97.08%

16. Publication of Statement of Ownership

☐ If the publication is a general publication, publication of this statement is required. Will be printed
in the October 2012 issue of this publication.

☐ Publication not required

17. Signature and Title of Editor, Publisher, Business Manager, or Owner

Stephen R. Bushing [signature]

Stephen R. Bushing — Inventory Distribution Coordinator

Date September 14, 2012

I certify that all information furnished on this form is true and complete. I understand that anyone who furnishes false or misleading information on this form or who omits material or information requested on the form may be subject to criminal sanctions (including fines and imprisonment) and/or civil sanctions (including civil penalties).

PS Form 3526, September 2007 (Page 2 of 3)

Moving?

Make sure your subscription moves with you!

To notify us of your new address, find your **Clinics Account Number** (located on your mailing label above your name), and contact customer service at:

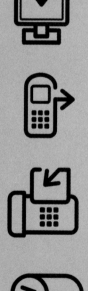

Email: journalscustomerservice-usa@elsevier.com

800-654-2452 (subscribers in the U.S. & Canada)
314-447-8871 (subscribers outside of the U.S. & Canada)

Fax number: 314-447-8029

Elsevier Health Sciences Division
Subscription Customer Service
3251 Riverport Lane
Maryland Heights, MO 63043

*To ensure uninterrupted delivery of your subscription, please notify us at least 4 weeks in advance of move.